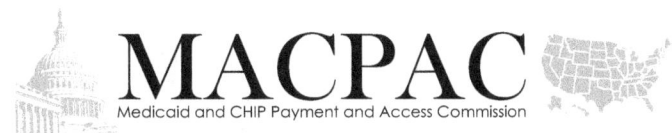

The Medicaid and CHIP Payment and Access Commission (MACPAC) was established in the Children's Health Insurance Program Reauthorization Act of 2009, and its charge was later revised in the Patient Protection and Affordable Care Act of 2010. Appointed by the U.S. Comptroller General, the 17 Commissioners have diverse backgrounds, offer broad perspectives on Medicaid and CHIP, and represent different regions across the United States.

The Commission is a non-partisan, federal, analytic resource for the Congress on Medicaid and CHIP. MACPAC is the first federal agency charged with providing policy and data analysis to the Congress on Medicaid and CHIP, and for making recommendations to the Congress and the Secretary of the U.S. Department of Health and Human Services on a wide range of issues affecting these programs. The Commission conducts independent policy analysis and health services research on key Medicaid and CHIP topics, including but not limited to:

- eligibility, enrollment, and benefits;
- payment;
- access to care;
- quality of care;
- interactions of Medicaid and CHIP with Medicare and the health care system generally; and
- data development to support policy analysis and program accountability.

As required in its statutory charge, the Commission will submit reports to the Congress by March 15 and June 15 of each year. As applicable, each member of the Commission will vote on recommendations contained in the reports. The Commission's reports provide the Congress with a better understanding of the Medicaid and CHIP programs, their roles in the U.S. health care system, and the key policy and data issues outlined in the Commission's statutory charge.

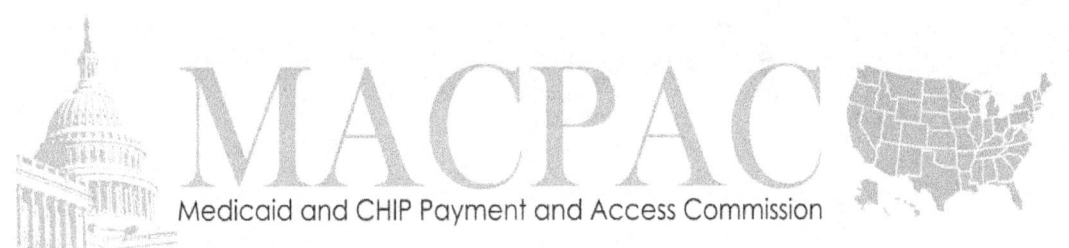

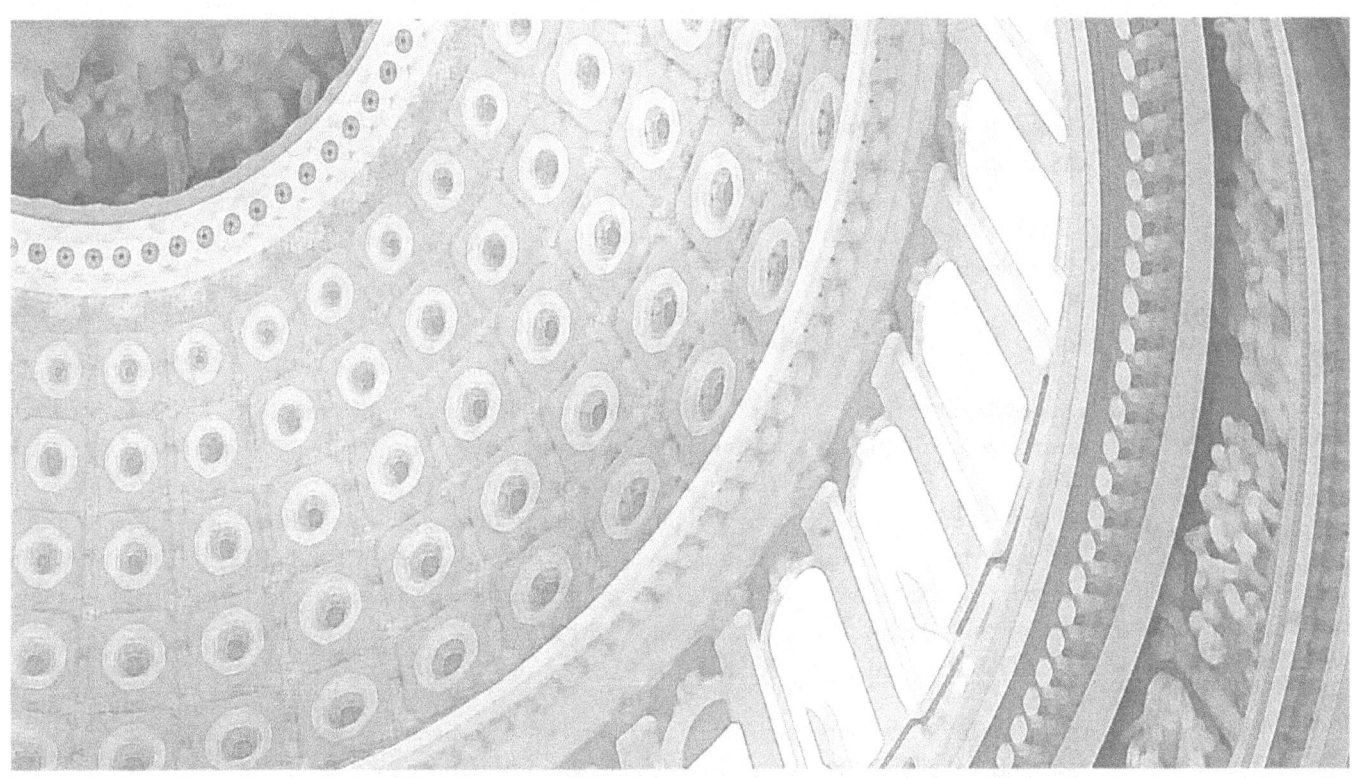

Report to the Congress on Medicaid and CHIP

June 2013

MACPAC
Medicaid and CHIP Payment and Access Commission

1800 M Street, NW
Suite 650 South
Washington, DC 20036
Phone: (202) 350-2000
Fax: (202) 273-2452
www.macpac.gov

Commissioners

Diane Rowland, ScD,
Chair

David Sundwall, MD,
Vice Chair

Sharon Carte, MHS
Richard Chambers
Donna Checkett, MPA, MSW
Andrea Cohen, JD
Burton Edelstein, DDS, MPH
Patricia Gabow, MD
Herman Gray, MD, MBA
Denise Henning, CNM, MSN
Mark Hoyt, FSA, MAAA
Norma Martinez Rogers, PhD, RN, FAAN
Judith Moore
Trish Riley, MS
Sara Rosenbaum, JD
Robin Smith
Steven Waldren, MD, MS

Anne L. Schwartz, PhD,
Executive Director

June 14, 2013

The Honorable Joseph R. Biden, Jr.
President of the Senate
U.S. Capitol
Washington, DC 20510

The Honorable John A. Boehner
Speaker of the House
U.S. House of Representatives
U.S. Capitol
H-232
Washington, DC 20515

Dear Mr. Vice President and Mr. Speaker:

On behalf of the Medicaid and CHIP Payment and Access Commission (MACPAC), I am pleased to submit this Congressionally mandated *Report to the Congress on Medicaid and CHIP*. MACPAC is a non-partisan commission that conducts objective policy and data analysis to assist the Congress in overseeing and improving these programs, which are major purchasers of health services. Currently, Medicaid covers about 73 million people and CHIP covers 8 million individuals. Although estimates vary, the size and reach of the Medicaid program is expected to increase substantially due to changes made by the Patient Protection and Affordable Care Act (ACA, P.L. 111-148, as amended).

In this report, the Commission examines several fundamental issues including Medicaid and CHIP eligibility and coverage for maternity services, the newly implemented increase in physician payment for primary care services, access to care for non-elderly persons with disabilities, the availability of Medicaid and CHIP data that can be used for oversight and program monitoring, and improving the effectiveness of program integrity activites.

As major purchasers of maternity services, Medicaid and CHIP paid for 1.8 million births in 2010, roughly half of all births in many states. States and the federal government have an interest in maximizing positive birth outcomes for all families, particularly those financed with taxpayer dollars. This chapter explores Medicaid and CHIP eligibility and coverage for these services, including enrollment and spending information. The chapter also highlights provisions of the ACA that affect eligibility for maternity services in Medicaid, CHIP, and health insurance exchanges.

The chapter on Medicaid primary care physician payment focuses on a specific provision of the ACA that became effective in January 2013: increasing Medicaid fees to Medicare payment levels for primary care services provided by primary care physicians. The provision is effective for 2013 and 2014 with the federal government paying 100 percent of the costs of the difference in fees. To better understand how the provision is being implemented by state Medicaid programs and its possible impact on beneficiary access and provider participation, we examined the relevant research literature and conducted interviews with states, providers, and other key stakeholders. The feedback we received, although early in the implementation process, highlights the challenges of implementing this provision and the need for broader investigation into various options to address access gaps in Medicaid.

In this report, the Commission builds on previous analyses related to persons with disabilities. Medicaid is an important source of coverage for these individuals, providing services not typically covered by Medicare or private insurers. This report includes a literature review on access to care for non-elderly adults with disabilities, highlights gaps in existing research, and suggests areas for additional research and analysis.

The report also focuses on the importance of having accurate, timely, and nationally comparable data on Medicaid and CHIP in order to answer key policy questions that affect enrollees, states, the federal government, health care providers, and others—and in ensuring accountability for taxpayer dollars. This chapter updates the Congress on progress that has been made in improving federal administrative data and identifies areas where additional improvements would benefit policymaking at the federal level.

In a related chapter, the Commission considers program integrity, a key Congressional priority for all publicly funded programs. Program integrity involves a discrete set of activities related to the detection and prevention of fraud, waste, and abuse, but is also an important part of day-to-day program administration activities such as beneficiary and provider enrollment, eligibility, service delivery, and payment. The chapter highlights two programs, Medicaid Eligibility Quality Control and Payment Error Rate Measurement (commonly known as MEQC and PERM). While both programs review the accuracy of individual Medicaid and CHIP eligibility determinations, the rules for the two programs overlap and do not align well with each other. This chapter lays the groundwork for future efforts to identify duplicative programs and strategies that provide the strongest return on investment.

As in each of our reports, this report includes the MACStats statistical supplement, which provides national and state-level data on enrollment, spending, health, and characteristics of Medicaid and CHIP populations and Medicaid managed care.

MACPAC is committed to being a source of in-depth, non-partisan analysis of Medicaid and CHIP, and their impact on beneficiaries, states, providers, and others. We hope our analytic work will continue to help inform and assist the Congress in identifying ways to strengthen the programs, particularly as implementation of ACA provisions continue.

Sincerely,

Diane Rowland

Diane Rowland, ScD
Chair

Enclosure

Commission Members and Terms

Diane Rowland, Sc.D., Chair
Washington, DC

David Sundwall, M.D., Vice Chair
Salt Lake City, UT

Term Expires December 2013

Sharon Carte, M.H.S.
South Charleston, WV

Andrea Cohen, J.D.
New York, NY

Herman Gray, M.D., M.B.A.
West Bloomfield, MI

Norma Martínez Rogers, Ph.D., R.N., F.A.A.N.
San Antonio, TX

Sara Rosenbaum, J.D.
Alexandria, VA

Term Expires December 2014

Richard Chambers
Palm Springs, CA

Burton Edelstein, D.D.S., M.P.H.
New York, NY

Denise Henning, C.N.M., M.S.N.
Ft. Myers, FL

Judith Moore
Annapolis, MD

Robin Smith
Awendaw, SC

David Sundwall, M.D.
Salt Lake City, UT

Term Expires December 2015

Donna Checkett, M.P.A., M.S.W.
Hartford, CT

Patricia Gabow, M.D.
Denver, CO

Mark Hoyt, F.S.A., M.A.A.A.
Phoenix, AZ

Patricia Riley, M.S.
Brunswick, ME

Diane Rowland, Sc.D.
Washington, DC

Steven Waldren, M.D., M.S.
Kansas City, MO

Commission Staff

Anne L. Schwartz, Ph.D.
Executive Director

Office of the Executive Director

Annie Andrianasolo, M.B.A.

Amy Bernstein, Sc.D.

Laura Diamond

Lindsay Hebert, M.S.P.H.

Mary Ellen Stahlman, M.H.S.A.

Analytic Staff

Benjamin Finder, M.P.H.

Moira Forbes, M.B.A.

April Grady, M.P.Aff.

Angela Lello, M.P.Aff.

Molly McGinn-Shapiro, M.P.P.

Chris Park, M.S.

Chris Peterson, M.P.P.

Lois Simon, M.H.S.

Anna Sommers, Ph.D.

James Teisl, M.P.H.

Operations and Management

Ricardo Villeta, M.B.A.
Deputy Director of Operations, Finance, and Management

Vincent Calvo

Mathew Chase

Benjamin Granata

Ken Pezzella

Eileen Wilkie

Acknowledgements

The Commission would like to thank the following people who provided valuable guidance in the development of the June 2013 *Report to the Congress on Medicaid and CHIP*.

The Commission was fortunate to receive insight from staff of the U.S. Department of Health and Human Services and the Government Accountability Office regarding this report. We would like to specifically thank Roxanne Andrews, Julie Boughn, Kenneth Campbell, Mary Cieslicki, Daniel Davis, Nancy De Lew, Chrissy Fowler, Elisabeth Handley, Timothy Hill, Paul Hughes, Katherine Iritani, Lyn Killman, Cindy Mann, Elaine Olin, Christie Peters, Jennifer Ryan, Loretta Schickner, Linda Tavener, Christopher Truffer, and Carolyn Yocom for their contributions and guidance.

We also received indispensible feedback from several state Medicaid officials and their representatives, including Jerry Dubberly, Darin Gordon, Aaron Larrimore, Andrea Maresca, Kathleen Nolan, Cathie Ott, Cindy Roberts, Matt Salo, and Jonas Schwartz.

Several research and policy experts provided the Commission with technical feedback, including Julie Bershadsky, Christina Bethell, Cheryl Camillo, Kavita Choudhry, Mary Lee Fay, Norma Gavin, Rebecca Gee, Marsha Gold, Elizabeth Hargrave, Gina Livermore, Tricia Morris, Chas Moseley, Mike Nordstrom, Susan Palsbo, James Scroggs, Kimberly Smith, Michelle Strollo, John Wachtel, and Steve Zuckerman.

The Commission received valuable programming and data support from Raja Gangopadhya, Martha Kelly, Sean MaCurdy, Emil Rusev, and colleagues from Acumen, LLC, and from Shamis Mahamoud, Cynthia Saiontz-Martinez, Lan Zhao, and colleagues from Social & Scientific Systems, Inc.

Finally, the Commission would like to thank Lynette Bertsche, Jason Coats, Imelda Demus, and the health care research staff at NORC at the University of Chicago for their assistance in editing and producing this report.

Table of Contents

Commission Members and Terms vii

Commission Staff ix

Acknowledgements xi

Executive Summary 1

Chapter 1: Maternity Services: Examining Eligibility and Coverage in Medicaid and CHIP 9
    Key Points 10
    Policy Context: Births in the United States 12
        Factors associated with pregnancy and birth outcomes 13
    Medicaid and CHIP Eligibility for Pregnant Women 13
        Medicaid eligibility for pregnant women through 2013 14
        CHIP 14
        Presumptive eligibility for pregnant women 17
        Non-citizens 17
        The ACA and eligibility for maternity services 17
    Covered Benefits for Maternity Services 18
        Pregnancy-related benefits through 2013 19
        Pregnancy-related benefits under the ACA 19
        Coverage for enhanced benefits during pregnancy 21
    Access to Maternity Care 21
    Utilization and Expenditures for Medicaid Maternity Services 22
        Medicaid spending 23
        Cost and prevalence of cesarean deliveries 23
    Programs to Improve the Effectiveness of Maternity Care 23
        Programs to enhance and increase use of prenatal care services 23
        Programs to target high-risk women 26
        Programs focused on preconception care 28
    Programs to reduce non-medically indicated deliveries 29
        Payment initiatives 29
        Quality improvement initiatives 30
        Performance measurement and public reporting 30
        Provider and patient education 35
    Issues and Next Steps 36
    Endnotes 37
    References 37
    Chapter 1 Appendix: Datasets used to Count Annual Number of Births in the Medicaid Program 41

Chapter 2: Medicaid Primary Care Physician Payment Increase 47
    Key Points 48
    Access to Primary Care and Physician Payment 50
    Statutory and Regulatory Requirements for the Primary Care Physician Payment Increase 51
        Eligibility for increased payments 51
        Payment amounts and frequency 52
    Issues Emerging from Early Implementation 54
    Implementation Issues Specific to Managed Care 56
    Evaluation 57
    Endnotes 58
    References 59

MACStats: Medicaid and CHIP Program Statistics 63
    MACStats Table of Contents 64
    Overview 67
    Section 1: Trends in Medicaid Enrollment and Spending 69
    Section 2: Health and Other Characteristics of Medicaid/CHIP Populations 75
    Section 3: Medicaid Enrollment and Benefit Spending 93
    Section 4: Medicaid Managed Care 107
    Section 5: Technical Guide to the June 2013 MACStats 119

Chapter 3: Access to Care for Persons with Disabilities 135
    Key Points 136
    Scope of Literature Review 138
    A Framework for Examining Access to Health Care 138
    Characteristics of the Population 138
        Health needs and risk factors 139
        Prevention and wellness 139
        Socioeconomic characteristics 139
    A Review of Research Findings on Access to Care 140
        Findings from large-scale population surveys 140
        Findings from provider and stakeholder data 144
        Findings from consumer interviews 146
        State Medicaid program data 149
    Further Research Needed 150
    Endnotes 153
    References 154

Chapter 4: Update on Medicaid and CHIP Data for Policy Analysis and Program Accountability **161**

    Key Points 162

    Brief Overview of Federal Administrative Data on Medicaid and CHIP 164

        State data systems 164

        Federal administrative data systems 165

    Recent Federal Efforts to Improve Data Timeliness, Quality, and Availability 167

    MACPro 167

    T-MSIS 168

    MITA 170

    Looking Forward 171

    References 172

Chapter 5: Update on Program Integrity in Medicaid **177**

    Key Points 178

    Previous Commission Review and Recommendations 180

    Current Status of Federal Medicaid Program Integrity Activities 181

    Key Programmatic Areas in Program Integrity 183

        Program integrity operations 183

        Individual and provider enrollment 186

        Service delivery 188

        Payment 188

        Post-payment review 189

        Reporting and follow-up 190

    PERM and MEQC: An Opportunity to Streamline 191

        Medicaid Eligibility Quality Control 191

        Payment Error Rate Measurement 192

    The Commission's Program Integrity Focus for the Coming Year 194

    Endnotes 195

    References 196

Appendix **199**

    Acronym List 201

    Authorizing Language from the Social Security Act (42 U.S.C. 1396) 205

    Biographies of Commissioners 213

    Biographies of Staff 219

List of Tables

TABLE 1-1. Legislative Milestones in Medicaid and CHIP Coverage of Pregnant Women 15

TABLE 1-2. Medicaid Spending 12 Months before and 2 Months after Delivery for Women with a Hospital Delivery in 2008 24

TABLE 1-3. Medicaid Births in Community Hospitals, by Type of Delivery, 2010 25

TABLE 1-4. Cost of Medicaid Births in Community Hospitals, by Type of Delivery, 2010 26

TABLE 1-5. Selected State-Based Payment Reform Initiatives to Reduce Induction, Cesarean Section, and Early Elective Deliveries 30

TABLE 1-6. Selected State-Based Quality Improvement Initiatives to Reduce Induction, Cesarean Section, and Early Elective Deliveries 31

TABLE 1-7. Performance Measurement and Public Reporting Initiatives to Reduce Induction, Cesarean Section, and Early Elective Deliveries 34

TABLE 1-8. Provider and Patient Education Initiatives to Reduce Induction, Cesarean Section, and Early Elective Deliveries 35

TABLE 1-A-1. Total and Medicaid Births Reported in Three Data Sources, 2008–2010 42

TABLE 4-1. Key Sources of Federal Administrative Data on Medicaid and CHIP 166

TABLE 5-1. Updates to CMS Medicaid Program Integrity Activities 182

TABLE 5-2. Overview of State and CMS Program Integrity Activities 184

TABLE 5-3. Comparison of Payment Error Rate Measurement (PERM) and Medicaid Eligibility Quality Control (MEQC) 193

Note: MACStats tables and figures are listed separately on pages 64 and 65.

List of Boxes

BOX 1-1.	Texas CHIP Perinatal Coverage	20
BOX 1-2.	North Carolina's Pregnancy Medical Home Model	27
BOX 1-3.	Florida's Healthy Start Legislation	27
BOX 3-1.	Other Large-Scale Surveys Supporting Analyses of Medicaid Enrollees with Disabilities Cited in This Chapter	141
BOX 5-1.	Regulatory Definitions of Fraud and Abuse	180

Executive Summary

The Medicaid and CHIP Payment and Access Commission's (MACPAC's) June 2013 *Report to the Congress on Medicaid and CHIP* examines several key policy issues, including Medicaid and State Children's Health Insurance Program (CHIP) eligibility and coverage for maternity services, the newly implemented increase in Medicaid physician payment for primary care services, access to care for persons with disabilities, the availability of Medicaid and CHIP data that can be used by the Congress for oversight and program monitoring, and improving the effectiveness of program integrity activities. The Commission's work in these areas is intended to help the Congress better understand the dynamics of two programs that are both in flux. While they continue to serve their long-standing purpose of providing health care coverage to millions of low-income children, pregnant women, seniors, and persons with disabilities, the size and reach of Medicaid, in particular, is expected to increase substantially over the next several years due to changes resulting from the Patient Protection and Affordable Care Act (ACA, P.L. 111-148, as amended).

The report is divided into five chapters and a statistical supplement:

- Maternity Services: Examining Eligibility and Coverage in Medicaid and CHIP
- Medicaid Primary Care Physician Payment Increase
- Access to Care for Persons with Disabilities
- Update on Medicaid and CHIP Data for Policy Analysis and Program Accountability
- Update on Program Integrity in Medicaid
- MACStats: Medicaid and CHIP Program Statistics

Maternity Services: Examining Eligibility and Coverage in Medicaid and CHIP

In 2010, Medicaid and CHIP paid for almost half of all births in the United States (about 1.8 million hospital births). Based on data for 2008 that identified 1.6 million Medicaid deliveries, Medicaid spending for women who delivered was over $11 billion during the 12 months before and 2 months following the delivery. The Congress has expanded Medicaid eligibility for poor and low-income pregnant women and children over the years, creating new mandatory and optional eligibility groups. While states are required to provide pregnancy-related coverage to pregnant women up to 133 percent of the federal poverty level (FPL), all but nine states have extended coverage to pregnant women above that level, and some states cover women with family incomes as high as 300 percent FPL. They may also offer CHIP-financed services to pregnant women through Section 1115 waivers, an option to cover services for unborn children (16 states in fiscal year (FY) 2012), or state plan amendments.

The ACA mandates maternity care for those covered by health insurance exchange plans and requires coverage of other pregnancy-related services. With respect to Medicaid, many states will have considerable discretion as to how they cover pregnant women above 138 percent FPL and may have the option to transition these individuals to exchange coverage. The separate eligibility pathways based on pregnancy may cause women to cycle among Medicaid, CHIP, and private coverage available through the exchanges, or to uninsured status. Churning among the different types of coverage could create challenges for enrollees. As networks and benefits change, enrollees may experience discontinuity of care and changes to their cost sharing. States, providers, and health plans could also experience administrative burdens as women change insurance status based on their pregnancy status.

For pregnant women, services covered under Medicaid and CHIP range from full Medicaid benefits (69 percent of Medicaid-covered births in 2008) to coverage of only pregnancy-related services (which are those necessary for the health of the pregnant woman and fetus) to emergency services only (for certain non-citizens). Most states also offer benefits to pregnant women that are not offered to other Medicaid adult enrollees. These benefits—aimed at improving pregnancy and birth outcomes—include dental services, prenatal risk assessments, home visiting programs, targeted case management, preconception counseling, psychosocial counseling, and substance abuse treatment.

Because Medicaid and CHIP are such important payers for maternity services, both programs have a stake in improving birth outcomes and in being prudent purchasers of care. Almost one-third of Medicaid deliveries (31 percent) were by cesarean section, a figure comparable to rates for all births. Cesarean deliveries cost more than vaginal deliveries and are associated with more adverse outcomes. Many states, in partnership with the federal government and private organizations, have initiated programs to reduce elective cesarean sections and non-medically indicated induced deliveries before 39 weeks gestation. The report details some of these efforts, including payment incentives and educational programs to help improve maternal and infant outcomes and reduce costs.

Medicaid Primary Care Physician Payment Increase

A provision in the ACA requires state Medicaid agencies to increase to Medicare levels the payment rates of primary care services furnished by primary care physicians in 2013 and 2014. The provision applies to services delivered by physicians paid under fee-for-service arrangements and by Medicaid managed care organizations (MCOs). The federal government will fund the full cost of the difference between the state's Medicaid fees as of July 1, 2009, and Medicare fees in 2013 and 2014. The inclusion of the provision reflects some concerns that the expansion of Medicaid eligibility to millions of additional enrollees could compromise access to primary care physicians for current Medicaid enrollees. There is also some evidence that Medicaid physician payment rates affect physician participation in Medicaid.

In an effort to understand the operational and policy issues surrounding implementation of the payment rate increase and its potential effects on access, MACPAC conducted semi-structured interviews with six states and the District of Columbia in late 2012 and early 2013. The findings from the interviews brought to light several issues, including some concerns about the time allotted to implement the provision and about the difficulty of identifying eligible providers. States also reported that the system modifications necessary for this increased payment are more complex than routine payment rate changes and require more time to implement. Some states and MCOs noted that they would need to amend their contracts and adjust capitation payments in order to ensure that payment increases are passed through to eligible physicians participating in Medicaid MCO networks. Several state Medicaid officials, as well as managed care and provider organizations, expressed concern that the effect of the provision on provider participation may be limited because it is set to expire after 2014.

A critical question for policymakers is how the payment increase will affect physician participation and enrollee access to care. In order to determine the provision's effect on access, evaluation efforts could use claims data to examine changes in service use. However, complete national claims data are not likely to be available until after the provision expires at the end of 2014. Surveys of physician attitudes or state-specific workforce data could provide useful information in evaluating the effect of the provision in a more timely fashion. In the months ahead, the Commission will continue to monitor implementation and will be looking at efforts of state, federal, and academic evaluators to understand what can be learned to inform future policy.

Access to Care for Persons with Disabilities

As part of MACPAC's ongoing charge to examine access to care for Medicaid enrollees, the report reviews the research literature on access to care for adults with disabilities under age 65 who are Medicaid-only enrollees living in the community. This group has a wide range of health care needs and functional limitations. The literature review found little research directly examining access to acute care for this population. Therefore, the Commission examined a wider range of studies based on large-scale population surveys, provider and stakeholder data, consumer interviews and other qualitative data, and state Medicaid program data.

Based on studies using large-scale population survey data, access to health care among Medicaid-only enrollees with disabilities is comparable to that of other insured persons with disabilities. Unmet need among Medicaid-only enrollees with disabilities is lower compared to individuals with disabilities covered by private insurance or Medicare only. However, preventive services are potentially underused among Medicaid enrollees with disabilities, though findings vary by service.

Studies that included interviews with providers, plans, and other stakeholders generally found three areas of concern for individuals with disabilities: (1) disability competency training in medical schools, (2) accessibility of equipment and services, and (3) access to dental services. Several access barriers figure prominently in qualitative studies of adults with disabilities, including scheduling appointments and receiving timely primary care, communicating with providers and staff, accessibility of health care facilities and services, finding a doctor who understands their disability, and transportation. However, the experiences of

Medicaid enrollees may vary from the general population of individuals with disabilities included in these studies.

Studies using state Medicaid program data provide little information on access to care for Medicaid enrollees with disabilities, because they often do not have comparison groups with other forms of coverage and include no data on service use prior to enrollment. Thus, they do not allow analysts to draw conclusions as to whether access levels are due to community factors that affect all individuals with disabilities or to program factors that affect only Medicaid enrollees.

Further research specific to Medicaid enrollees with disabilities is needed to inform state and federal policymakers about the nature of access for the population. Topics of particular interest include: the impact of enabling services on access to care, disability competency and accessibility in Medicaid provider networks, and evaluation and best practices in risk-based managed care. Future research should also focus on the role of non-physician practitioners in access to care for subpopulations with disabilities and on best practices in service delivery for enrollees with disabilities.

Update on Medicaid and CHIP Data for Policy Analysis and Program Accountability

Data on Medicaid and CHIP play a key role in answering policy questions that affect program enrollees, states, the federal government, health care providers, and others. They also help to ensure accountability for taxpayer dollars. Federal administrative data on Medicaid and CHIP are meant to provide comparable information across states, which maintain their own disparate data systems. This chapter provides an update on recent efforts by the Centers for Medicare & Medicaid Services (CMS) to improve the timeliness, quality, and availability of federal administrative data on Medicaid and CHIP, which MACPAC first addressed in its March 2011 report to the Congress.

Three CMS initiatives are described in the chapter. MACPro, a web-based system designed to collect state plan, waiver, and other programmatic documents in a structured format, will provide more consistent and comprehensive information on state activities for use by CMS, states, and analysts. The Transformed Medicaid Statistical Information System (T-MSIS), a data source that builds on existing person-level and claims-level MSIS data submitted by states, will include changes designed to address several concerns about current MSIS data, including its timeliness, reliability, and completeness. A third CMS effort, the Medicaid Information Technology Architecture (MITA) initiative, establishes national guidelines and standards for state-operated Medicaid and CHIP data systems that are funded with federal dollars.

Improvements to Medicaid and CHIP data require significant federal and state resource investments and will take several years to realize. MACPro and T-MSIS are scheduled for roll-out in 2013, with full implementation expected to take at least two years. MITA is an ongoing effort with states, whose data systems are at varying levels of modernization. The Commission supports CMS efforts to improve federal administrative data on Medicaid and CHIP and encourages the agency to continue seeking input on its initiatives from states and other stakeholders.

Update on Program Integrity in Medicaid

Program integrity activities are intended to ensure that public dollars are spent appropriately on delivering high-quality, medically necessary care. An effective program integrity approach should prevent improper payments, reduce waste and abuse particularly when it leads to patient harm, and help achieve value. First addressed in our March 2012 report, this report continues the Commission's focus on analyzing ways to improve the effectiveness of Medicaid and CHIP program integrity efforts.

A successful Medicaid program integrity strategy requires coordination among state and federal agencies—a task complicated by the fact that current activities are governed by multiple federal statutes and regulations. Each state develops its own approach to program integrity, while federal program integrity activities are guided by a comprehensive Medicaid integrity plan, which is expected to be updated later in 2013.

Program integrity includes both a discrete set of activities related specifically to the detection and prevention of fraud, waste, and abuse (such as post-payment review) and activities embedded in general program administration, such as individual enrollment (eligibility), provider enrollment, service delivery, and payment. In some programmatic areas, such as eligibility determination, there are multiple program integrity initiatives at both the federal and state levels that are duplicative, while other areas, such as managed care, receive comparatively little attention.

Potential opportunities exist to reconsider the state-federal division of responsibility and to examine where responsibilities align well and where they overlap. The Medicaid Eligibility Quality Control (MEQC) and Payment Error Rate Measurement (PERM) eligibility reviews are an example of duplicative program integrity initiatives. While both programs review the accuracy of individual Medicaid and CHIP eligibility determinations, the rules for the two programs overlap and do not align well with each other.

Future Commission analysis of these issues will help policymakers identify opportunities to streamline regulatory requirements, eliminate redundant functions, promote greater integration of state and federal activities, or invest additional resources.

MACStats: Medicaid and CHIP Program Statistics

MACStats, a standing section in all MACPAC reports to the Congress, presents data and information on Medicaid and CHIP that otherwise can be difficult to find. The June 2013 edition of MACStats is divided into five sections: (1) trends in Medicaid enrollment and spending, (2) health and other characteristics of Medicaid and CHIP populations, (3) Medicaid enrollment and benefit spending, (4) Medicaid managed care, and (5) a technical guide to the June 2013 MACStats.

Key points include:

- Individuals qualifying for Medicaid on the basis of a disability accounted for half of real Medicaid spending growth since FY 1975. About three-quarters of the growth for this group was driven by increased enrollment; the remainder was attributable to growth in per capita spending.

- Non-disabled children accounted for the largest Medicaid enrollment increase in absolute numbers since FY 1975, from 9.6 million in that year to 30 million in FY 2010.

- Medicaid and CHIP enrollees generally report being in poorer health and using more services than individuals who have other health insurance or who are uninsured.

- Children enrolled in Medicaid or CHIP were more likely than privately insured or uninsured children to have had a visit to the emergency department (ED) in the past year and to have been regularly taking prescription medications for at least three months.

- Adults younger than 65 enrolled in Medicaid were more likely than those with private insurance to have had four or more visits to a doctor or other health professional in the past 12 months.

- Medicaid enrollees aged 65 and older were more likely than those with private or Medicare coverage to have received at-home care, to have had multiple visits to a doctor or other health professional, and to have visited an ED in the past 12 months.

- Individuals eligible on the basis of a disability and those aged 65 and older account for about a quarter of Medicaid enrollees but about two-thirds of program spending in FY 2010.

- A large share of Medicaid spending for enrollees eligible on the basis of a disability and enrollees aged 65 and older is for long-term services and supports, while a substantial portion of spending for non-disabled children and adults is for capitation payments to managed care plans.

- The use of managed care varies widely by state, both in the arrangements used and the populations served. In 2011, all but three states reported using some form of managed care, including comprehensive risk-based plans, limited-benefit plans, or primary care case management programs.

- The share of enrollees in comprehensive risk-based plans in FY 2010 was 62 percent among non-disabled children, 47 percent among non-disabled adults, 29 percent among individuals eligible on the basis of a disability, and 12 percent among those aged 65 and older.

CHAPTER 1

Maternity Services: Examining Eligibility and Coverage in Medicaid and CHIP

Key Points

Maternity Services: Examining Eligibility and Coverage in Medicaid and CHIP

- In 2010, Medicaid and the State Children's Health Insurance Program (CHIP) paid for almost half of all births in the United States (about 1.8 million hospital births). Medicaid spending in the 12 months before and 2 months following deliveries for women in 2008 was about $11 billion.

- Between 1984 and 1990, the Congress expanded Medicaid eligibility for poor and low-income pregnant women and children, creating new mandatory and optional eligibility groups. States are required to provide pregnancy-related coverage to pregnant women below 133 percent of the federal poverty level (FPL); a majority of states provide coverage to women above that level.

- The Patient Protection and Affordable Care Act (ACA) has several provisions affecting pregnant women, including mandating maternity care and other pregnancy-related services. Under the ACA in 2014, states have considerable discretion whether or not they will cover pregnant women above 138 percent FPL, and many have the option to reduce Medicaid or CHIP eligibility to this group in favor of exchange coverage. Because separate eligibility pathways based on pregnancy will continue, the possibility of churning exists as women gain and lose eligibility based on their pregnancy status and cycle among Medicaid, CHIP, and private coverage available through health insurance exchanges, or to an uninsured status.

- Although CHIP originally did not include coverage for pregnant women, states can offer CHIP-financed services to pregnant women through Section 1115 waivers or through an option to cover services for unborn children. A law enacted in 2009 allowed states to cover pregnant women through state plan amendments.

- Depending on the eligibility pathway, services covered under Medicaid and CHIP range from full Medicaid benefits to coverage of only services related to the pregnancy to emergency coverage for labor and delivery.

- Many states offer benefits to pregnant women that are not offered to other Medicaid adult enrollees, including dental services, prenatal risk assessments, home visiting programs, targeted case management, preconception counseling, psychosocial counseling, and substance abuse treatment.

- Almost one-third of Medicaid deliveries (31 percent) were by cesarean section, a figure comparable to rates for all births. Cesarean deliveries cost more than vaginal deliveries and are associated with more adverse outcomes. Many states, in partnership with the federal government and private organizations, have initiated programs to reduce elective cesarean sections and non-medically indicated induced deliveries before 39 weeks of gestation to help improve maternal and infant outcomes and to reduce costs.

CHAPTER 1

Maternity Services: Examining Eligibility and Coverage in Medicaid and CHIP

In 2010, Medicaid and the State Children's Health Insurance Program (CHIP) together paid for nearly half of the nearly 4 million live births in the United States.[1] Maternity-related services covered by the programs include prenatal care, labor and delivery services, and 60 days of postpartum care.

There is room for improvement in the delivery of maternity services and related outcomes in the United States—overall and within Medicaid and CHIP. About one in eight of all babies born in the United States in 2011 were preterm (born before 37 weeks gestation), and 8 percent of babies born in that year were considered to have low birth weight (LBW, defined as less than 2,500 grams or 5 pounds, 8 ounces; Hamilton et al. 2012). As a major payer of maternity services, Medicaid plays a key role in reducing preterm births and improving care and outcomes for women and babies. Current efforts by state Medicaid programs to reduce unnecessary or potentially harmful procedures—such as non-medically indicated inductions or scheduled cesarean sections prior to 39 weeks of gestation—include both payment incentives and educational programs. Other efforts promote medical homes, tobacco cessation, obesity management, oral health, and early prenatal care.

The Patient Protection and Affordable Care Act (ACA, P.L. 111–148, as amended) includes many provisions that could benefit pregnant women, including the streamlining of Medicaid eligibility, the creation of health insurance exchanges with subsidized coverage, and the establishment of essential health benefit packages. However, issues remain related to transitions in eligibility due to changes in pregnancy status that create discontinuities in coverage, as well as discrepancies in covered benefits between Medicaid, CHIP, and insurance plans offered through the exchanges.

This chapter describes the role of Medicaid and CHIP in covering maternity care. It begins by presenting general statistics about births in the United States in order to put Medicaid and CHIP's role in a broader context. It then provides an overview of current eligibility pathways to Medicaid and CHIP for pregnant women, the packages of services offered to women who become eligible via each pathway, and how the ACA could affect the pathways and benefit packages. Next, the chapter describes Medicaid initiatives designed to improve maternal and perinatal outcomes. Finally, it concludes with a discussion of several policy issues, including those relating to ACA implementation, which MACPAC will follow over the next few years.

Policy Context: Births in the United States

Birth rates in the United States have been declining over time, as have births to teenage and unmarried mothers. There also have been recent declines in the share of births that are preterm or LBW babies, and in infant mortality.

Birth rate. The birth rate for 2011 was the lowest rate ever reported in the United States (63.2 births per 1,000 women aged 15 to 44). Birth rates vary considerably by state, ranging from 51.5 births per 1,000 women aged 15 to 44 in Rhode Island, to 83.6 births per 1,000 women aged 15 to 44 in Utah (Hamilton et al. 2012).

Teenage birth rate. The teenage birth rate fell to a historic low in 2011—31.3 births per 1,000 women aged 15 to 19—down 8 percent from 2010 (34.2 per 1,000). The birth rate for teenagers has declined more than 3 percent per year since the most recent peak in 1991 (61.8 per 1,000), and the rate of decline has accelerated since 2007 (Hamilton et al. 2012). Six percent of Medicaid deliveries in 2008 were to women under age 18 (MACPAC analysis of Medicaid Statistical Information System (MSIS) data, 2013).

Non-marital birth rate. Over two-fifths of all births (40.7 percent) in 2011 were to unmarried women. The percentage of births to unmarried women increased in 4 states and declined in 10 states between 2010 and 2011. Unmarried teenagers accounted for 18 percent of all non-marital births in 2011, the lowest percentage ever reported (Hamilton et al. 2012).

Preterm birth rate. The preterm birth rate (the percentage of births delivered at less than 37 completed weeks of gestation) fell for the fifth straight year in 2011 to 11.7 percent, from its 2006 peak of 12.8 percent (Hamilton et al. 2012). Rates declined in 47 states and the District of Columbia between 2010 and 2011, while remaining essentially unchanged in the remaining states.

The preterm birth rate rose by more than one-third from 1981 to 2006. Although at its lowest level in more than a decade, the 2011 preterm birth rate is still higher than rates reported during the 1980s and most of the 1990s (Martin et al. 2010).

Infant mortality rate. There were 26,408 infant deaths in the United States in 2009—a 6 percent decline from 2008. The U.S. infant mortality rate was 6.4 infant deaths per 1,000 live births in 2009 compared to 6.6 in 2008. Infant mortality was higher for male infants, infants born preterm, infants born with LBW (who were more likely to be twins or higher order births), and to mothers who were unmarried. From 2007 to 2009, infant mortality rates ranged from a high of 11.5 per 1,000 live births for the District of Columbia to a low of 4.8 per 1,000 live births for New Hampshire (Mathews and MacDorman 2013).

Low birth weight rate. The 2011 LBW rate was 8.1 percent (Hamilton et al. 2012). The LBW rate had increased more than 20 percent from the mid-1980s through 2006, but declined slowly from 2006 to 2011. In 2010, the jurisdictions with the highest percentages of LBW babies were Alabama, the District of Columbia, Louisiana, and Mississippi; each had more than 10 percent of newborns in this category. The lowest percentages were in Alaska, New Hampshire, North Dakota, Vermont, and Washington—all with a LBW rate lower than 7 percent (Martin et al. 2012b).

Low-income births. In 2010, 48 percent of children under age five lived in households whose incomes were below 200 percent of the federal poverty level (FPL) (U.S. Census Bureau 2011). Over the past four decades, nearly half of children born to poor parents were poor for at least half their childhoods—that is, persistently poor—and there have not been significant improvements for recent generations (Ratcliffe and McKernan 2012).

Factors associated with pregnancy and birth outcomes

Most births occur without adverse outcomes. The problems that do occur for mothers and infants during pregnancy and the birth process often stem from preventable causes. Maternal behaviors known to be related to poor birth outcomes include tobacco use, alcohol and drug use, and failure to consume adequate folic acid. Other conditions associated with poor pregnancy outcomes include unintended pregnancy, suboptimal birth spacing, physical abuse, and high levels of stress (Bailey and Byrom 2007, D'Angelo et al. 2007).

Certain maternal health conditions (e.g., diabetes, hypertension, and obesity), if uncontrolled, can have a long-term negative impact on a woman's health and can lead to poor infant outcomes. Uncontrolled diabetes during pregnancy, for example, raises the risk of maternal health problems and birth defects threefold (D'Angelo et al. 2007). Persons living below 200 percent FPL are almost twice as likely to have diabetes as persons above 400 percent FPL and are also significantly more likely to be obese (NCHS 2012). Obesity before and during the early months of pregnancy is closely linked to diabetes and is also associated with stillbirth, early neonatal death, fetal macrosomia (big baby, or large for gestational age, syndrome), birth defects, preeclampsia, and hypertensive and thromboembolic disease. In addition to these conditions, having had a previous preterm, LBW infant is a predictor of poor birth outcomes for subsequent pregnancies (D'Angelo et al. 2007).

Preterm births and low birth weight. Preterm birth and LBW babies are more likely than other infants to spend time in a neonatal intensive care unit (NICU) or a neonatal intermediate care unit (NINT). These special nursery hospital units or facilities are staffed and equipped to provide continuous specialized support for newborns requiring intensive care. According to a study commissioned by the March of Dimes, the average NICU stay at reporting hospitals cost about $76,000 for 13.2 days (March of Dimes 2011).[2] Nearly 7 percent of U.S. newborns were admitted to a NINT or a NICU in 2008, and about half of NICU stays at children's hospitals were paid for by Medicaid (Children's Hospital Association 2013, Osterman et al. 2011).

Medicaid and CHIP Eligibility for Pregnant Women

Historically, to be eligible for Medicaid or CHIP, an individual must fall into an eligibility category, such as pregnant women, and must meet certain financial and non-financial requirements. Generally, each category includes mandatory and optional eligibility groups. Because states can choose whether or not to adopt optional groups as part of their state plans, eligibility varies from state to state.

States can also receive approval from the Centers for Medicare & Medicaid Services (CMS) to expand eligibility via a Section 1115 demonstration waiver to individuals who would not otherwise be eligible for Medicaid or CHIP. Section 1115 demonstrations are initially approved for a five-year period, but can be renewed for additional years.

This section describes the various pathways through which pregnant women may become eligible for Medicaid or CHIP. The next section describes Medicaid or CHIP coverage provided to pregnant women by eligibility group.

Medicaid eligibility for pregnant women through 2013

Before 1984, the only pregnant women states were required to cover in Medicaid were eligible through two pathways: (1) as parents or caretaker relatives of dependent children receiving cash assistance under the Aid to Families with Dependent Children (AFDC) program, or (2) as disabled individuals. Today, most become eligible under more recent eligibility categories created specifically for pregnant women.

In 1984, the Congress added a mandatory eligibility category for certain low-income pregnant women who would be eligible for AFDC if their child were born and living with them. Between 1984 and 1990, the Congress repeatedly expanded Medicaid eligibility for low-income pregnant women, creating new mandatory and optional eligibility groups.

Pregnant women up to 133 percent FPL. Since 1989, pregnant women with incomes at or below 133 percent FPL have been a mandatory Medicaid eligibility group (Table 1-1). Because their eligibility is related to their income relative to the FPL, this pathway is referred to as mandatory poverty-related pregnant women. States are only required to cover pregnancy-related services for this group, but may cover full Medicaid benefits at the state option. Most states define such services broadly enough to equal full Medicaid coverage (CMS 2012).

Pregnant women with incomes above 133 percent FPL. All but nine states have extended Medicaid coverage to pregnant women above the required level of 133 percent FPL. Among those states, a majority (36 states and the District of Columbia) have raised their eligibility threshold for pregnant women to 185 percent FPL or higher. Iowa, Wisconsin, and the District of Columbia cover pregnancy-related services for optional poverty-related pregnant women with incomes as high as 300 percent FPL (MACPAC 2013).

CHIP

Compared to Medicaid, CHIP covers far fewer pregnant women. In 2012 there were about 10,000 pregnant women and 318,000 unborn children covered by CHIP (MACPAC analysis of CHIP enrollment data 2013). CHIP originally did not permit any coverage of pregnant adults. However, CMS later issued guidance allowing states to provide CHIP-financed services to pregnant women through Section 1115 demonstration waivers, or through an option to cover services for unborn children. The Children's Health Insurance Program Reauthorization Act of 2009 (CHIPRA, P.L. 111–3) created additional CHIP eligibility pathways for pregnant women.

Section 1115 waivers. In 2000, CMS issued guidance announcing it would use the authority under Section 1115 of the Social Security Act (the Act) to approve waivers of federal CHIP law to enroll uninsured pregnant women in CHIP under certain prescribed circumstances (CMS 2000). CHIP Section 1115 waivers give states the flexibility to provide comprehensive health benefits to pregnant women throughout

TABLE 1-1. Legislative Milestones in Medicaid and CHIP Coverage of Pregnant Women

1984   Deficit Reduction Act of 1984 (DRA, P.L. 98–369)
- Required states to provide Medicaid to pregnant women with no other dependent children who would be a single parent (or a parent with the other parent incapacitated) and eligible for Aid to Families with Dependent Children (AFDC) if the child were born.
- Required states to provide Medicaid to pregnant women who would be in a family with two able-bodied parents (one of whom must be unemployed) and who would be eligible for AFDC if the child were born.

1986   Consolidated Omnibus Budget Reconciliation Act of 1985 (COBRA, P.L. 99–272)
- Required states to cover pregnant women meeting state AFDC income and resource standards, regardless of the employment or martial status of the family.
- Required 60 days postpartum coverage for pregnant women.
- Provided that pregnancy-related services available to covered women need not be available to other Medicaid enrollees.

1986   Omnibus Budget Reconciliation Act of 1986 (OBRA '86, P.L. 99–509)
- Allowed states the option to cover all pregnant women (and young children up to age 5) in families with incomes at or below 100 percent of the federal poverty level (FPL), regardless of their AFDC eligibility status or assets.
- Permitted states to provide ambulatory prenatal care to women during a presumptive eligibility period of up to 45 days, if:
  - the woman has begun maternity care with a qualified provider;
  - the provider determines that the woman's family income falls below the applicable Medicaid standard and notifies the state of the woman's eligibility within five working days; and
  - the woman applies for such benefits within 14 days of being presumed eligible.

1987   Omnibus Budget Reconciliation Act of 1987 (OBRA '87, P.L. 100–203)
- Allowed states the option to extend Medicaid coverage to pregnant women and infants up to 185 percent FPL.

1988   Medicare Catastrophic Coverage Act of 1988 (MCCA, P.L. 100–360)
- Required states to phase in Medicaid coverage for all pregnant women and infants in families with income up to 100 percent FPL. (Much of MCCA was repealed in 1989, but provisions related to pregnant women were retained.)

1989   Omnibus Budget Reconciliation Act of 1989 (OBRA '89, P.L. 101–239)
- Required Medicaid coverage for all pregnant women (and children under age 6) in families with incomes at or below 133 percent FPL.

TABLE 1-1, Continued

1996 Personal Responsibility and Work Opportunity Reconciliation Act of 1996 (PRWORA, P.L. 104–193)
- ▸ Prohibited Medicaid coverage for non-emergency services to otherwise eligible legal non-citizens entering the United States on or after August 22, 1996 (including pregnant women), until they have resided in the United States for five years. Permitted coverage after the five-year ban at state option.

2009 Children's Health Insurance Program Reauthorization Act of 2009 (CHIPRA, P.L. 111–3)
- ▸ Permitted states to cover lawfully residing pregnant women and children through Medicaid and CHIP without regard to the five-year residency requirement.
- ▸ Allowed states to cover low-income pregnant women under CHIP through a state plan amendment.

2010 Patient Protection and Affordable Care Act of 2010 (ACA, P.L. 111–148)
- ▸ Added tobacco cessation programs for pregnant women and services provided at freestanding birth centers as mandatory benefits.

---

pregnancy, as well as during a 60-day postpartum period (CMS 2009). However, CHIP funding is capped, and states are required to prioritize coverage for children over coverage for adults. In fiscal year (FY) 2012, Colorado covered 4,873 pregnant women and Virginia covered 4,101 pregnant women under a CHIP waiver (MACPAC 2013).

Unborn child state plan option. In 2002, CMS provided a means of covering prenatal care under a CHIP state plan by revising the definition of the term child in federal regulations to include the period from conception to birth (CMS 2002). States that elect this option provide coverage to the unborn child, not the pregnant woman herself. Therefore, only services related to pregnancy or conditions that could complicate pregnancy may be covered using this option, although states have broad flexibility in defining these services. A pregnant woman may receive prenatal care under this option, regardless of her immigration status, because the fetus will be a citizen once born (CMS 2009, CMS 2002). Postpartum services for mothers are not covered under any circumstance. In FY 2012, 16 states enrolled approximately 318,000 unborn children in CHIP (MACPAC analysis of CHIP enrollment data 2013).

CHIP state plan coverage of pregnant women. CHIPRA allows states to provide health care coverage for uninsured, targeted low-income pregnant women under the CHIP state plan. Unlike the unborn child option, the CHIPRA option covers the pregnant woman—providing comprehensive benefits that include prenatal and delivery care, as well as 60 days of postpartum care. Cost sharing and benefit rules under this option must be comparable to the rules for children in CHIP. In FY 2012, New Jersey covered 312 women under this option, and Rhode Island covered 379 (MACPAC 2013).

Coverage provided through this option must not replace existing Medicaid coverage for pregnant women, and states must provide Medicaid to pregnant women with incomes up to at least 185 percent FPL. States must also provide CHIP to children with family incomes up to at least

200 percent FPL in order to cover targeted low-income pregnant women (CMS 2009).

Presumptive eligibility for pregnant women

As described in Table 1-1, the Omnibus Budget Reconciliation Act of 1986 (P.L.99-509) allowed states to permit certain qualified providers to provide ambulatory prenatal care to pregnant women on the basis of preliminary eligibility information, even if they have not formally been determined eligible. This mechanism of presumptive eligibility allows women to obtain Medicaid-covered prenatal care immediately. This ensures that providers are paid for any services they deliver during the presumptive eligibility period, even if the pregnant woman is not subsequently determined eligible. Under current law, a presumptive eligibility period lasts for up to 60 days, when the full eligibility determination must be completed for coverage to continue. Currently 31 states allow presumptive eligibility for pregnant women (KFF 2013).

Non-citizens

Eligibility for Medicaid maternity benefits and services differs by immigration status of the pregnant woman. Medicaid eligibility for non-citizens who are unauthorized or illegally present is limited to coverage for the treatment of an emergency medical condition, including labor and delivery. These individuals must meet all of Medicaid's financial and non-financial eligibility criteria, other than immigration status, in order to qualify for emergency coverage.

Under the Personal Responsibility and Work Opportunity Reconciliation Act of 1996 (P.L. 104–193), most legal immigrants (referred to as qualified aliens in that law) are subject to a five-year bar on regular Medicaid eligibility, at which point their coverage becomes a state option.

As with non-citizens who are unauthorized or illegally present, these qualified aliens are eligible for emergency Medicaid during their five-year waiting period (and beyond, if a state opts not to provide them with regular Medicaid coverage), but only if they meet all other eligibility criteria for the program. In 2009, CHIPRA permitted states to provide regular Medicaid and CHIP coverage to all lawfully residing pregnant women and children, including those otherwise subject to the five-year waiting period (CMS 2010).

In 2008, there were about 295,000 deliveries paid for by Medicaid under the restricted emergency benefit for non-citizens (Table 1-2).

The ACA and eligibility for maternity services

Pregnant women will be affected by ACA provisions that change Medicaid eligibility for many adults and create subsidies for private coverage through health insurance exchanges.

Under the ACA, states must maintain eligibility and enrollment policies for Medicaid that were in place for pregnant women (and all adults) at the time the law was enacted until new health insurance exchanges are operational in 2014. At that time, all states must determine eligibility for pregnant women (and certain other populations) using the new national income counting methodology, modified adjusted gross income (MAGI). As part of MAGI-based eligibility determinations, states will be required to disregard income equal to 5 percent FPL. For this reason, income eligibility in 2014 for populations including pregnant women is often referred to at its effective level of 138 percent FPL, even though federal statute specifies 133 percent FPL.

With the expiration of the maintenance of effort for adults in 2014, many states will have the option to transition pregnant women with incomes above 138 percent FPL from Medicaid to private coverage available through health insurance exchanges. However, states that had a higher income standard in effect for pregnant women in 1989 must keep their higher standard (§1902(l)(2)(A) of the Act); this long-standing maintenance of effort appears to apply to 19 states (NGA 1990).

Pregnant women and the new adult group. The ACA called for expanding Medicaid eligibility in 2014 to nearly all non-elderly adults with income up to 138 percent FPL. Newly eligible individuals in this expansion group are funded with a 100 percent federal match in 2014, 2015, and 2016, with the rate declining to 90 percent for 2020 and beyond. The ACA specifies that pregnant women with incomes below 138 percent FPL are not eligible for coverage under the new adult group. Because states are not required to track the pregnancy status of women enrolled through the new adult group, women who enroll in this group and later become pregnant are likely to stay enrolled in the adult group (CMS 2013). It is possible that some pregnant women would request that the state move them to a pregnancy-related eligibility group if they need specific benefits that are not available under the adult group benefit package. However, if a woman indicates on the application that she is pregnant, and is therefore enrolled in Medicaid coverage as a pregnant woman, the state will receive federal funds at the normal match rate (CMS 2012).

Pregnant women with incomes above 138 percent FPL. Under the ACA, states have considerable discretion as to how they will cover pregnant women above 138 percent FPL. For example, a state might provide full Medicaid benefits for pregnant women up to 185 percent FPL and provide only pregnancy-related coverage through the pregnant women group for those who have incomes up to a higher state-defined level. Alternatively, a state might provide full Medicaid for pregnant women with incomes at or below 138 percent FPL and CHIP waiver coverage for those with incomes up to 200 percent FPL. In this scenario, premium tax credits and cost-sharing reductions associated with private coverage available through health insurance exchanges may be accessible to eligible women above 200 percent FPL and below 400 percent FPL.

Concerns related to churning. Churning occurs when individuals enroll and disenroll in different health insurance programs, or to uninsured status, often within a relatively short period of time. Because separate eligibility pathways based on pregnancy will continue, the possibility of churning still exists as women gain and lose eligibility based on their pregnancy status and cycle between Medicaid, CHIP, and private coverage available through health insurance exchanges, or to uninsured status. This could create challenges as enrollees may experience discontinuity of care and changes in what they must pay for care if provider networks or benefits differ among programs. States, providers, and health plans could also experience administrative burdens as women change insurance status based on their pregnancy status.

Covered Benefits for Maternity Services

Depending on the eligibility group, as described above, pregnant women may qualify for different levels of coverage.

▶ **Full Medicaid or CHIP coverage.** Full Medicaid coverage includes all medically necessary hospital and physician services, as well as family planning, nurse midwife, and freestanding birth center services. Full CHIP coverage for pregnant women could consist of a Medicaid look-alike package, or benchmark or benchmark-equivalent coverage.

- **Pregnancy-related services only.** For Medicaid, pregnancy-related services are only services related to pregnancy, labor and delivery, and any complications that may occur during pregnancy, as well as prenatal and postpartum care.
- **Services for an unborn child.** State CHIP programs may cover the unborn children of pregnant women. In this instance, services related to prenatal care and other care to ensure a healthy baby and safe delivery are covered (CMS 2002).
- **Medicaid emergency medical services.** This includes labor and delivery, but not any prenatal or postpartum care.

This section discusses what services are included in pregnancy-related benefits in current Medicaid programs, and what will be required under the ACA. It also discusses some enhanced benefits that states offer and additional benefits required by the ACA that will be relevant for pregnant women.

Pregnancy-related benefits through 2013

Federal law permits states to limit coverage to pregnancy-related services for women with family incomes above the May 1, 1988, AFDC levels. Women below the 1988 AFDC levels must receive full Medicaid benefits; above this level, it is a state option whether to cover only pregnancy-related benefits or full benefits.

Pregnancy-related services are those that are necessary for the health of the pregnant woman and fetus, including:

- prenatal care;
- delivery;
- postpartum care;
- family planning services; and
- services for other conditions that might complicate the pregnancy, threaten carrying the fetus to full term, or create problems for the safe delivery of the fetus (42 CFR 440.210).

For eligibility groups entitled to only pregnancy-related services, most states define such services broadly enough to equal full Medicaid coverage (42CFR 435.116(d)(1); CMS 2012). It is not clear how many states define pregnancy-related services more narrowly and whether this has any impact on maternal or birth outcomes. Box 1-1 provides an example: Texas' CHIP perinatal coverage for unborn children through its state plan amendment (SPA).

Across all births covered by Medicaid in 2008, about 1.1 million (69 percent) were to women with full Medicaid benefits, while about 174,000 (11 percent) were to women categorized as having only pregnancy-related benefits (Table 1-2).

Pregnancy-related benefits under the ACA

Federal regulations issued under the ACA clarify that states can continue to choose to provide full Medicaid benefits to all pregnant women in Medicaid (42 CFR 435.116(d)(1)). As mentioned above, for eligibility groups entitled to only pregnancy-related services, most states define such services broadly enough to equal full Medicaid coverage, and the assumption is that full Medicaid coverage is the default for these groups (42 CFR 435.116(d)(1)). However, if a state chooses to limit coverage to pregnancy-related services, CMS will require a SPA that explains the state's basis for determining which services are not pregnancy-related, and the rationale for not covering them (CMS 2012).

This creates a situation in which women who are pregnant may be eligible for fewer Medicaid benefits than women of the same or higher income

> **BOX 1-1. Texas CHIP Perinatal Coverage**
>
> The Texas CHIP perinatal program pays for care to unborn children of pregnant women with household income up to 200 percent of the federal poverty level (FPL) and who are not eligible for Medicaid. Once born, the child will receive benefits that are similar to the traditional CHIP benefits for the duration of the 12-month coverage period.
>
> Benefits for the unborn child include:
>
> - up to 20 prenatal visits
>   - during the first 28 weeks of pregnancy: one visit every four weeks;
>   - during 28 to 36 weeks of pregnancy: one visit every two to three weeks;
>   - from 36 weeks to delivery: one visit per week;
>   - additional prenatal visits allowed if medically necessary;
> - some laboratory testing, assessments, planning services, education, and counseling;
> - prescription drug coverage based on the current CHIP formulary; and
> - hospital facility charges and professional services charges related to the delivery.
>
> False labor and preterm labor that does not result in a birth are not covered benefits.
>
> For families with income from 186 to 200 percent FPL:
>
> - qualifying hospital facility charges paid through the CHIP perinatal health plan; and
> - qualifying professional service charges paid through the CHIP perinatal health plan.
>
> For families with income at or below 185 percent FPL (the majority of CHIP perinatal clients):
>
> - hospital facility charges paid through Emergency Medicaid; and
> - professional service charges paid through CHIP.
>
> **Source:** Texas HHSC 2013.

levels. While women in the new adult group or in exchange coverage will have coverage for 10 broad categories of essential health benefits specified in the ACA, poverty-related pregnant women may have coverage for only pregnancy-related care.[3]

The ACA mandates that both Medicaid and exchange plans cover a number of preventive health services that the Institute of Medicine identifies as critical, including several related to healthy pregnancy and birth. No copayment, coinsurance, or deductible can be charged for maternity care or the following additional services:

- smoking cessation;
- screening for gestational diabetes;
- human papillomavirus (HPV) DNA testing for women 30 years and older;
- sexually transmitted infection counseling;

- Food and Drug Administration-approved contraception methods and contraceptive counseling;
- HIV screening and counseling;
- domestic violence screening and counseling;
- well women visits; and
- breastfeeding support and supplies (CMS 2011).[4]

The ACA also requires that Medicaid cover services provided in freestanding birth centers. States have discretion over the specific types of practitioners that can perform services at these birth centers.

Coverage for enhanced benefits during pregnancy

Some states offer benefits to pregnant women that are not offered to other Medicaid enrollees. While they are not mandated as pregnancy-related services, states have sought to improve pregnancy and birth outcomes with these enhanced benefits.

Dental services. Recent studies have reported an emerging link between periodontal disease and an increased risk for preterm birth and LBW infants. Some studies indicate that treatment for periodontal disease during pregnancy can improve birth outcomes. Other studies disagree; however, there appears to be an emerging consensus that preventive dental care during pregnancy is desirable (Boggess et al. 2013, Albert et al. 2011, Detman et al. 2010, Offenbacher et al. 2006). In 2004, data from the Pregnancy Risk Assessment Monitoring System showed that pregnant women covered by Medicaid prior to their pregnancy were significantly less likely to have had a dental visit (73 percent) during their pregnancy than privately insured women (85 percent) (D'Angelo et al. 2007).

Dental services for adults (age 21 and over) are an optional Medicaid benefit; most states provide limited, or no, coverage of adult oral health services. However, several states extend dental coverage only to pregnant women. In recent years, due in part to budget constraints, there has been considerable activity in state legislatures to either add or remove dental coverage for this group. For example, Louisiana removed dental coverage for pregnant women effective January 31, 2013 (Louisiana DHH 2012).

Other enhanced benefits. Enrollment in Medicaid or CHIP does not guarantee that pregnant women will receive recommended maternity care, such as early prenatal care. Most states cover some enhanced benefits for pregnant women that are designed to improve compliance with early prenatal care, encourage healthy behavior and nutrition in both the preconception period and during pregnancy, and to screen for, diagnose, and treat conditions that may complicate pregnancy (Johnson and Witgert 2010).

The extent of enhanced benefits coverage offered by states has changed over time. More states provided prenatal risk assessments, nutritional counseling, home visiting programs, health education, targeted case management, and preconception counseling in the 1990s than in 2007. However, other pregnancy benefits were more prevalent in 2007, including smoking cessation, transportation services, psychosocial counseling, dental coverage, and substance abuse treatment (Hill et al. 2009).

Access to Maternity Care

Having coverage for maternity services does not guarantee access to care. Access to obstetricians and gynecologists (OB/GYNs), who provide a majority of maternity care, is a significant issue in many areas of the country, possibly due to falling numbers of practicing maternity care providers (Anderson et al. 2008). Many OB/GYNs have either stopped delivering babies or plan to stop in the near future (Loafman and Nanda 2009).

In 2010, nearly 50 percent of U.S. counties had no OB/GYNs providing direct patient care (ACOG 2013). As another indication that OB/GYNs are not well distributed, 15 percent of counties have above-average concentrations of OB/GYNs relative to their population, while 85 percent of counties are below the national average. Relative to population, non-metropolitan counties have fewer than half as many OB/GYNs as metropolitan counties (1.4 versus 3.3 per 10,000 females 15 years of age and over). Almost all (93 percent) of the counties that had no OB/GYNs also had no certified nurse midwives in 2003 (NCHS 2008).

Shortages of OB/GYNs can result in long waiting times for appointments or long travel times to appointments. Obstetrics and gynecology have become particularly prone to workforce challenges due to concerns surrounding professional liability, unpredictable working hours, declining medical student interest, reductions in the numbers of OB/GYN residency programs, and increasing subspecialization by graduating residents. These factors have contributed to inadequate access to maternal and reproductive care, especially in underserved communities (Anderson et al. 2008).

The number of hospitals offering obstetric services has also been declining over time, particularly in non-metropolitan counties that may already have a shortage of OB/GYNs (Zhao 2007). Forty-four percent of non-metropolitan counties lacked hospital-based obstetric services in 2002, compared with 24 percent in 1985. In the mid-1980s, residents in about half of these counties had access to obstetric services in a local hospital; by the early 2000s, only about one-fifth of the most rural counties had at least one hospital providing obstetric services.

As the number of practicing OB/GYNs has declined, other practitioners are providing maternity care. In areas with few obstetricians, much of this care is delivered by family physicians and by nurse midwives or nurse practitioners. However, fewer family physicians have been providing maternity care over time (Tong et al. 2012). The trend is reversed for nurse midwives; in 2010, 8.4 percent all U.S. births were midwife-attended, up from 7.8 percent in 2000 and 1 percent in 1975 (Martin et al. 2012a, 2002). However, nurse midwives face potential barriers, including lower Medicaid payments relative to OB/GYNs in many states, restricted hospital privilege policies regarding non-physician practitioners practicing in inpatient settings, and state scope of practice laws (Brassard and Smolenski 2011, Reed and Roberts 2000).

Some states have implemented programs to increase access to obstetric providers in underserved areas for their Medicaid and CHIP enrollees. For example, New York's Medicaid Obstetrical and Maternal Services Program provides complete pregnancy care services (medical and health supportive) in areas of the state without prenatal care health centers. Medical services are provided in private physicians' offices. Health supportive services such as nutrition and psychosocial services, health education, HIV counseling and testing, and assistance with the Medicaid and Special Supplemental Nutrition Program for Women, Infants, and Children applications are provided by approved providers.

Utilization and Expenditures for Medicaid Maternity Services

In 2010, there were about 1.8 million births in community hospitals to women enrolled in Medicaid (or in some cases CHIP) at the time of their delivery. (See Chapter 1 Appendix for a description of data sources used and data limitations.) Almost half (46 percent) of all deliveries were paid by Medicaid in 2010 (Table 1-3). States varied in the percentage of total births paid by Medicaid from a low of 20 percent in Minnesota to a high of 61 percent in Oklahoma.

Medicaid spending

Medicaid spent about $11 billion on health care for women who delivered a baby in a hospital while enrolled in Medicaid in 2008 (Table 1-2). This includes all Medicaid costs billed for the mother for the 12 months before and 2 months following delivery, which could include costs not associated with the pregnancy. Sixty-nine percent of total spending was for women with full Medicaid benefits.[5] Using Healthcare Cost and Utilization Project (HCUP) data, which estimates costs based on charges for the hospitalization during which the deliveries occurred, the estimated cost of deliveries to Medicaid-covered women in 2010 was approximately $7.1 billion.

Cost and prevalence of cesarean deliveries

In general, cesarean deliveries are more expensive than vaginal deliveries. Comparing the most common types of deliveries, which do not have complicating conditions, the average cost of a hospitalization with a cesarean delivery paid by Medicaid was $5,162 in 2010 compared to $3,081 for a vaginal delivery with no complicating conditions (Table 1-4). Cesarean deliveries with complications also generate higher costs than vaginal deliveries with complications.

Cesarean deliveries also have more adverse outcomes than do vaginal deliveries, including complications of anesthesia and surgery, as well as infections (Risser and King 2010). Despite the risks and costs of cesarean deliveries, the percentage of births by cesarean rose nearly 60 percent from 1996 through 2011. However, the percentage of cesarean deliveries has stabilized over the past few years, remaining unchanged at 32.8 percent since 2009 (Martin et al. 2012a).

Almost one-third of Medicaid deliveries (31 percent) were by cesarean section (Table 1-3), though rates vary by state. For example, 21 percent of Medicaid deliveries in New Mexico were by cesarean whereas 36 percent of Medicaid deliveries in Florida were by cesarean. Medicaid cesarean rates did not differ from the total cesarean rate by more than a few percentage points in any of the reporting states.

Programs to Improve the Effectiveness of Maternity Care

State Medicaid programs have implemented a large number of initiatives designed to help women enroll into prenatal care programs as early as possible, to increase compliance with prenatal care protocols, and to increase access to needed services, as well as other interventions designed to improve maternal and infant outcomes while constraining costs.

Programs to enhance and increase use of prenatal care services

Research has shown that receiving prenatal care, especially during the first trimester, is a critical step toward having a healthy pregnancy and baby. Early prenatal visits can identify babies or mothers at risk for complications and give health care providers the opportunity to educate pregnant women. Early prenatal care also allows for appropriate first trimester screening tests that cannot be done at later stages of gestation. Women who receive prenatal care have consistently shown

TABLE 1-2. Medicaid Spending 12 Months before and 2 Months after Delivery for Women with a Hospital Delivery in 2008

	Number of Medicaid Deliveries	Percent of Medicaid Deliveries	Total Medicaid Spending for 12 months before and 2 Months after Delivery	Percent of Total Medicaid Spending for Women with Delivery in 2008	Average Medicaid Spending per Woman for 12 Months before and 2 Months after Delivery
Total Medicaid Deliveries	1,577,433	100%	$11,483,587,674	100%	$7,280
Benefit Status[1]					
Full benefit package	1,096,044	69[2]	8,395,765,887	73[2]	7,660
Pregnancy-related coverage only	174,151	11[2]	1,282,625,186	11[2]	7,365
Emergency coverage only, due to non-citizen status	294,508	19[2]	1,707,259,262	15[2]	5,797

Notes: Total federal and state spending. Includes spending on behalf of Medicaid-expansion CHIP enrollees. Excludes deliveries and spending in the territories. Medicaid Statistical Information System spending has not been adjusted to match totals in CMS-64 accounting data. Births may be undercounted in states whose managed care encounter data are incomplete, or whose inpatient hospital claims or encounter records have missing or non-standard diagnosis and procedure codes. See Chapter 1 Appendix for additional methodological information.

[1] Columns do not sum to 100 percent because a small number of women (about 13,000) with deliveries classified as having other types of restricted benefits are not included here.

[2] As noted above, managed care births may be undercounted in this analysis. Given that women with emergency coverage are unlikely to be enrolled in managed care, their shares of Medicaid deliveries (19 percent) and spending (15 percent) may be overestimates. Conversely, the Medicaid deliveries and spending for women with full or pregnancy-related coverage may be underestimates.

Source: MACPAC analysis of Medicaid Statistical Information System (MSIS) data.

better outcomes than those who did not receive prenatal care (Alexander and Kotelchuck 2001, McCormick 2001).

At the federal level, the Strong Start for Mothers and Newborns initiative is a joint effort between CMS, the Health Resources and Services Administration (HRSA), and the Administration on Children and Families. With the goals of reducing preterm births and improving outcomes for newborns and pregnant women enrolled in Medicaid and CHIP, this initiative will test four evidence-based maternity care service approaches. These include:

- prenatal care in group settings that incorporates peer-to-peer interaction in a facilitated setting for health assessment, education, and psychosocial support;
- comprehensive prenatal care facilitated by teams of health professionals, including peer counselors, with services such as collaborative practice, intensive case management, counseling, and psychosocial support; and
- enhanced prenatal care, including psychosocial support, education, and health promotion. Services provided will expand access to care, improve care coordination, and provide a broader array of health services.

TABLE 1-3. Medicaid Births in Community Hospitals, by Type of Delivery, 2010

State	Medicaid Births	Medicaid Births as Percent of Total Births	Total Cesareans as Percent of Singleton Births	Medicaid Cesareans as Percent of Singleton Births
United States	1,812,129	46%	32%	31%
Arizona	43,505	51	28	26
Arkansas	20,763	56	35	34
California	244,358	49	32	31
Colorado	23,761	39	26	23
Florida	115,145	55	38	36
Hawaii	6,609	42	27	27
Illinois	67,524	43	30	28
Iowa	15,282	40	29	28
Kansas	12,023	31	30	30
Kentucky	24,900	50	35	34
Maine	5,322	43	30	30
Maryland	29,638	44	34	31
Massachusetts	23,573	33	32	30
Michigan	51,630	46	32	30
Minnesota	12,454	20	27	25
Missouri	35,750	48	31	30
Nebraska	9,710	38	30	29
Nevada	12,922	38	35	32
New Jersey	25,444	25	37	32
New Mexico	15,037	60	23	21
New York	104,641	44	34	31
North Carolina	59,800	52	31	28
Oklahoma	29,590	61	34	33
Oregon	19,851	46	29	28
Rhode Island	5,341	45	32	29
South Carolina	25,102	46	34	33
Tennessee	38,462	52	35	32
Texas	191,496	52	36	34
Utah	17,581	34	22	23
Vermont	2,594	46	27	26
Washington	31,482	40	30	28
West Virginia	11,653	59	35	34
Wisconsin	24,954	38	25	23
Wyoming	2,045	33	28	29

Notes: Singleton births are defined as delivering one baby, meaning not twins or other multiple births. In the 2010 Healthcare Cost and Utilization Project (HCUP), states reported 48,981 Medicaid multiple births in community hospitals. Statistics are based in ICD-9-CM V30 codes that indicate delivery type for the newborn. Only liveborn singleton infants are counted in the percentages. All deliveries (including multiple births and non-liveborn infants) are counted in the total number of deliveries and the percentage of Medicaid deliveries. As discussed in Chapter 1 Appendix, Medicaid births may also include CHIP births. Not all states provide public use data for HCUP, however, the U.S. total reflects data for all states.

Source: MACPAC analysis of 2010 Healthcare Cost and Utilization Project (HCUP), Nationwide Inpatient Sample and State Inpatient Databases.

TABLE 1-4. Cost of Medicaid Births in Community Hospitals, by Type of Delivery, 2010

Delivery Type (DRG)	Number of Medicaid Deliveries	Average Length of Stay (days)	Average Cost
Cesarean Deliveries	548,006		
Without comorbidities or major complications (766)	345,667	3.0	$5,162
With comorbidities or major complications (765)	202,339	4.3	$7,018
Vaginal Deliveries	1,195,450		
Without complicating diagnoses (775)	987,770	2.1	$3,081
With complicating diagnoses (774)	159,046	2.8	$4,126

Notes: Healthcare Cost and Utilization Project (HCUP) converts total charges into costs using cost-to-charge ratios based on hospital accounting reports from the Centers for Medicare & Medicaid Services. In general, costs are less than charges. For each hospital, a hospital-wide cost-to-charge ratio is used because detailed charges are not available across all HCUP states. The costs presented here are estimates of the costs to the hospital of producing the entire hospital stay and not the amount billed to the Medicaid program or costs to the Medicaid program. DRGs 767 (Vaginal delivery w sterilization &/or d&c) and 768 (Vaginal delivery w O.R. proc except steril &/or d&c) are not included here; total vaginal deliveries include these cases.

Source: MACPAC analysis of 2010 Healthcare Cost and Utilization Project (HCUP).

The fourth approach to prevent preterm births, currently being evaluated, is enhanced prenatal care through home visiting. This approach is being evaluated as part of the evaluation of evidence-based models under the Maternal, Infant, and Early Childhood Home Visiting program, Nurse Family Partnership, and Healthy Families America programs.

To date, CMS has made 27 Strong Start program awards using the first three models to organizations such as universities, health care authorities, health plans, and associations that coordinate the program for participating health care providers. Awardees in total can spend up to $41.4 million and cannot use grant funds to supplement or supplant any funding sources, including Medicaid and CHIP reimbursement.

Many states have their own programs to increase use of prenatal care services, or they contract with health plans that have prenatal care initiatives. For example, Washington State's First Steps program, run by the Washington State Health Care Authority, is designed to promote healthy birth outcomes, increase access to early prenatal care, and reduce infant morbidity and mortality. Horizon Health, a managed care organization that contracts with the New Jersey Medicaid program, created Moms Getting Early Maternity Services (GEMS) to ensure that expecting mothers get proper prenatal care and education regarding having a healthy pregnancy and baby. Boxes 1-2 and 1-3 describe programs in place in North Carolina and Florida to improve pregnancy outcomes.

Programs to target high-risk women

Many state Medicaid programs, often in partnership with other state, federal, or private organizations, have implemented programs to

BOX 1-2. North Carolina's Pregnancy Medical Home Model

North Carolina's Pregnancy Home Model is a three-way partnership between Community Care of North Carolina, North Carolina's Medicaid program, and the North Carolina Division of Public Health to improve the quality of perinatal care given to Medicaid recipients, thereby improving birth outcomes and reducing Medicaid spending. First implemented in 2011, the partnership oversees a combined network of 14 regional networks that recruit and support participating providers. These providers agree to complete a risk assessment for each pregnant enrollee, collaborate with a care manager assigned to high-risk pregnancies, adhere to certain process and performance standards, and designate a practice champion. Participating primary care practices receive per member per month payments from Medicaid (in addition to standard fee-for-service payments). The partnership's central office supports the networks through analysis of claims, birth certificates, and care management data; technical assistance; and quality improvement support. The initiative has enhanced access to comprehensive care for pregnant Medicaid enrollees, including access to care coordination for those facing high-risk pregnancies. Preliminary data suggest the program has also increased provider adherence to evidence-based care standards and has begun to have a positive impact on the incidence of low birth weight and rates of primary cesarean sections. Providers participating in the Pregnancy Medical Home will receive the following:

- exemption from prior approval on ultrasounds;
- $50 for completing a high-risk screening tool at initial visit;
- $150 incentive for a postpartum visit for each woman; and
- higher payment rates for a vaginal delivery.

Source: AHRQ 2013.

BOX 1-3. Florida's Healthy Start Legislation

Florida's Healthy Start program provides for universal risk screening of all pregnant women and newborns in the state to identify those at risk of poor outcomes. Healthy Start includes targeted support services that address identified risks. The range of Healthy Start services available to pregnant women, infants, and children up to age three include:

- information and referral;
- comprehensive assessment of service needs in light of family and community resources;
- ongoing care coordination and support to assure access to needed services;
- psychosocial, nutritional, and smoking cessation counseling;
- childbirth, breastfeeding, and parenting support and education; and
- home visiting.

Source: Florida DOH 2013.

target women at greatest risk of premature delivery and poor birth outcomes. These programs include identifying high-risk women in areas with high rates of infant mortality, out-of-wedlock births, late or no prenatal care, teen pregnancies and births, and births to low-income women. They may also identify high-risk populations by conducting risk assessments at initial prenatal care visits. The prenatal risk assessment is often considered an integral part of care coordination and case management because it provides the mechanism by which states target high-risk mothers to receive additional services (Johnson and Witgert 2010). Targeted case management (called care coordination in some settings) is central to many states' enhanced prenatal benefits programs and typically determines a woman's needs by assessing risk factors, developing a plan of care to address those needs, coordinating referrals to appropriate service providers, and ensuring that the woman receives services (Hill and Breyel 1989).

Targeted case management may target high-risk women based on multiple socioeconomic, health, or behavioral risk factors, or women with a specific condition or risk factor. Programs can target pregnant women with specific diseases, including sexually transmitted diseases (STDs) and HIV; women with multiple risk factors; or women with specific health behaviors such as smoking, alcohol or drug abuse, or obesity. Counseling for smoking cessation, now a required health benefit in Medicaid under the ACA, must be provided with no cost sharing to women.

Programs focused on preconception care

Preconception care is defined as evidence-based risk screening, health promotion, and interventions that enable women to enter pregnancy in optimal health (Johnson et al. 2006). The American Congress of Obstetricians and Gynecologists (ACOG), the American Academy of Pediatrics, and the American College of Nurse-Midwives (ACNM) identify four key categories of preconception care interventions:

- maternal assessment (e.g., family history, behaviors, obstetric history, general physical exam);
- vaccinations (e.g., rubella, varicella, and hepatitis B);
- screening (e.g., HIV, STD, genetic disorders); and
- counseling (e.g., folic acid consumption, smoking and alcohol cessation, weight management) (Atrash et al. 2006).

Clinical practice guidelines have been developed based on evidence demonstrating the effectiveness of certain preconception practices, such as provision of folic acid; treatment of diabetes, HIV/AIDS, maternal phenylketonuria, epilepsy, and STDs; and counseling for smoking, alcohol use, and obesity.

Medicaid does not recognize preconception care services as a defined category of covered services, and only a handful of states include many of the elements of preconception care in family planning services. In a survey of 44 responding states and the District of Columbia, 26 of the states covered preconception counseling in 2007, but only 7 states routinely consider it to be a family planning service, in contrast to contraceptive counseling (29 states and the District of Columbia) and reproductive health education (20 states) (Ranji et al. 2009).

Programs to reduce non-medically indicated deliveries

Recently, policymakers and payers have begun focusing on the impact of non-medically indicated deliveries prior to 39 weeks gestation on health outcomes and costs. Early non-medically indicated deliveries include both inductions of labor and cesarean births scheduled before 39 weeks of gestation. These types of deliveries are associated with an increase in premature births, respiratory problems of the infant, and admissions to NICUs (Smith et al. 2012, Tita et al. 2009, NIH 2006). Although it is difficult to determine from administrative data whether deliveries are elective or not, a study conducted in 27 hospitals found that 71 percent of planned deliveries via labor induction or cesarean section occurred for no clear medical reason (Clark et al. 2009).

Although there is substantial literature that non-medically indicated early deliveries are associated with several adverse outcomes (King et al. 2010; Risser and King 2010), little available literature focuses on the Medicaid population or the specific initiatives being undertaken by state Medicaid agencies to reduce the number of these deliveries. In June 2012, MACPAC convened an expert roundtable to discuss the issue of early elective deliveries in Medicaid and commissioned a background paper on ongoing and proposed Medicaid programs to reduce non-medically indicated deliveries. Meeting participants and the background paper analysis concluded that this apparent gap in the current literature is likely due to analytic limitations of Medicaid administrative data and to the procedure coding system with respect to measuring maternity care processes, procedures, and outcomes, as well as to challenges associated with obtaining timely vital records data and linking these data to Medicaid data. In addition, several of the programs designed to reduce early elective deliveries have been implemented relatively recently and have yet to be evaluated. The large shifts in mode of delivery and use of obstetric procedures in the United States over the last two decades have significant implications for Medicaid.

ACOG, ACNM, the March of Dimes, CMS, and others have all called for reducing rates of non-medically indicated deliveries (both cesareans and medically induced deliveries) prior to 39 weeks gestation. In addition, these organizations also call for approaches to reduce non-medically indicated elective cesarean sections at any time. States have begun to respond to this call by changing payments and educating providers.

Payment initiatives

Several types of state Medicaid payment reforms are being proposed and tested to reduce or eliminate financial incentives for potentially unnecessary and costly procedures during childbirth (Table 1-5). One approach involves using penalties to discourage—or payments to reward—use of certain clinical procedures. Such an approach may involve offering additional payments or higher reimbursement rates to providers that meet a benchmark indicating provision of high-quality care. Another payment reform approach involves providing one blended payment for all deliveries, where the payment is set at a level greater than the current payment rate of a vaginal delivery and less than that for a cesarean delivery. A third approach involves providing bundled payments that encourage care coordination and discourage unnecessary use of services. Bundled payments may take the form of a single, combined payment for both hospital and provider services, a single payment for both maternal and infant care, or a single payment for all care provided during pregnancy.

TABLE 1-5. Selected State-Based Payment Reform Initiatives to Reduce Induction, Cesarean Section, and Early Elective Deliveries

State	Description of Initiative
Georgia	Starting July 1, 2013, the initiative eliminates Medicaid payments for elective cesarean deliveries and induced deliveries before 39 weeks (Williams 2013).
Minnesota	Minnesota's Medicaid program offers a single blended payment for all deliveries, whether vaginal or cesarean. The program intends to lower the cesarean delivery rate by 5 percent.
Nevada	As of March 2012, Nevada Medicaid pays the lower vaginal delivery payment rate for elective cesarean section.
South Carolina	As of January 1, 2013, South Carolina no longer provides payment to hospitals and physicians for elective inductions or non-medically indicated deliveries prior to 39 weeks gestational age. This applies to both inductions of labor and cesarean sections.
Texas	Texas Medicaid no longer pays providers (physicians or hospitals) for elective inductions and cesarean deliveries prior to 39 weeks of gestation (Texas Human Resources Code §32.0313).
Washington	Washington state offers a 1 percent Medicaid quality incentive payment to hospitals that maintain a rate of elective deliveries prior to 39 weeks below a given benchmark (7 percent).

Source: Smith et al. 2012.

Several states have undertaken payment reforms aimed at improving the quality of perinatal care. For example, Medicaid programs in South Carolina and Texas no longer pay for early non-medically indicated elective deliveries. Other states are relying on provider and enrollee feedback and education in an attempt to reduce these rates.

Quality improvement initiatives

Quality improvement initiatives generally establish health care processes and procedures to discourage elective inductions and cesarean deliveries, with many initiatives focused primarily on deliveries before 39 weeks of gestation (Table 1-6). Common elements of these initiatives include internal audit and feedback procedures, patient and provider education, policies limiting circumstances under which elective deliveries prior to 39 weeks can take place (for example, only when medically indicated or after peer review), and changes in delivery scheduling processes. Quality improvement initiatives have been implemented by statewide collaboratives, state agencies (including Medicaid), and health systems, with some supported by state legislation or occurring within a learning network, where hospitals or other organizations learn from their peers while implementing systems changes at the same time (Main et al. 2010). The Louisiana Institute for Healthcare Improvement, for example, is working with 28 of the state's 58 maternity hospitals to engage providers in quality improvement programs.

Performance measurement and public reporting

Performance measurement and public reporting of perinatal health clinical quality measures is another

TABLE 1-6. Selected State-Based Quality Improvement Initiatives to Reduce Induction, Cesarean Section, and Early Elective Deliveries

State and Initiative	Description of Initiative	Evidence of Effects
Louisiana 39-Week Initiative	In this initiative, which is led by the Institute for Healthcare Improvement Perinatal Improvement Community Collaborative, hospitals establish quality improvement policies to end early elective deliveries. The program uses the Elimination of Non-medically Indicated (Elective) Deliveries Before 39 Weeks Gestational Age toolkit created by the California Maternal Quality Care Collaborative, the March of Dimes, and the California Department of Public Health. As of January 2012, all 58 of Louisiana's birthing hospitals were involved. The state medical society and the state chapter of the American Congress of Obstetricians and Gynecologists (ACOG) are also partners on the project.	Program participation has been associated with decreases in the rates of neonatal intensive care unit admissions.
Minnesota	Beginning January 1, 2012, Minnesota requires hospitals to implement policies and processes to minimize inductions prior to 39 weeks without a medical reason and to report labor induction data for all births covered by Minnesota Health Care Programs, including Medical Assistance (Minnesota's Medicaid program) and MinnesotaCare (another publicly subsidized program for those without access to affordable health coverage). Obstetric providers will not need to submit additional information with delivery claims if the following are included in hospital policies and quality improvement programs: ▸ "hard stop" policies restricting elective inductions prior to 39 weeks; ▸ policy encouraging documentation of final estimated date of delivery by 20 weeks of gestation and sharing that information with the patients; ▸ policy encouraging patient education about elective inductions with documentation of that education; and ▸ ongoing quality improvement review of facility-level data, with required audits if the rate of elective deliveries between 37 and 39 weeks is higher than 25 percent, and required peer review of labor inductions prior to 39 weeks.	Unknown

TABLE 1-6, Continued

State and Initiative	Description of Initiative	Evidence of Effects
North Carolina Pregnancy Medical Home (PMH) Initiative	In this Medicaid-based program, PMHs (physician practices and health clinics) employ care managers (nurses and social workers) from local health departments to provide case management for high-risk pregnant Medicaid enrollees in the practice. The provided services include a comprehensive assessment on each enrollee who screens as high risk for poor birth outcomes and follow-up or referral for necessary services. To qualify for participation as a PMH, providers must agree to: (1) ensure that no elective deliveries (induction and cesarean section) are performed before 39 weeks of gestation, (2) use 17 alpha hydroxyprogesterone to prevent recurrent preterm birth, and (3) maintain a primary (first birth) cesarean section rate at or below 20 percent. PMHs, in turn, receive a higher rate of payment for vaginal deliveries to equal that of cesarean deliveries.	Unknown
Ohio Perinatal Quality Collaborative's (OPQC) 39-Week Project	Under the 39-Week Project, the collaborative (which includes state government, providers, and other policymakers and leaders in perinatal health) works to reduce elective deliveries prior to 39 weeks by ensuring hospital access to best methods of care, increasing hospital collaboration, and providing research and evidence to leaders and providers. From September 2008 to June 2010, OPQC worked with 20 maternity hospitals to implement quality improvement activities to reduce early elective delivery. Strategies included: documenting reasons for a scheduled delivery prior to 39 weeks, discussing with patients the risks of delivery earlier than 39 weeks, and implementing a form for scheduled deliveries to reduce scheduled births. Additional strategies included: pregnancy dating with an ultrasound before 20 weeks of gestation; producing peer reviewed guidelines and criteria about when deliveries can be scheduled; recruiting physician champions for the program's new policies; and publicly sharing hospital-level data on the prevalence of scheduled deliveries less than 39 weeks.	A recent study suggests that OPQC's 39-Week Project led to a decline in the rate of early elective deliveries from 25 percent to less than 5 percent over a 14-month period from 2008 to 2009.

TABLE 1-6, Continued

State and Initiative	Description of Initiative	Evidence of Effects
Washington State Perinatal Collaborative: Reducing Elective Delivery Before 39 Weeks	The collaborative (which includes state government, hospitals and other providers, the March of Dimes, and other organizations) is conducting several initiatives, including the Reducing Elective Delivery Before 39 Weeks initiative. The goal of the program is to reduce elective deliveries before 39 weeks to 7 percent or less. Participating hospitals are provided with support as they establish various policies to decrease early elective deliveries. The policies vary by hospital, but include requiring documentation of medical reason when scheduling a delivery prior to 39 weeks, requiring approval of the chief of obstetrics prior to scheduling a delivery, and physician and patient education about risks from elective deliveries prior to 39 weeks. In addition, hospitals submit performance measurement data consistent with the Leapfrog Group and the Joint Commission submission requirements.	Project reports indicate that from the third quarter of 2010 to the fourth quarter of 2011, the rate of early elective deliveries decreased by 65 percent from 15.3 percent to 5.4 percent.*
West Virginia Elective Delivery Quality Collaborative	The collaborative was developed to reduce the rate of elective deliveries prior to 39 weeks of gestation. In 2009, 14 of the state's 30 hospitals participated in a 6-month learning collaborative that involved monthly reporting on quality measures, technical assistance, and web-based and face-to-face sessions to share lessons learned with other participants. Participating hospitals were provided with evidence-based change packets that included communication and education materials for patients, providers, administrators, and the broader community, as well as best practices for quality improvement policies, procedures, and documentation. Partners included the WV Health Care Authority, the WV Health Improvement Institute, the WV Perinatal Partnership, and the March of Dimes.	At the end of the 6-month initiative, there was a 50 percent decrease in the rate of non-medically indicated elective deliveries prior to 39 weeks, and the rate had been maintained one year after the collaborative ended.

Notes: * The rate is calculated by dividing number of patients with elective deliveries between 37 and 39 weeks by number of patients who delivered babies between 37 and 39 weeks. This rate does not include births for most medical exclusions (Washington SHA 2013).

Sources: Smith et al. 2012; Louisiana DHH 2012; Minnesota DHS 2011; North Carolina DHHS 2011; OPQC 2012a, 2012b, and 2010; Washington SHA 2013; West Virginia HCA 2011.

TABLE 1-7. Performance Measurement and Public Reporting Initiatives to Reduce Induction, Cesarean Section, and Early Elective Deliveries

Organization and Initiative	Description of Initiative
California Maternal Quality Care Collaborative (MQCC)	The California MQCC is rolling out a statewide data center initiative to create rapid-cycle performance measures about maternity services and outcomes. The project is supported by the Centers for Disease Control and Prevention and the California HealthCare Foundation, and is overseen by a multistakeholder collaborative. Partnering agencies include state government, public groups, professional groups, health systems, and universities. Participating hospitals will submit performance data, and the collaborative envisions that some performance measures will be publicly reported in the future. There are currently six reporting sets, including elective deliveries prior to 39 weeks. The Joint Commission's measure of cesarean deliveries (see row below) is an updated version of a similar measure created by the California MQCC.
Centers for Medicare & Medicaid Services (CMS), Core Set of Children's Health Care Quality Measures	The Children's Health Insurance Program Reauthorization Act required the Secretary of the Department of Health and Human Services to identify an initial core set of recommended pediatric quality measures for voluntary use by state Medicaid and CHIP programs. The 25 measures include one on the percentage of women who had a cesarean section among women with first live singleton births (also known as nulliparous term singleton vertex (NTSV) births) at 37 weeks of gestation or later.
The Joint Commission, Perinatal Care Core Quality Measures	The Joint Commission has a core set of five perinatal care core quality measures endorsed by the National Quality Forum (NQF). This set includes a measure of elective deliveries between 37 and 39 weeks of gestation and a measure of cesarean deliveries for NTSV births. Beginning in 2010, Joint Commission-accredited hospitals could choose to report on the Perinatal Care Core set of measures to meet accreditation requirements.
The Leapfrog Group, Public Reporting on Early Elective Deliveries	The Leapfrog Group, a non-profit organization that compares hospitals on national standards of safety and quality, collects and publicly reports hospital performance data on early elective deliveries using the NQF-endorsed measure. In 2010, Leapfrog became the first national organization to make hospital-specific information about early elective deliveries available to the public. In addition, Leapfrog is partnering with the Institute for Healthcare Improvement, Childbirth Connection, Catalyst for Payment Reform, and employer and regional business coalition members to educate healthcare consumers, employers, health plans, hospitals, and policymakers about this issue. Rates of early elective delivery among reporting hospitals improved in the second year of reporting, from 17 percent in 2010 to 14 percent in 2011.

Sources: Smith et al. 2012; California MQCC 2013; Leapfrog Group 2013, 2012.

strategy payers and providers can use to facilitate and monitor reductions in labor inductions, cesarean deliveries, and early elective deliveries. While the use of quality measures in health care has expanded rapidly, there are still relatively few valid measures of labor and delivery care processes and outcomes. In addition, performance reporting on maternity care remains relatively limited and inconsistent across the country and among various entities, including health plans, health systems, and facilities.

However, some notable efforts have been made in recent years to develop and promote reporting on measures of elective deliveries (Table 1-7). The National Quality Forum endorses a set of 14 clinical quality measures related to perinatal care, including a measure of elective delivery between 37 and 39 weeks of gestation and a measure of the cesarean delivery rate in low-risk, first-birth women. One or both of these measures has been adopted by the Joint Commission, the Leapfrog Group, and CMS (as part CMS's Core Set of 25 Children's Health Care Quality Measures). In August of 2012, ACOG convened the reVITALize conference to assist in clarifying existing data definitions and in streamlining measurement for obstetrical outcomes nationwide (ACOG 2013).

Provider and patient education

Many organizations are funding, conducting, and disseminating research to increase knowledge and use of evidence-based maternity care (Table 1-8). Recent efforts include disseminating tools that providers can use for quality improvement

TABLE 1-8. Provider and Patient Education Initiatives to Reduce Induction, Cesarean Section, and Early Elective Deliveries

Organization	Name of Initiative	Description of Initiative
California Maternal Quality Care Collaborative, California Department of Public Health, March of Dimes	Elimination of Non-medically Indicated (Elective) Deliveries Before 39 Weeks Gestational Age Quality Improvement Toolkit	This quality improvement toolkit aims to help groups decrease elective deliveries before 39 weeks and to identify and disseminate best practices related to preventing elective early deliveries.
March of Dimes	Healthy Babies are Worth the Wait	This initiative provides an implementation toolkit to states that aim to decrease preventable preterm birth. The implementation manual helps states think about the "Five P's": partnerships and collaborations, provider initiatives, patient support, public engagement, and measuring progress. The March of Dimes has been working with Kentucky on this initiative since 2006, and Texas and New Jersey more recently to implement prematurity prevention programs.

Sources: Smith et al. 2012; California MQCC 2011.

initiatives and reaching out to non-physician practitioners and allied health professionals to provide education and support to pregnant women. One recent study that examined childbirth-related outcomes for Medicaid enrollees who received prenatal education and childbirth support from trained doulas found that after controlling for clinical and sociodemographic factors, the odds of cesarean delivery were 40.9 percent lower for doula-supported births (Kozhimannil et al. 2013). Potential cost savings to Medicaid programs associated with such cesarean rate reductions are substantial but depend on states' payment rates, birth volume, and current cesarean rates.

Issues and Next Steps

Medicaid and CHIP pay for nearly half of all deliveries in the United States; therefore, both the states and the federal government have a strong interest in creating the proper incentives to provide high-quality maternity care in the most effective and cost-efficient manner possible. Doing so will likely require efforts that touch on eligibility and enrollment, benefit design, payment, and program monitoring. Activities that will inform MACPAC's future work in this area may include:

- conducting analyses that describe the experiences of pregnant women served by Medicaid and CHIP, including spending, use of different types of services, site of service, and financing arrangement (managed care versus fee for service);

- developing a more thorough understanding of the effectiveness of targeted case management and other efforts to reduce risks associated with poor birth outcomes;

- tracking federal, state, and private-sector efforts to reduce rates of elective cesarean deliveries and non-medically indicated early-induced deliveries;

- examining how changes in eligibility under the ACA will affect pregnant women, including the potential for unnecessary churning among Medicaid, CHIP, and subsidized private coverage available through exchanges;

- tracking the number of states that reduce Medicaid eligibility levels for pregnant women due to the availability of exchange coverage; and

- better understanding the supply of providers available to serve pregnant Medicaid and CHIP enrollees and possible barriers to practice created by state and federal law and other regulations or licensing practices.

Moving forward, the Commission will track and document trends in utilization and expenditures, as well as programs and initiatives to improve care to almost two million women who receive maternity care through Medicaid and CHIP each year.

Endnotes

[1] Estimates of the number of Medicaid and CHIP births vary by data source, due to factors including non-reporting by hospitals, non-reporting or underreporting of managed care encounter data by states, and differential reporting of waiver and expansion program data. See Chapter 1 Appendix to this chapter for a comparison of estimates of the annual number of Medicaid births by state.

[2] Reporting hospitals are members of the National Perinatal Information Center/Quality Analytic Services, a non-profit organization which began in 1985 with a charter membership of major perinatal centers across the United States.

[3] Essential health benefits include ambulatory services, emergency services, hospitalization, maternity and newborn care, mental health and substance abuse services, prescription drugs, rehabilitative and habilitative services and devices, laboratory services, preventive and wellness services and chronic disease management, and pediatric services, including oral and vision care (§1302(b)(1) of the ACA).

[4] Covered preventive benefits include services for women established in health plan coverage guidelines supported by HRSA (45 CFR 147.130(a)(1)(iv)).

[5] Women had an average of about seven months of pre-delivery Medicaid eligibility months. For women with multiple deliveries in the 14-month period, expenditures for both deliveries are included.

References

Agency for Healthcare Research and Quality (AHRQ). U.S. Department of Health and Human Services. 2013. *Statewide medical home program for low-income pregnant women enhances access to comprehensive prenatal care and case management, improves outcomes.* Rockville, MD: AHRQ. http://www.innovations.ahrq.gov/content.aspx?id=3778.

Albert, D.A., M.D. Begg, et al. 2011. An examination of periodontal treatment, dental care, and pregnancy outcomes in an insured population in the United States. *American Journal of Public Health* 101, no. 1: 151–156.

Alexander, G.R., and M. Kotelchuck. 2001. Assessing the role and effectiveness of prenatal care: History, challenges, and directions for future research. *Public Health Reports* 116, no. 4: 306–316.

American Congress of Obstetrics and Gynecology (ACOG). 2013. *The obstetrician-gynecologist distribution atlas.* Washington, DC: ACOG. http://www.acog.org/Resources_And_Publications/The_Ob-Gyn_Workforce.

Anderson, B.L., R.W. Hale, et al. 2008. Outlook for the future of the obstetrician-gynecologist workforce. *American Journal of Obstetrics and Gynecology* 199, no. 1: 88.e1–88.e8.

Atrash, H.K., K. Johnson, M. Adams, et al. 2006. Preconception care for improving perinatal outcomes: The time to act. *Maternal and Child Health Journal* 10, no. 1: S3–S11. http://www.ncbi.nlm.nih.gov/pmc/articles/PMC1592246/#CR17.

Bailey, B.A., and A.R. Byrom. 2007. Factors predicting birth weight in a low-risk sample: The role of modifiable pregnancy health behaviors. *Maternal and Child Health Journal* 11, no. 2: 173–179.

Boggess, K., E.K. Berggren, V. Koskenoja, et al. 2013. Severe preeclampsia and maternal self-report of oral health, hygiene, and dental care. *Journal of Periodontology* 84, no. 2: 143–151.

Brassard, A., and M. Smolenski. 2011. *Removing barriers to advanced practice registered nurse care: Hospital privileges.* Washington, DC: AARP. http://assets.aarp.org/rgcenter/ppi/health-care/insight55.pdf.

Byrd, V., and A. Dodd. 2013. Assessing the usability of MAX 2008 encounter data for comprehensive managed care. *Medicare & Medicaid Research Review* 3, no. 1: e1–e19. http://www.cms.gov/Research-Statistics-Data-and-Systems/Research/MMRR/Downloads/MMRR2013_003_01_b01.pdf.

California Maternal Quality Care Collaborative (MQCC). 2013. California Maternal Data Center (CMDC). http://www.cmqcc.org/california_maternal_data_center_cmdc.

California Maternal Quality Care Collaborative (MQCC). 2011. <39 weeks toolkit. http://www.cmqcc.org/_39_week_toolkit.

Centers for Medicare & Medicaid Services (CMS), U.S. Department of Health and Human Services. 2013. *Questions and answers: Medicaid and the Affordable Care Act.* Baltimore, MD: CMS. http://medicaid.gov/State-Resource-Center/FAQ-Medicaid-and-CHIP-Affordable-Care-Act-ACA-Implementation/Downloads/ACA-FAQ-BHP.pdf.

Centers for Medicare & Medicaid Services (CMS), U.S. Department of Health and Human Services. 2012. Medicaid program; Eligibility changes under the Affordable Care Act of 2010. Final rule. *Federal Register* 77, no. 57 (March 23): 17143–17217. http://www.gpo.gov/fdsys/pkg/FR-2012-03-23/html/2012-6560.htm.

Centers for Medicare & Medicaid Services (CMS), U.S. Department of Health and Human Services. 2011. Group health plans and health insurance issuers relating to coverage of preventive services under the Patient Protection and Affordable Care Act. Interim final rules with request for comments. *Federal Register* 76, no. 149 (August 3): 46621–46625. http://www.gpo.gov/fdsys/pkg/FR-200-08-03/pdf/2001-19684.pdf.

Centers for Medicare & Medicaid Services (CMS), U.S. Department of Health and Human Services. 2010. Letter from Cindy Mann to State Health Officials regarding "Medicaid and CHIP coverage of 'lawfully residing' children and pregnant women." July 1, 2010. http://downloads.cms.gov/cmsgov/archived-downloads/SMDL/downloads/SHO10006.pdf.

Centers for Medicare & Medicaid Services (CMS), U.S. Department of Health and Human Services. 2009. Letter from Jackie Garner to State Health Officials regarding "General information concerning the new option and guidance on amending your CHIP plan to reflect the coverage of pregnant women." May 11, 2009. http://downloads.cms.gov/cmsgov/archived-downloads/SMDL/downloads/SHO051109.pdf.

Centers for Medicare & Medicaid Services (CMS), U.S. Department of Health and Human Services. 2002. State Children's Health Insurance Program; Eligibility for prenatal care and other health services for unborn children. Final rule. *Federal Register* 67, no. 191 (October 2): 61956–61974. http://www.cms.gov/Regulations-and-Guidance/Regulations-and-Policies/QuarterlyProviderUpdates/downloads/cms2127f.pdf.

Centers for Medicare & Medicaid Services (CMS), U.S. Department of Health and Human Services. 2000. Letter from Timothy M. Westmoreland to State Health Officials regarding "Guidance on proposed demonstration projects under Section 1115 Authority." July 31, 2000. http://www.cms.hhs.gov/smdl/downloads/sho073100.pdf.

Children's Hospital Association. 2013. Communication with MACPAC staff, April 17.

Clark, S.L., D.D. Miller, M.A. Belfort, et al. 2009. Neonatal and maternal outcomes associated with elective term delivery. *American Journal of Obstetrics and Gynecology* 200, no. 2: 156.e1–156.e4.

D'Angelo, D., L. Williams, B. Morrow, et al. 2007. Preconception and interconception health status of women who recently gave birth to a live-born infant—pregnancy risk assessment monitoring system (PRAMS), United States, 26 reporting areas, 2004. *MMWR Surveillance Summaries* 56, no. 10: 1–35. http://www.cdc.gov/mmwr/preview/mmwrhtml/ss5610a1.htm.

Detman, L.A., B.H. Cottrell, and M.F. Denis-Luque. 2010. Exploring dental care misconceptions and barriers in pregnancy. *Birth* 37, no. 4: 318–324.

Florida Department of Health (DOH). 2013. Florida's Healthy Start Initiative. Tallahassee, FL: Florida DOH. http://www.doh.state.fl.us/family/mch/hs/hs.html.

Hamilton, B.E., J.A. Martin, and S.J. Ventura. 2012. *Births: Preliminary data for 2011.* National Vital Statistics Reports 61, no. 5. Hyattsville, MD: National Center for Health Statistics. http://www.cdc.gov/nchs/data/nvsr/nvsr61/nvsr61_05.pdf.

Hill, I.T., S. Hogan, L. Palmer, et al. 2009. *Medicaid outreach and enrollment for pregnant women: What is the state of the art?* Washington, DC: Urban Institute. http://www.urban.org/UploadedPDF/411898_pregnant_women.pdf.

Hill, I.T., and J. Breyel. 1989. Coordinating prenatal care. Washington, DC: National Governors Association.

Johnson, C.F., and K.E. Witgert. 2010. *Enhanced pregnancy benefit packages: Worth another look.* Washington, DC: National Academy for State Health Policy. http://www.nashp.org/sites/default/files/PregBenefits.pdf.

Johnson, K., S.F. Posner, J. Biermann, et al. 2006. Recommendations to improve preconception health and health care—United States. A report of the CDC/ATSDR Preconception Care Work Group and the Select Panel on Preconception Care. *MMWR Recommendations and Reports* 55, no. RR-6: 1–23.

Kaiser Family Foundation (KFF). 2013. State health facts: Has presumptive eligibility for children in Medicaid and CHIP. Washington, DC: KFF. http://statehealthfacts.org/comparetable.jsp?cat=4&ind=229.

King, V., R. Pilliod, and A. Little. 2010. *Rapid review: Elective induction of labor*. Portland, OR: Center for Evidence-based Policy. http://www.ohsu.edu/xd/research/centers-institutes/evidence-based-policy-center/med/upload/Elective-Induction-of-Labor_PUBLIC_RR_Final_12_10.pdf.

Kozhimannil, K.B., R.R. Hardeman, L.B. Attanasio, et al. 2013. Doula care, birth outcomes, and costs among Medicaid beneficiaries. *American Journal of Public Health* 103, no. 4: e113–e121.

Leapfrog Group. 2013. Hospital rates of early scheduled deliveries. Washington, DC: Leapfrog Group. http://www.leapfroggroup.org/tooearlydeliveries.

Leapfrog Group. 2012. Hospitals make progress in eliminating early elective deliveries: Good news, but more work needs to be done. January 25, 2012, press release. http://www.leapfroggroup.org/policy_leadership/leapfrog_news/4827337.

Loafman, M., and S. Nanda. 2009. Who will deliver our babies?: Crisis in the physician workforce. *American Journal of Clinical Medicine* 6, no. 2: 11–16. http://www.aapsus.org/articles/10.pdf.

Louisiana Department of Health and Hospitals (DHH). 2012. Health department announces response to mid-year budget reductions. December 14, 2012, press release. http://new.dhh.louisiana.gov/index.cfm/newsroom/detail/2727.

Main, E., B. Oshiro, B. Chagolla, et al. 2010. *Elimination of non-medically indicated (elective) deliveries before 39 weeks gestational age*. Developed under contract no. 08-85012 with the California Department of Public Health, Maternal, Child and Adolescent Health Division. Stanford, CA: California Maternal Quality Care Collaborative. http://www.cdph.ca.gov/programs/mcah/Documents/MCAH-EliminationOfNon-MedicallyIndicatedDeliveries.pdf.

March of Dimes Perinatal Data Center (March of Dimes). 2011. *Special care nursery admissions*. White Plains, NY: March of Dimes. http://www.marchofdimes.com/peristats/pdfdocs/nicu_summary_final.pdf.

Martin, J.A., B.E. Hamilton, S.J. Ventura, et al. 2012a. *Births: Final data for 2010*. National Vital Statistics Reports 61, no. 1. Hyattsville, MD: National Center for Health Statistics. http://www.cdc.gov/nchs/data/nvsr/nvsr61_01.pdf.

Martin, J.A., B.E. Hamilton, S.J. Ventura, et al. 2012b. *Births: Final data for 2010. Supplemental Tables*. National Vital Statistics Reports 61, no. 1. Hyattsville, MD: National Center for Health Statistics. http://www.cdc.gov/nchs/data/nvsr/nvsr61/nvsr61_01_tables.pdf#102.

Martin, J.A., M.J.K. Osterman, and P.D. Sutton. 2010. *Are preterm births on the decline in the United States? Recent data from the National Vital Statistics System*. National Center for Health Statistics Data Brief, no 39. Hyattsville, MD: National Center for Health Statistics. http://www.cdc.gov/nchs/data/databriefs/db39.htm.

Martin, J.A., B.E. Hamilton, S.J. Ventura, et al. 2002. *Births: Final data for 2000*. National Vital Statistics Reports 50, no. 5. Hyattsville, MD: National Center for Health Statistics. http://www.cdc.gov/nchs/data/nvsr/nvsr50/nvsr50_05.pdf.

Mathews, T.J., and M.F. MacDorman. 2013. *Infant mortality statistics from the 2009 period linked birth/infant death data set*. National Vital Statistics Reports 61, no. 8. Hyattsville, MD: National Center for Health Statistics. http://www.cdc.gov/nchs/data/nvsr/nvsr61/nvsr61_08.pdf.

McCormick, M.C. 2001. Prenatal care—necessary but not sufficient. *Health Services Research* 36, no 2: 399–403.

Medicaid and CHIP Payment and Access Commission (MACPAC). 2013. *Report to the Congress on Medicaid and CHIP*. March 2013. Washington, DC: MACPAC.

Minnesota Department of Human Services (DHS). 2011. Evidence-based Childbirth Program. St. Paul, MN: Minnesota DHS. http://www.dhs.state.mn.us/main/idcplg?IdcService=GET_DYNAMIC_CONVERSION&RevisionSelectionMethod=LatestReleased&dDocName=dhs16_165841.

National Center for Health Statistics (NCHS), Centers for Disease Control and Prevention, U.S. Department of Health and Human Services. 2012. *Health, United States, 2011*. Hyattsville, MD: NCHS. http://www.cdc.gov/nchs/hus.htm.

National Center for Health Statistics (NCHS), Centers for Disease Control and Prevention, U.S. Department of Health and Human Services. 2008. *Health, United States, 2007*. Hyattsville, MD: NCHS. http://www.cdc.gov/nchs/data/hus/hus07.pdf.

National Governors Association (NGA), Center for Best Practices. 2011. 2010 *Maternal and child health update: States make progress towards improving systems of care*. Washington, DC: NGA. http://www.nga.org/files/live/sites/NGA/files/pdf/MCHUPDATE2010.PDF.

National Governors Association (NGA). 1990. *State coverage of pregnant women and children—January 1990*. Washington, DC: NGA. http://www.nga.org/files/live/sites/NGA/files/pdf/MCHUPDATE0190.pdf.

National Institutes of Health (NIH), U.S. Department of Health and Human Services. 2006. NIH state-of-the-science conference statement on cesarean delivery on maternal request. *NIH Consensus and State-of-the-Science Statements* 23, no. 1 : 1–29. Bethesda, MD: NIH. http://consensus.nih.gov/2006/cesareanstatement.pdf.

North Carolina Department of Health and Human Services (DHHS). 2012. Pregnancy medical home. Raleigh, NC: North Carolina DHHS. http://www.ncdhhs.gov/dma/services/pmh.htm.

Offenbacher, S., D. Lin, R. Strauss, et al. 2006. Effects of periodontal therapy during pregnancy on periodontal status, biologic parameters, and pregnancy outcomes: A pilot study. *Journal of Periodontology* 77, no. 12: 2011–2024.

Ohio Perinatal Quality Collaborative (OPQC). 2012a. Welcome to OPQC. Cincinnati, OH: OPQC. https://opqc.net/.

Ohio Perinatal Quality Collaborative (OPQC). 2012b. Ohio's 39-week project: Collaborating to deliver quality care and healthy babies. Cincinnati, OH: OPQC. https://opqc.net/webfm_send/277.

Ohio Perinatal Quality Collaborative Writing Committee. 2010. A statewide initiative to reduce inappropriate scheduled births at 360/7-386/7 weeks' gestation. *American Journal of Obstetrics & Gynecology* 202, no. 3: 243.e1–243.e8.

Osterman, M.J.K., J.A. Martin, T.J. Mathews, et al. 2011. *Expanded data from the new birth certificate, 2008*. National Vital Statistics Reports 59, no 7. Hyattsville, MD: National Center for Health Statistics. http://www.cdc.gov/nchs/data/nvsr/nvsr59/nvsr59_07.pdf.

Ranji, U., A. Salganicoff, A. Stewart, et al. 2009. *State Medicaid coverage of family planning services: Summary of state survey findings*. Menlo Park, CA: Kaiser Family Foundation. http://www.kff.org/womenshealth/upload/8015.pdf.

Ratcliffe, C., and S. McKernan. 2012. *Child poverty and its lasting consequence: Low-income working families*. Washington, DC: Urban Institute. http://www.urban.org/UploadedPDF/412659-Child-Poverty-and-Its-Lasting-Consequence-Paper.pdf.

Reed, A., and J.E. Roberts. 2000. State regulation of midwives: Issues and options. *Journal of Midwifery & Women's Health* 45, no. 2: 130–149.

Risser, A., and V. King. 2010. *Rapid review: Elective cesarean section*. Portland, OR: Center for Evidence-based Policy. http://www.ohsu.edu/xd/research/centers-institutes/evidence-based-policy-center/med/upload/Elective-Delivery-Elective-Cesarean_PUBLIC_Rapid-Review_Final_12_1_10.pdf.

Smith, K., B. Natzke, and A. Christensen. 2012. Rising rates of labor induction and cesarean delivery: Issues, implications, and current initiatives to reduce rates. Unpublished white paper for MACPAC. Princeton, NJ: Mathematica Policy Research.

Texas Health and Human Services Commission (HHSC). 2013. CHIP perinatal coverage: Provider fact sheet. Austin, TX: HHSC. http://www.hhsc.state.tx.us/chip/perinatal/InfoForProvidersAndCBOs.htm#b1.

Tita, A.T., M.B. Landon, C.Y. Spong, et al. 2009. Timing of elective repeat cesarean delivery at term and neonatal outcomes. *New England Journal of Medicine* 360, no. 2: 111–120.

Tong, S.T., L.A. Makaroff, I.M. Xierali, et al. 2012. Proportion of family physicians providing maternity care continues to decline. *Journal of the American Board of Family Medicine* 25, no. 3: 270–271.

U.S. Census Bureau, U.S. Department of Commerce (DOC). 2011. Current Population Survey. 2010 poverty table of contents. Washington, DC: DOC. http://www.census.gov/hhes/www/cpstables/032011/pov/POV01_200.htm.

Washington State Hospital Association (SHA). 2013. Quality indicators search page. Safe deliveries. Seattle, WA: Washington SHA. http://www.wahospitalquality.org/.

West Virginia Health Care Authority (HCA). 2011. *West Virginia quality collaborative for eliminating non-medically indicated elective deliveries prior to 39 weeks gestation*. Charleston, WV: West Virginia HCA. http://www.wvperinatal.org/downloads/OBCollaborative0211.pdf.

Williams, M. 2013. State to end Medicaid payments for elective early births. *Atlanta Journal-Constitution*. March 24, 2013. http://www.myajc.com/news/news/state-regional-govt-politics/state-to-end-medicaid-payments-for-elective-early-/nW2WM/.

Zhao, L. 2007. *Why are fewer hospitals in the delivery business?* Chicago, IL: Walsh Center for Rural Health Analysis, NORC at the University of Chicago. http://www.norc.org/PDFs/Walsh%20Center/Links%20Out/DecliningAccesstoHospitalbased ObstetricServicesin RuralCounties.pdf.

Chapter 1 Appendix

Datasets Used to Count Annual Number of Births in the Medicaid Program

Data on births in the Medicaid program are available from multiple sources, and each source gives a somewhat different number of births for each state. This appendix provides information on Medicaid births from three sources: Healthcare Cost and Utilization Project (HCUP) data, the National Governors Association (NGA), and a MACPAC analysis of Medicaid Statistical Information System (MSIS) data (Table 1-A-1). The number of states with data available in each source varies, and we report the most recent year of data available when the analysis began.

Differences among the three data sources reflect a variety of factors, including how Medicaid and the State Children's Health Insurance Program (CHIP) are identified and defined, the underlying data used in each source (claims, vital statistics, or other source), and underreporting or non-reporting of data. For example, some states do not report Medicaid managed care encounter data in MSIS and some hospitals do not submit discharge data to states that can be used for HCUP.

Healthcare Cost and Utilization Project

The HCUP is a family of health care databases and related software tools and products developed through a federal, state, and industry partnership and sponsored by the Agency for Healthcare Research and Quality (AHRQ). HCUP databases bring together the data collection efforts of state data organizations, hospital associations, private data organizations, and the federal government to create a national information resource of patient-level health care data. The Nationwide Inpatient Sample (NIS) contains data from approximately 8 million hospital stays from roughly 1,000 hospitals; this approximates a stratified sample of 20 percent of U.S. community hospitals. The State Inpatient Databases (SID) contains the universe of inpatient discharge abstracts from data organizations. Currently 44 states participate in the SID; not all allow their data to be made available to the public but estimates can be generated by AHRQ.

Insurance status information in HCUP is based on primary expected source of payment reported on the discharge abstract. Patients covered by CHIP may be included under Medicaid, private insurance, or other insurance, depending on the structure of the state program.

TABLE 1-A-1. Total and Medicaid Births Reported in Three Data Sources, 2008–2010

States	HCUP (2010)			NGA (2009)		MSIS (2008)
	Total births	Medicaid births	Percent Medicaid births	Medicaid births	Percent Medicaid births	Medicaid births
Alabama	–	–	–	–	–	27,570
Alaska	–	–	–	5,891	53%	3,609
Arizona	84,805	43,505	51%	49,538	54	52,137
Arkansas	37,235	20,763	56	25,337	64	20,125
California	495,252	244,358	49	–	–	215,704
Colorado	60,266	23,761	39	26,101[1]	38	22,731
Connecticut	–	–	–	14,500[2]	–	5,822
Delaware	–	–	–	6,202	–	2,561
District of Columbia	–	–	–	–	–	1,771
Florida	209,525	115,145	55	–	–	69,570
Georgia	–	–	–	–	–	66,607
Hawaii	15,804	6,609	42	–	–	2,310
Idaho	–	–	–	–	–	9,618
Illinois	157,019	67,524	43	81,104	–	58,844
Indiana	–	–	–	41,793	–	36,861
Iowa	38,043	15,282	40	15,732	–	14,228
Kansas	38,951	12,023	31	–	–	14,429
Kentucky	50,343	24,900	50	24,604	44	28,739
Louisiana	–	–	–	–	–	37,722
Maine	12,463	5,322	43	5,400	40	6,252
Maryland	68,089	29,638	44	30,267	40	28,285
Massachusetts	71,810	23,573	33	12,913[3]	–	7,725
Michigan	112,481	51,630	46	–	–	28,197
Minnesota	63,563	12,454	20	31,209[4]	–	12,484
Mississippi	–	–	–	–	–	27,142
Missouri	75,278	35,750	48	31,326	48	34,994
Montana	–	–	–	12,076[5]	–	4,098
Nebraska	25,667	9,710	38	11,668	43	2,922
Nevada	34,458	12,922	38	17,753	48	6,602
New Hampshire	–	–	–	3,912	32	3,726
New Jersey	103,130	25,444	25	–	–	14,941
New Mexico	24,917	15,037	60	–	–	17,691
New York	239,999	104,641	44	–	–	116,913

TABLE 1-A-1, Continued

States	HCUP (2010) Total births	HCUP (2010) Medicaid births	HCUP (2010) Percent Medicaid births	NGA (2009) Medicaid births	NGA (2009) Percent Medicaid births	MSIS (2008) Medicaid births
North Carolina	116,184	59,800	52%	64,439	51%	65,701
North Dakota	–	–	–	–	–	2,424
Ohio	–	–	–	–	–	10,391
Oklahoma	48,758	29,590	61	33,898	64	30,399
Oregon	43,538	19,851	46	19,664[6]	43	18,119
Pennsylvania	–	–	–	57,371	–	17,479
Rhode Island	11,815	5,341	45	–	–	3,947
South Carolina	54,510	25,102	46	–	–	26,467
South Dakota	–	–	–	4,662	39	4,459
Tennessee	73,816	38,462	52	43,000	49	36,277
Texas	369,475	191,496	52	–	–	216,452
Utah	51,941	17,581	34	15,045	34	15,615
Vermont	5,630	2,594	46	2,827	44	2,642
Virginia	–	–	–	28,047[7]	27	31,193
Washington	79,463	31,482	40	–	–	20,607
West Virginia	19,753	11,653	59	12,001	–	2,415
Wisconsin	66,037	24,954	38	–	–	19,031
Wyoming	6,234	2,045	33	3,401	43	3,222
U.S. Total	**3,905,481**	**1,812,129**	**46%**	–	–	**1,529,770**

Notes: See text for additional methodological information. In HCUP data, Medicaid is based on primary expected source of payment reported on the discharge abstract. Several states have non-reporting hospitals which makes their estimates underreports. States with the highest underreporting (compared to American Hospital Association data) are Minnesota (14.1%), Tennessee (8.5%), Kansas (6.3%), and Nebraska (4.6%). Although not all states provide public use data for HCUP, the U.S. total reflects data for all states because estimates from the Nationwide Inpatient Sample are weighted to reflect all discharges from community hospitals. Dashes indicate data that are not available or not provided.

NGA data are gathered from U.S. states and territories in an annual maternal and child health survey.

MSIS data include Medicaid-expansion CHIP enrollees and exclude separate CHIP program enrollees. Low numbers of births in some states may indicate that the state has incomplete reporting of managed care encounter data or has inpatient hospital claims or encounter records with missing or non-standard diagnosis and procedure codes.

[1] Colorado data are from the Inpatient Utilization Reports created by the Colorado Foundation of Medical Care. Colorado's total births are from the U.S. Census Bureau, State Population Estimates by Component of Change.

[2] Connecticut calendar year matches Department of Social Services claims data with Department of Public Health Vital Records. 2009 data is an estimate.

[3] Massachusetts' birth data include CHIP births.

[4] Medicaid births for Minnesota include births in Minnesota's 1115 Medicaid expansion program (MinnesotaCare).

[5] Montana's definition of a Medicaid birth is any child that had a paid Medicaid claim indicating delivery or a paid Medicaid claim in the first month of life, or a child that has been matched to a mother eligible for Medicaid and the mother had a paid Medicaid claim indicating a delivery.

[6] Oregon bases the number of Medicaid births on Medicaid claims data.

[7] Virginia data is based on the state fiscal year and is derived from the Virginia Department of Health, Office of Vital Statistics.

Sources: MACPAC analysis of Healthcare Cost and Utilization Project (HCUP) Nationwide Inpatient Sample and State Inpatient Databases; National Governors Association (NGA) Center for Best Practices 2010 Maternal and Child Health Update; and Medicaid Statistical Information System (MSIS) data.

Several states have non-reporting hospitals, which makes their estimates lower than they would be if full data were available. States with the highest number of hospital discharges that are underreported (compared to American Hospital Association data) are Minnesota (14.1 percent), Tennessee (8.5 percent), Kansas (6.3 percent), and Nebraska (4.6 percent). For statistics reported at the national level, available data in the NIS are weighted to obtain a nationally representative estimate of all discharges from community hospitals.

National Governors Association

NGA's 2010 Maternal and Child Health Update presents data for 2009 and prior years gathered from U.S. states and territories in an annual maternal and child health survey (NGA 2011). The survey was sent out to state governments; states report births at the state level. The number of states reporting data on Medicaid births varies from year to year and, as indicated in state-specific notes, sometimes includes separate CHIP-financed births.

Medicaid Statistical Information System

MSIS is a data source compiled by the Centers for Medicare & Medicaid Services (CMS) from detailed Medicaid eligibility and claims information reported on a quarterly basis by the 50 states and the District of Columbia since fiscal year 1999. These raw data are processed and made available by CMS in a number of formats including the online State Summary Datamart that provides state-level statistics for months, quarters, and fiscal years; Annual Person Summary files with person-level summary information for each fiscal year; and Medicaid Analytic eXtract (MAX) data files that have been enhanced for research purposes (e.g., through the creation of final action claims by date of service that incorporate information from original submissions and any subsequent adjustments). For this analysis, MACPAC used a file similar to the MAX that was created by Acumen, LLC from raw MSIS data.

The analysis identified Medicaid births in the MSIS by the presence of specific procedure and diagnosis codes on an inpatient fee-for-service claim or inpatient encounter record with a date of service in calendar year 2008. The following specific codes, listed on inpatient claims and inpatient encounter records, were used to identify women with deliveries:

- ICD-9-CM codes 650, 651-659, 660-669, 669.5x-669.7x, V27.x;
- DRG codes 370-371, 372-375, 765-766, 767-768, 774-775; and
- CPT codes 59514, 59620, 59409, 59612, 59515, 59622, 59410, 59614.

Most states with managed care report at least some encounter data in MSIS, but births may be undercounted in states whose encounter data are incomplete or of low quality (Byrd and Dodd 2013). Births may also be undercounted in states whose inpatient hospital claims or encounter records have missing or non-standard diagnosis and procedure codes.

Total Medicaid spending in the 12 months before and 2 months after the birth date was obtained by summing the Medicaid paid amounts for claims with dates of service within this period surrounding and including the birth. Although a woman's length of Medicaid enrollment prior to giving birth may vary for a number of reasons, including her pathway to eligibility, all pregnant women remain eligible for Medicaid for at least 60 days postpartum.

The MSIS analysis includes Medicaid-expansion CHIP enrollees and spending, although other

MACPAC Medicaid analyses (e.g., most MACStats tables and figures where Medicaid and CHIP tend to be reported separately) may exclude them. It excludes separate CHIP enrollees and spending. Readers should note that MSIS data are known to undercount total U.S. Medicaid spending relative to CMS-64 data submitted by states to obtain federal matching funds, with variation by state and type of service. Medicaid spending amounts from MSIS presented in this chapter have not been adjusted to address this issue, as done in other MACPAC analyses.

CHAPTER 2

Medicaid Primary Care Physician Payment Increase

Key Points
Medicaid Primary Care Physician Payment Increase

- The Patient Protection and Affordable Care Act (ACA, P.L. 111-148, as amended) includes a provision that requires state Medicaid agencies to increase the payment rates of services furnished by certain primary care physicians in 2013 and 2014 to Medicare levels. The provision applies to fee-for-service fee schedules and Medicaid managed care organizations (MCOs). The federal government will fund the full cost of the difference between the prevailing fee schedule on July 1, 2009 and the 2013 and 2014 Medicare rates.

- In an effort to understand the operational and policy issues surrounding implementation of this provision and its potential effects on access, MACPAC conducted semi-structured interviews with six states (Alabama, California, Indiana, Massachusetts, Oregon, and Rhode Island) and the District of Columbia in late 2012 and early 2013. Several issues emerged during early implementation of the provision including:

    - Some states reported difficulty in identifying eligible providers.
    - States reported that the system modifications necessary for claims payment are more complex than routine payment rate changes, and require more time to implement.
    - Some states and MCOs noted that they would need to amend their contracts and adjust capitation payments in order to ensure that payment increases were passed through to physicians participating in Medicaid MCO networks.

- Several state Medicaid officials, Medicaid managed care staff, and provider organizations expressed concern that the effect of the provision on provider participation may be limited because it is set to expire after 2014.

- Six months into implementation, questions are already being raised about the effect of the payment increase. Evaluation efforts could use claims data to examine changes in service use. However, complete national claims data are not likely to be available until after the provision expires at the end of 2014. Surveys of physician attitudes or state-specific workforce data could provide useful information in a more timely fashion.

CHAPTER 2

Medicaid Primary Care Physician Payment Increase

The Patient Protection and Affordable Care Act (ACA, P.L. 111-148, as amended) includes a provision that requires Medicaid to increase the payment rates of services furnished by certain primary care physicians in 2013 and 2014 to Medicare levels. This requirement is projected to increase Medicaid rates for these services by 73 percent on average in 2013, although there is significant variation around this average (Zuckerman and Goin 2012). Primary care rates in six states (Rhode Island, New York, California, Michigan, New Jersey, and Florida) are expected to double. On the other hand, rates in three states (Wyoming, Oklahoma, and Delaware) are likely to increase by less than 5 percent and rates in two other states (Alaska and North Dakota) are expected to remain the same. The federal government will fully fund the increase in payment rates.[1]

The Commission's interest in this provision relates both to its work focusing on the implementation of the ACA and to more general issues of payment and access that are referenced in its statutory mandate. To better understand issues in implementation, we undertook a series of semi-structured interviews in several states with state Medicaid officials, Medicaid managed care organizations (MCOs), and provider organizations. Because these interviews took place in fall 2012 and early winter 2013, they primarily focused on state planning efforts and early issues encountered in implementation, concerns mirrored in official comments to the Centers for Medicare & Medicaid Services (CMS) in the rulemaking process. We also took the opportunity to explore state and stakeholder perspectives on the effect the payment increase might have on enrollee access to primary care and plans for evaluating its impact.

This chapter begins by describing the concerns that led to the inclusion of the payment rate increase in the ACA, including a review of previous research on the effect of payment increases on physician participation and enrollee access to care. Subsequent sections provide an overview of both statutory and regulatory requirements for states, and discuss some of the concerns that have surfaced as states proceed with implementation. The chapter concludes with a brief discussion of evaluation strategies.

Access to Primary Care and Physician Payment

Inclusion of the primary care rate increase in the ACA reflects two related concerns about access to care for Medicaid enrollees. First, there were particular concerns that the expansion of Medicaid eligibility to millions of additional enrollees could compromise access to primary care physicians for current Medicaid enrollees and result in higher levels of unmet need (Ku et al. 2011). For example, after Massachusetts enacted health insurance reforms in 2006, individuals reported longer wait times for office visits and more difficulty finding a doctor than they experienced prior to the reforms (KFF 2012, Long 2010).[2] But the provision also reflects more general concerns that low Medicaid physician payment rates (relative to other payers) affect physician participation in Medicaid, and thus access to care (Decker 2012, Cunningham and May 2006). While other factors, such as administrative burden, are also known to affect physician participation, the following section reviews what is known about the relationship between fee-for-service (FFS) payment rates and physician participation in Medicaid. The provision also affects managed care payments to physicians, an area that has been subject to less study.

Medicaid FFS physician payment rates are, on average, two-thirds of the rates that Medicare pays, although this varies by state and by service. In 2012, 38 states and the District of Columbia paid 85 percent of the Medicare rate or less for all physician services, while only 3 states offered rates that were higher than Medicare for all physician services on average (Zuckerman and Goin 2012).[3]

The disparity between Medicaid and Medicare payment rates is even larger for primary care services. In 2012, Medicaid payment rates for a representative sample of primary care services eligible for the ACA payment increase were 58 percent of Medicare rates. This disparity has increased recently: payments for these primary care services were 65 percent of Medicare's rates in 2008. However, the difference over time is due primarily to increases in Medicare's payments for certain physician services (Zuckerman and Goin 2012).

Because states have the authority to establish payment rates within broad federal parameters, Medicaid FFS physician rates vary across states. Nine states and the District of Columbia have reduced physician payment rates since July 1, 2009 (Ollove 2013).

The rate of physician participation in Medicaid has historically been considered an indicator of access. In a survey from 2004 and 2005, 21 percent of all physicians reported that they were not accepting new Medicaid patients (Cunningham and May 2006). In contrast, 4.3 percent reported that they were not accepting new privately insured patients, and 3.4 percent reported that they were not accepting new Medicare patients.

Lower rates relative to other payers are also associated with lower levels of physician participation. A 2012 study found that about 70 percent (69.4 percent) of physicians accepted new Medicaid patients in 2011. In contrast, 81.7 percent of physicians accepted new privately insured patients, and 83 percent accepted new Medicare enrollees. New Jersey (40.4 percent) and California (57.1 percent) had the lowest percentage of physicians accepting new Medicaid patients, and Minnesota (96.3 percent) and Wyoming (99.3 percent) had the highest. The study compared the share of physicians accepting new patients with the Medicaid-to-Medicare fee ratio in each state, and found that a 10 percentage point increase in the fee ratio correlated with a 4 percentage point increase in the acceptance of new Medicaid patients (Decker 2012).

Medicaid enrollees are more likely to see a physician in an outpatient setting or emergency room than a physician's office in states where rates are low relative to Medicare. One study found that as the Medicaid-to-Medicare fee ratio decreased (from 1 to 0.64), the likelihood of Medicaid enrollees receiving physician care in an outpatient hospital department or emergency department increased by 10.7 percentage points (Decker 2009). On the other hand, researchers have also demonstrated that higher payments increase the probability of Medicaid enrollees having a visit with a doctor or other health professional (Shen and Zuckerman 2005).

Payment rates are just one of several factors that affect physician participation in Medicaid. Physicians typically cite low rates as a major factor in not accepting new patients, but other factors—such as patient non-compliance, delayed payment, and paperwork requirements—rank close behind (Cunningham 2011, KFF 2011, Cunningham and Nichols 2005). About 70 percent of physicians said that billing requirements and paperwork were a moderate or very important reason for not accepting new Medicaid patients in a 2004 and 2005 survey, ranked second behind low payment rates (84 percent) (Cunningham and May 2006). In the same survey, physicians reported that Medicaid required more prior authorizations than private insurance carriers.[4] Close to two-thirds (64.8 percent) of all physicians reported that delayed payment was a moderately or very important reason for not accepting new Medicaid patients.

Statutory and Regulatory Requirements for the Primary Care Physician Payment Increase

As noted above, the ACA requires that state Medicaid programs pay rates at least as high as Medicare rates for primary care services furnished by certain physicians in 2013 and 2014 (§1202). It also requires that states implement the rate increase in their Medicaid managed care programs as well as in FFS Medicaid. The federal government will fund the cost of the difference between the state's Medicaid fees as of July 1, 2009, and Medicare fees in 2013 and 2014 at a 100 percent federal matching rate. The nine states and the District of Columbia that reduced Medicaid physician rates since July 1, 2009, must fund the difference between their current rates and the prevailing rates on that date, at their usual federal medical assistance percentage (FMAP). The payment rate increase is expected to cost the federal government nearly $11.9 billion over the two-year period and save state governments over $500 million in provider payments for those states that have increased rates since July 1, 2009 (CMS 2012b).[5] Costs incurred to Medicaid agencies in implementing the provision are not eligible for enhanced match.

CMS published a final rule for the implementation of the provision on November 6, 2012 (CMS 2012b), and has issued six further clarifying documents since then.[6] Selected regulatory requirements are described below.

Eligibility for increased payments

Not all providers are eligible for increased payment rates under the ACA, nor are all services included. Eligibility requirements and the process for verification are described below.

Eligible services. The payment increase applies to evaluation and management services and some vaccine administration services. Evaluation and management services primarily include physician visits in which the physician takes a patient's history, examines the patient, and engages in medical decisionmaking or counseling.[7]

Eligible providers. The statute limits increased payment to physicians with a primary specialty designation of family medicine, general internal medicine, or pediatric medicine. The final rule identifies eligible providers to include physicians practicing primary care with a subspecialty recognized by the American Board of Medical Specialties (ABMS), the American Board of Physician Specialties, or the American Osteopathic Association (AOA).[8] The rule also extends eligibility to physicians who are not board certified in a primary care field if they show that 60 percent of their Medicaid billed claims for the prior year (or previous month, for newly participating physicians) were for eligible services.[9]

Non-physician practitioners, such as advanced practice nurses and physician assistants, may be eligible for the payment increase if they provide primary care services under the supervision of an eligible provider. Physicians practicing in rural health clinics and federally qualified health centers are not eligible for the higher payments because these entities are governed by special payment rules and are classified under a different benefit category than specified in the Social Security Act.

Verification of eligibility. Physicians are required to self-attest to their eligibility by providing evidence of either board certification in one of the specialty or subspecialty designations, or an eligible claims history. The proposed rule had included a requirement that states verify the eligibility and self-attestation of each physician. Some states commented that this would be administratively burdensome and require costly modifications to their Medicaid Management Information Systems (MMIS) used to process and adjudicate claims. In response, CMS amended the final rule and instead required states to retrospectively review a statistically valid sample of physicians receiving the higher payments in calendar year (CY) 2013 and CY 2014 to verify their eligibility for the payment.

CMS provided additional details and guidelines for the self-attestation process in further sub-regulatory guidance:

- States may establish reasonable time frames for providers to submit self-attestations (CMS 2013c). All providers will be eligible for increased rates on the date that they make their self-attestation but may also be eligible for services already provided dating back to January 1, 2013. Many states required that providers make their attestations prior to March 31, 2013, in order to receive retroactive payments. Other states will not provide retroactive eligibility (AAP 2013).
- States may require providers to resubmit self-attestations each year (CMS 2013c).
- Providers who participate in both Medicaid FFS and managed care are required to self-attest only once, effectively requiring state agencies to coordinate sharing of self-attestation information with managed care plans (CMS 2013a).
- States may delegate self-attestation collection to their contracted MCOs (CMS 2013a).

Payment amounts and frequency

States were required to submit a state plan amendment (SPA) with their proposed implementation procedures by March 31, 2013.[10] This must include information on their payment amounts, payment type, and managed care methodologies, as described below.

Payment amount. The final rule provided some flexibility to states in determining their payment rates for eligible primary care services in 2013 and 2014. Medicare fees vary by geographic area and site of service (e.g., physician office versus hospital outpatient department). In response to state concerns about administrative complexity, CMS does not require states to vary their new Medicaid rates to the same extent. In their SPAs, states were required to indicate how they will address the following options in rate setting:

- **Geography.** States may pay the region-specific Medicare physician fee schedule rate or use an average rate for all counties.
- **Site of service.** States may implement site-of-service rate adjustments or pay one rate for each code, based on Medicare's rate for office-based services.
- **Provider type.** Some states also vary rates based on provider type, paying mid-level professionals a lower rate than physicians—for example, paying physician assistants providing services under the supervision of a physician 80 percent of the physician rate. The final rule stipulates that a state's mid-level professional payment methodology in place on July 1, 2009, must also be used for covered services and eligible providers under the primary care payment increase provision.

In addition to updating the rates paid for vaccine administration codes, the rule also updates the maximum regional administration fee that a provider may charge to administer vaccines to children eligible for the Vaccines for Children (VFC) program.[11]

Payment type and frequency. The final rule provides states two alternatives for making payments to physicians:

- **Add-on to the existing fee schedule.** Under this option, states would adjust their fee schedule to include the 2013 or 2014 Medicare rates and would provide the payment increase to physicians on a claim-by-claim basis.
- **Lump-sum supplemental payment.** If states do not wish to adjust payments for each claim, they may calculate the additional amount owed to each physician and pay the amount in a lump sum quarterly or more frequently.

States were required to specify in their SPAs which methodology they will use. And while CMS may adjust the Medicare physician fee schedule more than once annually, the final rule allows states the option to adjust their fee schedule each time a new Medicare physician fee schedule is published or once annually.

Managed care. Medicaid MCOs must comply with the ACA primary care payment provision in 2013 and 2014. This obligation must be specified in the states' contracts with the MCOs. For each MCO contract, the state is required to submit to CMS the methodologies the state will use to identify the services covered by the payment, to calculate the amounts owed, and to verify that MCOs delivered the enhanced primary care rate to eligible providers.

CMS developed a framework for states that could assist them in this process. CMS has also issued two additional question and answer documents for implementation in managed care settings that answer eligible provider, eligible payment, and operational questions specific to MCOs (CMS 2013b, CMS 2012d).

Interaction with Medicare payments for dual eligibles. The payment increase will also affect physicians who provide care to individuals dually eligible for both Medicare and Medicaid. Medicare is the primary payer for primary care services for these individuals, and Medicaid covers cost sharing. However, in many states, Medicaid pays the lesser of the Medicare cost-sharing amount or the difference between the Medicaid rate and the amount already paid by Medicare—effectively limiting the physician's total payment to the Medicaid rate when it is lower than Medicare's rate. (For a more complete discussion of these lesser-of policies, see MACPAC's March 2013 report to the Congress.) When Medicaid physician fees are paid at Medicare rates in 2013 and 2014, primary care physicians serving dual eligibles under lesser-of policies should receive full payment of Medicare coinsurance.

Issues Emerging from Early Implementation

The primary care payment increase provision is simple in concept, but has proven difficult to operationalize. Although states routinely make changes to their fee schedules and payment policies, this provision is distinguished by the fact that the changes are federally mandated for specific services provided by specific physicians. States must make administrative changes in order to comply with these requirements— changes that are not easy to make, particularly within the short time frame between the publication of the final rule and the effective date of the provision. The requirement that the payment increase also apply to managed care represents an additional layer of complexity.

In order to better understand the challenges associated with implementation, MACPAC conducted semi-structured interviews with officials from six states (Alabama, California, Indiana, Massachusetts, Oregon, and Rhode Island) and the District of Columbia.[12] Interviews were conducted from mid-October 2012 through January 2013, and most state Medicaid policy officials were interviewed around the time the final rule was published in November. This meant that state Medicaid officials were either anticipating or analyzing the final rule, and staff responded to our interviews with some uncertainty about how to proceed with implementation issues such as site-of-service and geographic adjustments to their fee schedules, proposed requirements that were eventually made optional in the final rule.

These interviews and subsequent conversations with Medicaid officials and other stakeholders brought to light concerns in six areas: modifying claims-processing systems, identifying eligible providers, the exclusion of mid-level and non-physician practitioners, aligning with current payment methodology, the time allotted to implement the provision, and the temporary nature of the provision. The discussion below highlights the themes raised in the interviews, many of which were reinforced by comments on CMS' proposed rule and more recent reports from states, provider associations, and others.

MMIS modifications. Although states make rate adjustments routinely, the MMIS changes required to implement the primary care payment increase are not routine, and the administrative costs of making them will be matched at the usual FMAP. The data systems changes essentially require new functions: flagging providers as eligible or ineligible for a rate increase based on self-attestation, paying two rates for a specific code depending on provider eligibility, and tracking and reporting the amount spent on the increased rates to CMS for enhanced federal match. Such changes have to be programmed into the MMIS system and then tested.

Identifying eligible providers. States consistently reported that determining which providers would be eligible for the rate increase based on specialty or subspecialty is both complex and burdensome. States must develop and implement a self-attestation process for providers that is unique to the primary care payment increase. Moreover, not all states routinely collect board certification information from their providers. Additionally, states reported not having complete encounter and FFS claims data to determine eligibility for providers who participate in both FFS Medicaid and MCOs and are seeking eligibility under the 60 percent billed code threshold. States must also coordinate the self-attestation process with their managed care contractors.

Non-physician providers. Some states interviewed indicated that the effect of the provision on access to care may be limited because the statute excludes independently practicing non-physician practitioners. Some states rely on these providers, particularly in underserved and rural areas.[13] And for non-physician practitioners practicing under the supervision of a physician, the state must verify that the supervising physician has self-attested to his or her eligibility, another possible layer of complexity.

Aligning alternative payment methods. Not all states use procedure codes in the same way, and aligning alternative payment methods with Medicare's payment rates can be a challenge. For example, some states will pay for pediatric vaccine administration using the service codes associated with the vaccines instead of the vaccine administration codes.[14] The requirement that states pay at Medicare rates for certain codes makes it necessary for states to crosswalk codes unique to their state with those used by Medicare, and, in some cases, amend their payment policy.

In some cases, states indicated that the provision conflicts with other efforts to implement alternative payment methods. For example, some states are considering accountable care organizations or bundled payments as alternatives to traditional FFS methods. Among states that are implementing alternative payment methods, the primary care rate increase means that while they are moving away from the traditional volume-based FFS system, they have to maintain some form of it to ensure their compliance with the primary care rate increase provisions.

Implementation time frame. Publication of the final rule on November 6, 2012, gave states little time to be ready for making increased payments on January 1, 2013. In addition to the systems changes and provider outreach activities described above (which may include additional steps in a managed care environment, discussed later), each state had to submit a SPA. All states were able to meet CMS' March 31, 2013, deadline to submit their SPA, and as of mid-June, SPAs had been approved for nearly half of the states. Thus, only these states were allowed to make increased payments five months after the effective date of the provision. At the time of our interviews, state Medicaid officials had anticipated delays and were planning to make at least some increased payments to providers retroactively, even in states that planned to implement the provision as an add-on to the standing fee schedule.

Primary care rates in 2015 and beyond. A consistent theme from MACPAC's interviews was a concern that the effect of the provision on provider participation may be limited because it is set to expire after 2014. Several of the states included in our interviews indicated that they are unlikely to be able to maintain the rates in 2015 and beyond without the enhanced federal matching funds. For example, the California legislature passed a law in June 2012 (AB 1467 [Monning], Chapter 23, Statutes of 2012), that mandated that rates return to pre-2013 levels in 2015 unless the enhanced federal match continues. Others voiced concern that rolling back rates in 2015 to pre-2013 levels would be perceived as a rate reduction rather than a discontinuation of the rate increase and could negatively affect provider recruitment efforts. Such concerns were also cited as a rationale for making lump-sum supplemental payments rather than incremental additional payments for each primary care claim. Similarly, some states reported concerns that because the rate increase is temporary, it will not provide enough incentive for non-participating physicians to become Medicaid providers.

Implementation Issues Specific to Managed Care

Many of the challenges reported by states in implementing the provision within FFS extend to managed care, including identifying eligible providers, modifying administrative systems, and coordinating attestation. In addition, states must develop a methodology to adjust payments to MCOs to account for the increase in spending on eligible services and report this amount for enhanced federal funding. This requires contracting with actuaries to calculate and certify rates, and then amending contracts with managed care plans to reflect new rates.

Managed care rate setting. States typically pay participating managed care plans through a capitation payment—a fixed payment for a defined package of benefits, usually paid on a per member per month basis.[15] The methodology that states use to determine these capitation rates must be certified by actuaries and approved by CMS. To meet the requirements of the statute, states must adjust those methodologies to pass the primary care increase through to eligible physicians and identify the payment amount eligible for full federal funding.

CMS published technical guidance that states could use for this task, proposing three risk models that would generally be considered reasonable and acceptable and would deliver enhanced payment to eligible physicians participating in managed care networks:

- **Full-risk prospective capitation.** The state calculates the capitation rates for 2013 and 2014 inclusive of the primary care rate increase. This model shifts financial risk entirely to the managed care plan because there would be no reconciliation to actual utilization.

- **Prospective capitation with risk sharing that incorporates retrospective reconciliation.** The state calculates the capitation rates for 2013 and 2014 inclusive of the primary care rate increase but retrospectively analyzes encounter data and reconciles payments to the plans to ensure that capitation payments were sufficient to cover the rate increase. States may reimburse plans for the full amount of any shortfall, or use a risk-sharing arrangement so that the state only gives the plan additional funds for costs outside of a specified risk corridor.

- **Non-risk reconciled payments for enhanced rates.** The state makes 2013 and 2014 capitation payments to managed care contractors without adjusting for the primary care rate increase. Instead, the managed care contractor reports primary care service utilization at some interval (e.g., quarterly), and the state reviews the report and pays accordingly.

According to CMS, every state has proposed to use one of these models (CMS 2013d). In some cases, states have customized the model to better fit their program (Mercer 2013).

Under any of these models, states must make a judgment about the share of capitation payments that is attributable to eligible primary care services at the Current Procedural Terminology (CPT) code level. This task is challenging because MCOs may use varying payment methods to compensate providers (Mercer 2013). For example, MCOs may employ salaried physicians or use sub-capitated agreements. Neither method is tied to the volume or type of services the physician provides. MCOs may also use a different coding system that would require a crosswalk, perhaps imperfect, to those used in the Medicare physician fee schedule.

When calculating the additional primary care payment for MCOs, states must also decide whether to calculate a single, average amount for all enrollees or to vary the payment across different subgroups to reflect differences in their utilization of the eligible primary care services. Calculating the impact at this rate-cell level might better align payment to take into account differences in plans' enrollment mix, but would likely be more difficult to administer (Mercer 2013).

Also at issue is the availability of data to conduct the provider and procedure-level analyses required to calculate the level of rate increases. Actuaries typically use plan encounter data and financial statements, which may not have sufficient detail for this purpose.

Managed care contract amendments. Finally, states must renegotiate contracts with MCOs, a source of concern among state officials in our interviews.[16] Some states anticipated this in late 2012 and either put contract changes on hold or put in placeholders for the payment increase during contract negotiations with MCOs. They anticipated amending those contracts upon receipt of formal guidance and approval of their plans from CMS. CMS will use approved SPAs and payment increase methodologies in their approval of contract amendments.

Evaluation

Given the limited two-year time period that the primary care payment increase will be in effect, questions are already being raised as to whether an extension of the policy is warranted. Although prior research suggests an association between relatively higher physician fees and physician participation, it is not clear whether this scenario will be borne out.

At the time of our interviews, state officials were more focused on implementation than evaluation. Moreover, complete national claims data that could be used to examine changes in service use will not be available until well after the payment increase expires at the end of 2014. On the other hand, surveys of physician attitudes or state-specific workforce data could provide useful information in a more timely fashion.

States are required to submit certain physician participation and utilization information, pre- and post-implementation, to CMS (42 CFR 447.400(d)). CMS will specify the format that states will use to submit data and when submissions are due, and is likely to elaborate on what information is expected at that time. The regulation requires CMS to make the information from states available on the Medicaid website. State-specific information that includes participation among non-physician practitioners, as well as provider specialty and subspecialty details, could prove useful in assessing the effect of the provision in advance of a more comprehensive and systematic evaluation.

Efforts to implement the primary care payment increase are ongoing, and we can expect more states to begin making increased payments as they receive SPA approval. As states transition to day-to-day operation, more information will become available. In the months ahead, the Commission will continue to monitor implementation and will be looking at efforts of state, federal, and academic evaluators to see what can be learned to inform future work.

Endnotes

[1] The increase, as described later in this chapter, is the difference between the prevailing fee schedule on July 1, 2009, and the 2013 and 2014 Medicare rates. This difference is fully funded by the federal government; administrative costs associated with implementing this change are funded at a state's usual FMAP.

[2] The Massachusetts reform had some positive effects: more people reported having a usual source of care, and the number of people who had one physician office visit in the past year increased (Long and Masi 2009). On the other hand, individuals' reported level of unmet need was nearly at the same level it was pre-reform.

[3] Published Medicaid FFS rates may not reflect total payments to physicians. In fiscal year 2012, 20 states made supplemental payments to physicians, typically those employed by state university hospitals (MACPAC 2013). These payments are made in addition to the standard fee schedule payments.

[4] Prior authorization is the requirement that a provider must obtain prior approval from a health insurer (including Medicaid) before providing a service to an enrollee. Without this approval, the insurer may deny a claim and not pay the provider for the service.

[5] These figures represent aggregate projections. The state savings come with two caveats. The first is that savings figures do not include administrative costs incurred by states as they operationalize the provision. Secondly, some states will have to pay the difference between current rates and the rates as of July 1, 2009, with their usual federal match.

[6] The first two documents came out at the same time as the final rule (CMS 2012c and 2012d). An additional set came out in 2012 (CMS 2012a), and three more have been published in 2013 (CMS 2013a, 2013b, and 2013c).

[7] Evaluation and management codes are designated as codes 99201 through 99499 in the CPT code set. The vaccine administration services covered by the payment provision are CPT codes 90460 and 90461 for administration and counseling related to children's vaccines, and 90471–90474 for other vaccine administration. For codes for which there is no Medicare rate, CMS will publish applicable rates. States with alternative methodologies for paying for vaccine administration may also be eligible to increase those rates in an equivalent manner, subject to CMS approval.

[8] The ABMS recognizes approximately five eligible family medicine subspecialties, and some examples include adolescent medicine, geriatric medicine, and sports medicine. Among the list of internal medicine subspecialties recognized by ABMS (19 total) and AOA (11 total), some examples include diabetes and metabolism, gastroenterology, and rheumatology. Among the list of pediatric subspecialties recognized by ABMS (20 total) and AOA (5 total), some examples include neonatology or neonatal-perinatal medicine, pediatric allergy and immunology, and pediatric pulmonology. CMS has published additional information in a question and answer document (CMS 2012b).

[9] Sub-regulatory guidance offered an example of a physician who is board certified in dermatology and who practices in the community as a family practitioner. This physician would be eligible if he or she could support his or her attestation with 60 percent claims history.

[10] SPAs may be made retroactive to the first day of the federal fiscal quarter in which they were submitted to CMS. For example, the primary care payment increase was scheduled to become effective on January 1, 2013. Therefore, states had until March 31, 2013, to submit the SPA so that they could make retroactive payments for services provided on or after January 1, 2013.

[11] The VFC program was authorized in the Omnibus Budget Reconciliation Act of 1993 (P.L. 103-66, as amended). The program makes vaccines available to providers at no cost, who must administer the vaccines to children who cannot otherwise pay. The final rule published for the primary care payment increase updates the amount that providers may charge for the administration of vaccines, although providers may not charge for the vaccines themselves.

[12] States were selected based on three criteria: (1) states with the potential to derive a significant benefit from the increase (i.e., those with a Medicaid-to-Medicare fee ratio of 0.9 or less based on 2008 data), (2) states with different potential challenges in implementing the payment increase, and (3) states from different regions of the country. To ensure inclusion of states facing different implementation challenges, we included states representing different levels of managed care penetration and with different physician payment arrangements.

[13] States have the authority to pay health care professionals other than physicians, such as certified nurse practitioners and nurse midwives, and states have differing requirements as to what extent these professionals are paid based on physician fee schedules.

[14] State health departments and other local and territorial public health agencies distribute vaccines to private providers at no charge through the VFC program. Under these circumstances, the vaccines are not eligible for payment. Because of this, some states may use the service codes associated with the vaccine to pay providers for the administration of the vaccine instead of the codes set aside for vaccine administration.

[15] For more discussion of managed care payment policy, see Section D of MACPAC's June 2011 report to the Congress.

[16] Contracts with MCOs serving Medicaid enrollees are required by CMS to include a provision that allows a state to amend the contract to come into compliance with a newly issued legislative mandate.

References

American Academy of Pediatrics (AAP). 2013. ACA 2013–2014 Medicaid payment increase state documents. Washington, DC: AAP. http://www.aap.org/en-us/advocacy-and-policy/state-advocacy/Documents/State_Md_Payment_Increase.pdf.

Centers for Medicare & Medicaid Services (CMS), U.S. Department of Health and Human Services. 2013a. *Qs & As on the increased Medicaid payment for primary care. CMS 2370-F (Set IV)*. Baltimore, MD: CMS. http://www.medicaid.gov/AffordableCareAct/Provisions/Downloads/Qs-and-As-on-the-Increased-Medicaid-Payment-for-Primary-Care-Set-IV.pdf.

Centers for Medicare & Medicaid Services (CMS), U.S. Department of Health and Human Services. 2013b. *Qs & As on the increased Medicaid payment for primary care. CMS 2370-F–Managed care (Set II)*. Baltimore, MD: CMS. http://www.medicaid.gov/AffordableCareAct/Provisions/Downloads/Qs-andAs-on-the-Increased-Medicaid-Payment-for-Primary-Care-MANAGED-CARE-Set-II.pdf.

Centers for Medicare & Medicaid Services (CMS), U.S. Department of Health and Human Services. 2013c. *Qs and As on the increased Medicaid payment for primary care. CMS 2370-F (Set III)*. Baltimore, MD: CMS. http://www.medicaid.gov/AffordableCareAct/Provisions/Downloads/Qs-and-As-on-1202-III-1-30-13.pdf.

Centers for Medicare & Medicaid Services (CMS), U.S. Department of Health and Human Services. 2013d. Communication with MACPAC staff, May 8.

Centers for Medicare & Medicaid Services (CMS), U.S. Department of Health and Human Services. 2012a. *Qs and As on the increased Medicaid payment for primary care. CMS 2370-F (Set I)*. Baltimore, MD: CMS. http://www.medicaid.gov/AffordableCareAct/Provisions/Downloads/QandA-Set-II-Increased-Payments-for-PCPs.pdf.

Centers for Medicare & Medicaid Services (CMS), U.S. Department of Health and Human Services. 2012b. Medicaid program; payments for services furnished by certain primary care physicians and charges for vaccine administration under the vaccines for children program. Final rule. *Federal Register* 77, no. 215 (November 6): 66670–66701.

Centers for Medicare & Medicaid Services (CMS), U.S. Department of Health and Human Services. 2012c. *Qs & As on the increased Medicaid payment for primary care. CMS 2370-F*. Baltimore, MD: CMS. http://www.medicaid.gov/AffordableCareAct/Provisions/Downloads/Q-andA-Managed-Care-Increased-Payments-for-PCPs.pdf.

Centers for Medicare & Medicaid Services (CMS), U.S. Department of Health and Human Services. 2012d. *Qs & As on the increased Medicaid payment for primary care. CMS 2370-F–Managed care.* Baltimore, MD: CMS. http://www.medicaid.gov/AffordableCareAct/Provisions/Downloads/Q-and-A-on-Increased-Medicaid-Payments-for-PCPs-managed-care.pdf.

Cunningham, P. 2011. *State variation in primary care physician supply: Implication for health reform Medicaid expansions.* Washington, DC: Center for Studying Health System Change. http://www.hschange.com/CONTENT/1192/.

Cunningham, P., and J. May. 2006. *Medicaid patients increasingly concentrated among physicians.* Washington, DC: Center for Studying Health System Change. http://www.hschange.com/CONTENT/866/.

Cunningham, P., and L. Nichols. 2005. The effects of Medicaid reimbursement on the access to care of Medicaid enrollees: A community perspective. *Medical Care Research and Review* 62, no. 6: 676–695.

Decker, S. 2012. In 2011 nearly one-third of physicians said they would not accept new Medicaid patients, but rising fees may help. *Health Affairs* 31, no. 8: 1673–1679.

Decker, S. 2009. Changes in Medicaid physician fees and patterns of ambulatory care. *Inquiry* 46, no. 3: 291–304.

Kaiser Family Foundation (KFF). 2012. *Massachusetts health care reform: Six years later.* Publication no. 8311. Washington, DC: KFF. http://www.kff.org/healthreform/8311.cfm.

Kaiser Family Foundation (KFF). 2011. *Physician willingness and resources to serve more Medicaid patients: Perspectives from primary care physicians.* Publication no. 8178. Washington, DC: KFF. http://www.kff.org/medicaid/8178.cfm.

Ku, L., Jones, K., et al. 2011. The states' next challenge—securing primary care for expanded Medicaid populations. *New England Journal of Medicine* 364, no. 6: 493–495.

Long, S. 2010. *What is the evidence on health reform in Massachusetts and how might the lessons from Massachusetts apply to national health reform?* Washington, DC: Urban Institute. http://www.urban.org/publications/412118.html.

Long, S, and P. Masi. 2009. Access and affordability: An update on health reform in Massachusetts. *Health Affairs* 28, no. 4: w578–w587.

Medicaid and CHIP Payment and Access Commission (MACPAC). 2013. *Report to the Congress on Medicaid and CHIP.* March 2013. Washington, DC: MACPAC. http://www.macpac.gov/reports.

Mercer Government Human Services Consulting. 2013. Communication with MACPAC staff. April 16.

Ollove, M. 2013. Medicaid expansion puts spotlight on access to primary care. Washington, DC: Kaiser Health News. http://www.kaiserhealthnews.org/Stories/2013/February/14/Medicaid-primary-care-doctor-payment.aspx.

Shen, Y., and S. Zuckerman. 2005. The effect of Medicaid payment generosity on access and use among beneficiaries. *Health Services Research* 40, no. 3: 723–744.

Zuckerman, S., and D. Goin. 2012. *How much will Medicaid physician fees for primary care rise in 2013? Evidence from a 2012 survey of Medicaid physician fees.* Publication no. #8398. Washington, DC: Kaiser Family Foundation. http://www.kff.org/medicaid/8398.cfm.

MACStats: Medicaid and CHIP Program Statistics

MACStats Table of Contents

Overview of MACStats 67

Section 1. Trends in Medicaid Enrollment and Spending 69

FIGURE 1. Medicaid Enrollment and Spending, FY 1966–FY 2012 70

FIGURE 2. Medicaid Spending in Nominal and Real Dollars, FY 1975–FY 2010 71

TABLE 1. Medicaid Beneficiaries (Persons Served) by Eligibility Group, FY 1975–FY 2010 (thousands) 72

TABLE 2. Components of Growth in Real Medicaid Benefit Spending, FY 1975–FY 2010 73

Section 2. Health and Other Characteristics of Medicaid/CHIP Populations 75

TABLE 3. Health Insurance and Demographic Characteristics of Non-Institutionalized Individuals Aged 0–18 by Source of Health Insurance, 2009–2011 80

TABLE 4. Health Characteristics of Non-Institutionalized Individuals Aged 0–18 by Source of Health Insurance, 2009–2011 81

TABLE 5. Use of Care by Non-Institutionalized Individuals Aged 0–18 by Source of Health Insurance, 2009–2011 82

TABLE 6. Health Insurance and Demographic Characteristics of Non-Institutionalized Individuals Aged 19–64 by Source of Health Insurance, 2009–2011 83

TABLE 7. Health Characteristics of Non-Institutionalized Individuals Aged 19–64 by Source of Health Insurance, 2009–2011 84

TABLE 8. Use of Care by Non-Institutionalized Individuals Aged 19–64 by Source of Health Insurance, 2009–2011 86

TABLE 9. Health Insurance and Demographic Characteristics of Non-Institutionalized Individuals Aged 65 and Older by Source of Health Insurance, 2009–2011 87

TABLE 10. Health Characteristics of Non-Institutionalized Individuals Aged 65 and Older by Source of Health Insurance, 2009–2011 88

TABLE 11. Use of Care by Non-Institutionalized Individuals Aged 65 and Older by Source of Health Insurance, 2009–2011 90

Section 3. Medicaid Enrollment and Benefit Spending 93

TABLE 12. Medicaid Enrollment by State, Eligibility Group, and Dual Eligible Status, FY 2010 (thousands) 94

TABLE 13.	Medicaid Benefit Spending by State, Eligibility Group, and Dual Eligible Status, FY 2010 (millions)	96
TABLE 14.	Medicaid Benefit Spending Per Full-Year Equivalent (FYE) Enrollee by State and Eligibility Group, FY 2010	98
FIGURE 3.	Distribution of Medicaid Benefit Spending by Eligibility Group and Service Category, FY 2010	100
FIGURE 4.	Medicaid Benefit Spending Per Full-Year Equivalent (FYE) Enrollee by Eligibility Group and Service Category, FY 2010	101
FIGURE 5.	Distribution of Medicaid Enrollment and Benefit Spending by Users and Non-Users of Long-Term Services and Supports, FY 2010	102
FIGURE 6.	Distribution of Medicaid Benefit Spending by Long-Term Services and Supports Use and Service Category, FY 2010	103
FIGURE 7.	Medicaid Benefit Spending Per Full-Year Equivalent (FYE) Enrollee by Long-Term Services and Supports Use and Service Category, FY 2010	104

Section 4. Medicaid Managed Care 107

TABLE 15.	Medicaid Enrollees in Managed Care by State, July 1, 2011	108
TABLE 16.	Number of Managed Care Entities by State and Type, July 1, 2011	110
TABLE 17.	Percentage of Medicaid Enrollees in Managed Care by State and Eligibility Group, FY 2010	112
TABLE 18.	Percentage of Medicaid Benefit Spending on Managed Care by State and Eligibility Group, FY 2010	116

Section 5. Technical Guide to the June 2013 MACStats 119

TABLE 19.	Medicaid and CHIP Enrollment by Data Source and Enrollment Period, 2010	120
TABLE 20.	Medicaid and CHIP Enrollment by Data Source and Enrollment Period Among Children Under Age 19, 2010	120
TABLE 21.	Medicaid and CHIP Enrollment by Data Source and Enrollment Period Among Adults Aged 19-64, 2010	121
TABLE 22.	Medicaid and CHIP Enrollment by Data Source and Enrollment Period Among Adults Aged 65 and Older, 2010	121
TABLE 23.	Medicaid Benefit Spending in MSIS and CMS-64 Data by State, FY 2010 (billions)	125
TABLE 24.	Service Categories Used to Adjust FY 2010 Medicaid Benefit Spending in MSIS to Match CMS-64 Totals	126

MAC Stats

Overview

MACStats, a standing section in all MACPAC reports to the Congress, presents data and information on Medicaid and the State Children's Health Insurance Program (CHIP) that otherwise can be difficult to find and are spread out across multiple sources. The June 2013 edition of MACStats is divided into five sections, each prefaced by key points.

Section 1: Trends in Medicaid Enrollment and Spending

- Growth in Medicaid spending and enrollment has varied over the years, reflecting shifts in federal and state policy along with changing economic conditions (Figure 1).
- Individuals qualifying for Medicaid on the basis of a disability accounted for half of real Medicaid spending growth since fiscal year (FY) 1975 (Table 2). Over the same period, non-disabled children accounted for the largest Medicaid enrollment increase in absolute numbers.

Section 2: Health and Other Characteristics of Medicaid/CHIP Populations

- The characteristics of individuals enrolled in Medicaid and CHIP differ from those with other types of coverage, but there is also great diversity within the Medicaid/CHIP population (Tables 3–11).
- Medicaid/CHIP enrollees generally report being in poorer health and using more services than individuals who have other health insurance or who are uninsured (Tables 4, 7, and 10).

Section 3: Medicaid Enrollment and Benefit Spending

- Individuals eligible on the basis of a disability and those aged 65 and older account for about a quarter of Medicaid enrollees, but about two-thirds of program spending (Tables 12 and 13).
- Medicaid spending per enrollee is affected by large numbers of individuals with limited benefits in some states (Table 14).
- Users of Medicaid long-term services and supports are a small but high-cost population (Figures 5–7).

Section 4: Medicaid Managed Care

▶ About half of Medicaid enrollees are in comprehensive risk-based managed care plans. When limited-benefit plans and primary care case management programs are also included, more than 70 percent of enrollees are in some form of managed care (Tables 15 and 17).

▶ The share of enrollees in comprehensive risk-based plans in FY 2010 was 62 percent among non-disabled children, 47 percent among non-disabled adults, 29 percent among individuals eligible on the basis of a disability, and 12 percent among those aged 65 and older (Table 17).

Section 5: Technical Guide to the June 2013 MACStats

This section provides supplemental information to accompany the tables and figures in Sections 1–4 of MACStats. It describes some of the data sources used in MACStats, the methods that MACPAC uses to analyze these data, and reasons why numbers in MACStats tables and figures—such as those on enrollment and spending—may differ from each other or from those published elsewhere.

SECTION 1

Key Points

Trends in Medicaid Enrollment and Spending

- Medicaid spending and enrollment are affected by both federal and state policy choices and economic factors. For example, the Congress made a number of changes that expanded eligibility for pregnant women and children between 1984 and 1990, with delayed effective dates or phase-in provisions that resulted in substantial enrollment growth through the mid-1990s (Figure 1). Economic recessions spurred enrollment growth at the beginning and end of the first decade of the 2000s.

- Individuals qualifying for Medicaid on the basis of a disability accounted for half of real Medicaid spending growth since fiscal year (FY) 1975. Of the real (adjusted for health care inflation) growth in Medicaid spending between FY 1975 and FY 2010, 50.9 percent was attributable to individuals qualifying for Medicaid on the basis of a disability. About three-quarters of the growth for this group was driven by increased enrollment, with the remainder being attributable to growth in per capita spending (Table 2).

- Enrollment trends vary by eligibility group. Children (excluding those eligible on the basis of a disability) experienced the largest enrollment increase in absolute numbers, from 9.6 million in FY 1975 to 30.0 million in FY 2010 (Table 2). However, enrollment among the smaller group of individuals qualifying for Medicaid on the basis of a disability showed the largest annual growth rate over this time period (3.9 percent).

FIGURE 1. Medicaid Enrollment and Spending, FY 1966–FY 2012

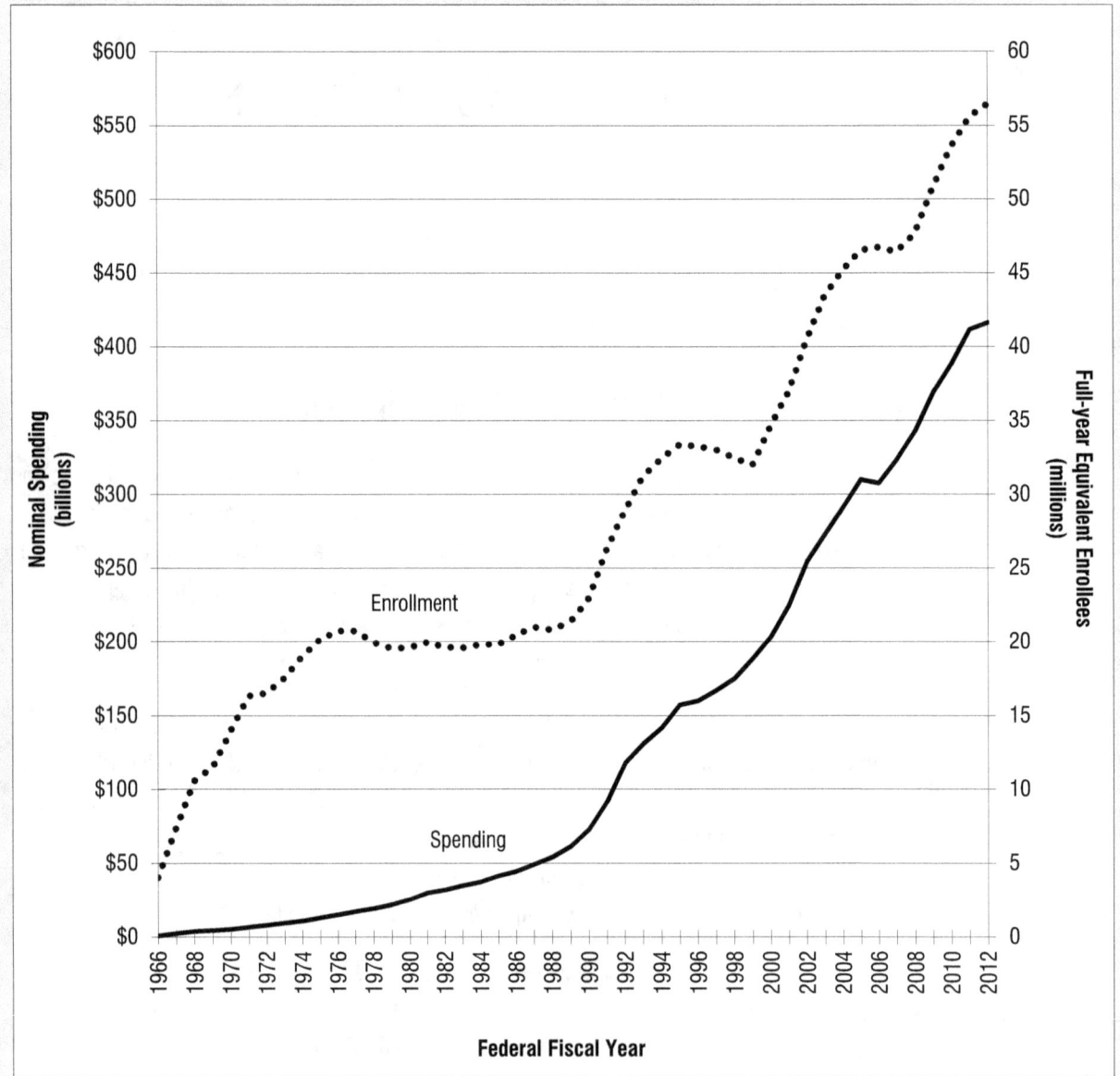

Notes: Spending consists of federal and state Medicaid expenditures for benefits and administration, excluding the Vaccines for Children program. Numbers exclude coverage financed by CHIP. Enrollment data for fiscal year (FY) 2010–2012 are projected. Data prior to FY 1977 have been adjusted to the current federal fiscal year basis (October 1 to September 30). The amounts in this figure may differ from those published elsewhere due to slight differences in the timing of data and the treatment of certain adjustments. Enrollment counts are full-year equivalents and, for fiscal years prior to FY 1990, have been estimated from counts of persons served. (See Section 5 of MACStats for a discussion of how enrollees are counted.)

Source: Data compilation provided to MACPAC by Centers for Medicare & Medicaid Services (CMS), Office of the Actuary, April 2013.

FIGURE 2. Medicaid Spending in Nominal and Real Dollars, FY 1975–FY 2010

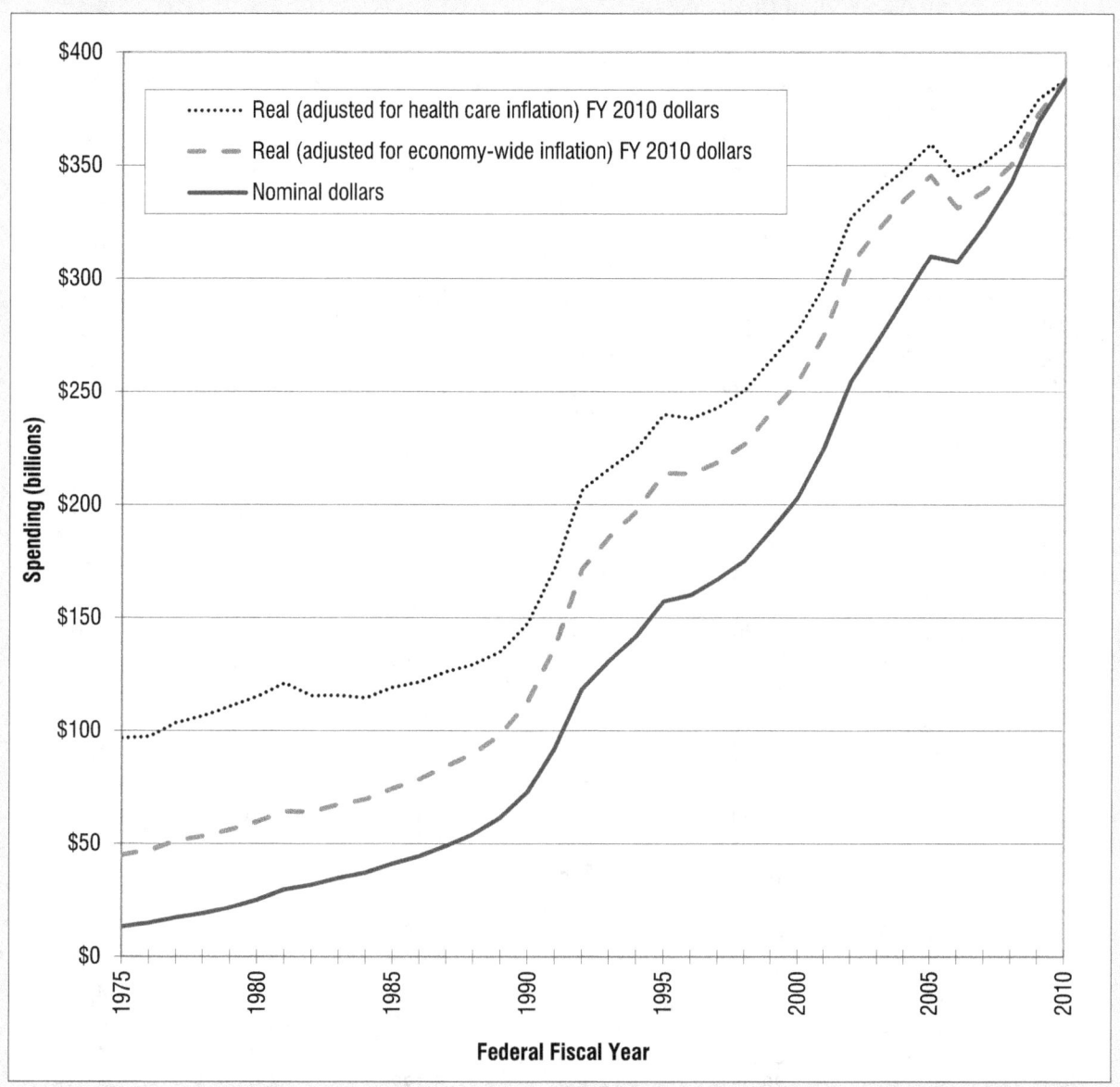

Notes: Spending includes benefits and administrative spending. The bottom line in the figure shows actual (nominal) spending. The middle line transforms nominal Medicaid spending to real fiscal year (FY) 2010 dollars by adjusting for economy-wide inflation, using the gross domestic product (GDP) price deflator. The top line also shows real FY 2010 dollars, but based on inflation for health care in particular. Real historical Medicaid spending adjusted for health care inflation is higher than when adjusted for economy-wide inflation, which reflects the long history of health care inflation in excess of economy-wide inflation. The drop in spending for FY 2006, compared to FY 2005, is the result of the implementation of Medicare Part D.

Sources: Nominal Medicaid spending based on data compilation from the Centers for Medicare & Medicaid Services (CMS), Office of the Actuary, April 2013; real spending based on MACPAC analysis of nominal spending and quarterly National Income and Product Account (NIPA) historical tables for Quarter 4 of 2012 from the Bureau of Economic Analysis, U.S. Department of Commerce (http://www.bea.gov/histdata/NIyear.asp).

TABLE 1. Medicaid Beneficiaries (Persons Served) by Eligibility Group, FY 1975–FY 2010 (thousands)

Year	Total	Children	Adults	Disabled	Aged	Unknown
1975	22,007	9,598	4,529	2,464	3,615	1,801
1976	22,815	9,924	4,773	2,669	3,612	1,837
1977	22,832	9,651	4,785	2,802	3,636	1,958
1978	21,965	9,376	4,643	2,718	3,376	1,852
1979	21,520	9,106	4,570	2,753	3,364	1,727
1980	21,605	9,333	4,877	2,911	3,440	1,044
1981	21,980	9,581	5,187	3,079	3,367	766
1982	21,603	9,563	5,356	2,891	3,240	553
1983	21,554	9,535	5,592	2,921	3,372	134
1984	21,607	9,684	5,600	2,913	3,238	172
1985	21,814	9,757	5,518	3,012	3,061	466
1986	22,515	10,029	5,647	3,182	3,140	517
1987	23,109	10,168	5,599	3,381	3,224	737
1988	22,907	10,037	5,503	3,487	3,159	721
1989	23,511	10,318	5,717	3,590	3,132	754
1990	25,255	11,220	6,010	3,718	3,202	1,105
1991	27,967	12,855	6,703	4,033	3,341	1,035
1992	31,150	15,200	7,040	4,487	3,749	674
1993	33,432	16,285	7,505	5,016	3,863	763
1994	35,053	17,194	7,586	5,458	4,035	780
1995	36,282	17,164	7,604	5,858	4,119	1,537
1996	36,118	16,739	7,127	6,221	4,285	1,746
1997	34,872	15,791	6,803	6,129	3,955	2,195
1998	40,096	18,969	7,895	6,637	3,964	2,631
1999	39,748	18,233	7,446	6,690	3,698	3,682
2000	41,212	18,528	8,538	6,688	3,640	3,817
2001	45,164	20,181	9,707	7,114	3,812	4,349
2002	46,839	21,487	10,847	7,182	3,789	3,534
2003	50,716	23,742	11,530	7,664	4,041	3,739
2004	54,250	25,415	12,325	8,123	4,349	4,037
2005	56,276	25,979	12,431	8,205	4,395	5,266
2006	56,264	26,358	12,495	8,334	4,374	4,703
2007	55,210	26,061	12,264	8,423	4,044	4,418
2008	56,962	26,479	12,739	8,685	4,147	4,912
2009	60,880	28,344	14,245	9,031	4,195	5,066
2010[1]	63,730	30,024	15,368	9,341	4,289	4,709

Notes: Beneficiaries (enrollees for whom payments are made) are shown here because they provide the only historical time series data directly available prior to fiscal year (FY) 1990. Most current analyses of individuals in Medicaid reflect enrollees. For additional discussion, see Section 5 of MACStats. The increase in FY 1998 reflects a change in how Medicaid beneficiaries are counted: beginning in FY 1998, a Medicaid-eligible person who received only coverage for managed care benefits was included in this series as a beneficiary. Excludes Medicaid-expansion CHIP enrollees.

Children and adults who qualify for Medicaid on the basis of a disability are included in the disabled category. In addition, although disability is not a basis of eligibility for aged individuals, states may also report some enrollees aged 65 and older in the disabled category. Unlike the majority of the June 2013 MACStats, this table (along with Table 2) does not recode individuals aged 65 and older who are reported as disabled, due to a lack of necessary detail in the historical data. Generally, individuals whose eligibility group is unknown are persons who were enrolled in the prior year but had a Medicaid claim paid in the current year.

[1] This table shows the number of beneficiaries. See Table 12 for the number of Medicaid enrollees in FY 2010, which is larger than the number of beneficiaries. FY 2010 unavailable for Idaho and Missouri; FY 2009 values used instead.

Sources: For FY 1999 to FY 2010: MACPAC analysis of Medicaid Statistical Information System (MSIS) data. For FY 1975 to FY 1998: CMS Medicare & Medicaid Statistical Supplement, 2010 edition, Table 13.4, http://www.cms.gov/Research-Statistics-Data-and-Systems/Statistics-Trends-and-Reports/MedicareMedicaidStatSupp/2010.html.

TABLE 2. Components of Growth in Real Medicaid Benefit Spending, FY 1975–FY 2010

	FY 1975 (in FY 2010 dollars)	FY 2010[1]	Annual Growth Rate	Relative Contribution to Real Spending Growth, FY 1975 to FY 2010
All eligibility groups				
Spending per beneficiary	$4,463	$6,588[2]	1.1%	29.7%
Number of beneficiaries (millions)	20.2	59.0	3.1	70.3
Total benefit spending (millions)	**$90,181**	**$388,611**	**4.3**	**100.0**
Children				
Spending per beneficiary	$1,748	$2,481[2]	1.0	3.2
Number of beneficiaries (millions)	9.6	30.0	3.3	16.1
Total benefit spending (millions)	**$16,776**	**$74,398**	**4.3**	**19.3**
Adults				
Spending per beneficiary	$3,494	$3,726[2]	0.2	0.4
Number of beneficiaries (millions)	4.5	15.4	3.6	13.5
Total benefit spending (millions)	**$15,825**	**$57,256**	**3.7**	**13.9**
Disabled				
Spending per beneficiary	$9,795	$18,857[2]	1.9	12.7
Number of beneficiaries (millions)	2.5	9.3	3.9	38.3
Total benefit spending (millions)	**$24,136**	**$176,143**[3]	**5.8**	**50.9**
Aged				
Spending per beneficiary	$9,252	$18,841[2]	2.1	13.4
Number of beneficiaries (millions)	3.6	4.3	0.5	2.4
Total benefit spending (millions)	**$33,445**	**$80,815**[3]	**2.6**	**15.9**

Notes: Beneficiaries are shown here because they provide the only historical time series data available prior to fiscal year (FY) 1990. Most current analyses of individuals in Medicaid reflect enrollees, as shown in Table 12. For additional discussion of the definitions of enrollees and beneficiaries, see Section 5 of MACStats.

Dollar amounts were adjusted for inflation using the gross domestic product (GDP) price deflator for health care. In this table, real Medicaid spending growth is attributed to spending per beneficiary and number of beneficiaries. The effect of the interaction between these two factors is allocated between them in proportion to each factor's contribution to spending growth.

The number of beneficiaries excludes individuals whose basis of Medicaid eligibility is unknown. In this analysis, FY 1975 benefit spending for these individuals with an unknown basis of eligibility was allocated proportionally to the four eligibility groups in the table. FY 2010 benefit spending reflects Medicaid Statistical Information System (MSIS) data that have been adjusted to match CMS-64 totals; see Section 5 of MACStats for a discussion of the methodology used.

Results can differ if using different years or eras. The period FY 1975 to FY 2010 is used here to examine factors driving growth over the Medicaid program's long history, rather than a particular time period (e.g., recent growth fueled by recessions in the early and late 2000s).

[1] FY 2010 data unavailable for Idaho and Missouri; FY 2009 values used instead.

[2] Benefit spending per beneficiary shown here differs from the FY 2010 benefit spending per full-year equivalent (FYE) enrollee shown in Table 14 and Figure 4. Per beneficiary numbers are used here because they are the only readily available data prior to FY 1990; they reflect the average amount spent on individuals for whom at least one Medicaid payment was made during the year. Per FYE numbers reflect the average amount spent on individuals enrolled in Medicaid for the entire year.

[3] Total benefit spending shown here differs from the FY 2010 benefit spending in Table 13 and Figure 3. Unlike the majority of the June 2013 MACStats, this table (along with Table 1) does not recode individuals aged 65 and older who are reported as eligible on the basis of a disability.

Sources: MACPAC analysis of CMS 2012 Medicare and Medicaid Statistical Supplement data from Tables 13.4 and 13.10 (for FY 1975) and Medicaid Statistical Information System (MSIS) annual person summary (APS) and CMS-64 net financial management report data as of May 2013 (for FY 2010).

MAC Stats

SECTION 2

Health and Other Characteristics of Medicaid/CHIP Populations

This section uses data from the federal National Health Interview Survey (NHIS) to describe how Medicaid and State Children's Health Insurance (CHIP) enrollees differ from individuals with other types of coverage in terms of their self-reported demographic, socioeconomic, and health characteristics as well as their use of care. It also explores how subpopulations of individuals enrolled in Medicaid or CHIP can differ markedly from one another, even within the same age group.

Our analysis divides the U.S. population into three age groups corresponding to key eligibility pathways in Medicaid and CHIP: children aged 0 to 18, adults aged 19 to 64, and adults aged 65 and older. Tables for each age group explore the following self-reported characteristics from the survey data: health insurance coverage and demographics, health characteristics, and use of health care. (See Section 5 for a discussion of how estimates of insurance coverage may vary depending on the data source and the time period examined.)

The data are presented in two parts. First, we provide comparisons of Medicaid/CHIP enrollees in that age group to individuals with other sources of health insurance. Second, we show estimates for selected subgroups of Medicaid/CHIP enrollees in that age group. The data presented are for the combined Medicaid/CHIP population because, as described in Section 5, surveys like the NHIS generally do not support valid estimates separately for Medicaid and CHIP enrollees.

Our analyses of subgroups of children are divided into three groups:

▶ children who receive Supplemental Security Income (SSI) benefits and are therefore disabled under that program's definition;

▶ children who do not receive SSI, but who are classified as children with special health care needs (CSHCN); and

▶ children who neither receive SSI nor are considered CSHCN.

Our analyses of Medicaid enrollees aged 19 to 64 years old are divided into three categories, the first two of which are primarily composed of persons with disabilities:

- individuals also enrolled in Medicare (dual eligibles), nearly all of whom have obtained their Medicare coverage after a two-year waiting period following their initial receipt of Social Security Disability Insurance (SSDI) benefits;
- Medicaid enrollees receiving SSI who are not enrolled in Medicare; and
- Medicaid enrollees who are neither SSI nor Medicare enrollees.

Our analyses of Medicaid enrollees aged 65 and older focus on the differences between those reporting a functional limitation, and those not reporting a functional limitation. Individuals with a functional limitation are those who reported any degree of difficulty—ranging from "only a little difficult" to "can't do at all"—performing any of a dozen activities (such as walking specified distances, moving objects such as a chair, or going out to do things like shopping) by themselves and without special equipment. It should be noted that individuals with functional limitations can vary substantially in their health needs—from being bedridden to being relatively healthy but responding that walking a quarter of a mile is "only a little difficult." (Individuals in institutions such as nursing homes or assisted living facilities are not interviewed in the NHIS.)

Key Points

Health and Other Characteristics of Medicaid/CHIP Populations

Children under age 19 (Tables 3-5)

- More than a third (36.2 percent) of children were reported to be Medicaid or CHIP enrollees at the time of the survey, while 54.5 percent of children were in private coverage, and 8 percent were uninsured.

- Children enrolled in Medicaid or CHIP were more likely to be Hispanic (34.4 percent) than are privately insured children (12.5 percent) and less likely to be Hispanic than are uninsured children (39.3 percent); Medicaid/CHIP children were more likely to be non-Hispanic black (23.7 percent) than are privately insured (10 percent) or uninsured children (12.3 percent).

- Children enrolled in Medicaid or CHIP were more likely than privately insured or uninsured children to be in fair or poor health and to have certain impairments and health conditions (e.g., attention deficit hyperactivity disorder/attention deficit disorder (ADHD/ADD), asthma, autism).

- Children enrolled in Medicaid or CHIP were more likely to have had a visit to the emergency department (ED) in the past year and to have been regularly taking prescription medications for at least three months.

- Differences in self-reported health status exist among children enrolled in Medicaid or CHIP. Among these children, 22.7 percent of those receiving Supplemental Security Income (SSI) were reported to be in fair or poor health, compared to 13.8 percent for non-SSI children with special health care needs (CSHCN) and less than 1 percent for children who are neither SSI nor CSHCN.

- Prevalence of specific health conditions varies among children enrolled in Medicaid or CHIP. The prevalence of ADHD/ADD among children enrolled in Medicaid or CHIP was 38.8 percent for children receiving SSI, 38.2 percent for non-SSI CSHCN, and 2.1 percent for children who were neither receiving SSI nor CSHCN. The prevalence of asthma for children receiving SSI was 32.3 percent, compared to 40.2 percent for non-SSI CSHCN and 11.1 percent for children who were neither SSI nor CSHCN.

- SSI children and non-SSI CSHCN were each nearly twice as likely to visit health care providers four or more times within a year as are children with Medicaid or CHIP who are neither SSI nor CSHCN.

Adults aged 19 to 64 (Tables 6-8)

- Nearly 1 in 10 (9.5 percent) of non-institutionalized adults aged 19 to 64 reported that they were enrolled in Medicaid.

- Medicaid enrollees in this age group were more likely to be female and to be the parent of a dependent child, compared to those with private insurance, Medicare, or no insurance.

- Adults younger than 65 enrolled in Medicaid (who are generally eligible on the basis of being the parent of a dependent child, pregnant, or disabled) reported that they were in worse health than were those enrolled in private coverage or the uninsured, but were in better health than those enrolled in Medicare (nearly all of whom are eligible for that program on the basis of a disability).

- Adults younger than 65 enrolled in Medicaid were more likely than those with private insurance to have had four or more visits to a doctor or other health professional in the past 12 months.

- Adults with Medicaid were more likely than those with private insurance or no insurance to have visited the ED during the past year. Even after controlling for differences in enrollees' health, demographic, and socioeconomic characteristics, adults younger than 65 enrolled in Medicaid were still more likely to have had an ED visit.

- Among 19- to 64-year-olds, nearly all individuals who are dually enrolled in both Medicaid and Medicare qualify for these programs on the basis of a disability.

- Among adults younger than 65 enrolled in Medicaid, 11.3 percent reported they were also enrolled in Medicare. Conversely, of the Medicare enrollees in this age group, 30.3 percent also were enrolled in Medicaid.

- Differences in self-reported health exist among 19- to 64-year-olds enrolled in Medicaid. Individuals dually enrolled in Medicaid and Medicare, as well as non-dual SSI beneficiaries report fair or poor health (61.2 and 56.5 percent, respectively) at much higher rates than do non-SSI, non-dual enrollees (19.9 percent).

- Among 19- to 64-year-olds enrolled in Medicaid, those who were also enrolled in Medicare or SSI were more likely to have limitations in activities of daily living (ADLs)—as well as the presence of chronic conditions such as heart disease, diabetes, depression, chronic bronchitis, and arthritis—than the overall Medicaid population for this age group.

- Persons with disabilities also had higher use of care—in particular, for at-home care and visits to a doctor or other health professional in the past 12 months—than 19- to 64-year-old Medicaid enrollees overall. Individuals dually enrolled in Medicaid and Medicare and non-dual SSI beneficiaries were also more likely than 19- to 64-year-old Medicaid enrollees overall to have had an ED visit in the past 12 months.

Adults aged 65 and older (Tables 9–11)

- Among non-institutionalized adults aged 65 and older, 7.5 percent reported being enrolled in Medicaid. Most of these Medicaid enrollees (92.1 percent) reported being dually eligible for Medicare, which covered nearly all individuals aged 65 and older.

- Medicaid enrollees aged 65 and older were more likely to be female and less likely to be white (non-Hispanic) than were those with Medicare or private coverage.

- Compared to those enrolled in private coverage or Medicare, Medicaid enrollees aged 65 and older were more likely to report being in fair or poor health, being in worse health compared to 12 months before, and having any of several limitations in their ADLs. Medicaid enrollees aged 65 and older were also more likely to have lost all of their natural teeth, or have any of a number of specific chronic conditions (e.g., depression, diabetes, chronic bronchitis).

- Medicaid enrollees aged 65 and older were also more likely than those with private or Medicare coverage to have received at-home care, to have had multiple visits to a doctor or other health professional, and to have visited an ED in the past 12 months.

- Because more than three-quarters of Medicaid enrollees aged 65 and older had functional limitations, these individuals drive the overall characteristics of enrollees in this age range, and thus do not show significant differences from the total as often as do those with no functional limitations.

- Compared to the overall group of Medicaid enrollees aged 65 and older, Medicaid enrollees who had no functional limitations were less likely to be 85 years old or older, to report being in fair or poor health, and to have any of several specific chronic health conditions. They were also less likely to have visited a doctor or other health professional, or to have visited an ED in the past 12 months.

SECTION 2

TABLE 3. Health Insurance and Demographic Characteristics of Non-Institutionalized Individuals Aged 0–18 by Source of Health Insurance, 2009–2011

	All Children	Selected Sources of Insurance[1]			Medicaid/ CHIP children	Medicaid/CHIP[2]		
		Medicaid/ CHIP[2]	Private[3]	Uninsured[4]		SSI	Non-SSI CSHCN[5]	Neither SSI nor CSHCN
Health Insurance Coverage	36.2%	36.2%	54.5%	8.0%	100.0%	3.3%	17.9%	78.8%
Age (categories sum to 100%)								
0–5	32.5%*	39.1%	29.3%*	23.7%*	39.1%	17.2%*	26.5%*	42.9%*
6–11	30.9	30.9	31.0	29.7	30.9	38.1*	36.1*	29.4
12–18	36.6*	30.0	39.6*	46.6*	30.0	44.7*	37.4*	27.7*
Gender (categories sum to 100%)								
Male	51.3%	50.9%	51.6%	52.4%	50.9%	61.7%*	59.2%*	48.6%*
Female	48.7	49.1	48.4	47.6	49.1	38.3*	40.8*	51.4*
Race (categories sum to 100%)								
Hispanic	22.7%*	34.4%	12.5%*	39.3%*	34.4%	24.3%*	23.4%*	37.4%*
White, non-Hispanic	56.3*	37.7	71.2*	41.4*	37.7	37.8	47.5*	35.4
Black, non-Hispanic	15.3*	23.7	10.0*	12.3*	23.7	34.7*	26.9*	22.4
Other and multiple races, non-Hispanic	5.6*	4.3	6.3*	6.9*	4.3	3.3	2.2*	4.8
Health insurance								
Medicaid/CHIP	36.2%*	100.0%	2.4%*	—	100.0%	100.0%	100.0%	100.0%
Private	54.5*	3.6	100.0*	—	3.6	7.9*	6.1*	2.9

See Table 5 for notes.
Source: MACPAC analysis of the 2009-2011 National Health Interview Survey (NHIS).

TABLE 4. Health Characteristics of Non-Institutionalized Individuals Aged 0–18 by Source of Health Insurance, 2009–2011

	All Children	Selected Sources of Insurance[1]			Medicaid/CHIP[2]			
		Medicaid/CHIP[2]	Private[3]	Uninsured[4]	Medicaid/CHIP children	SSI	Non-SSI CSHCN[5]	Neither SSI nor CSHCN
Children with disabilities or with special health care needs								
Receives Supplemental Security Income (SSI)	1.4%*	3.3%	0.4%*	0.4%*	3.3%	100.0%*	—	—
Children with special health care needs (CSHCN)[5]	15.3*	20.4	13.0*	10.7*	20.4	76.4*[6]	100.0%*	—
Current health status (categories sum to 100%)								
Excellent or very good	82.7%*	73.2%	89.2%*	79.1%*	73.2%	42.0%*	53.6%*	79.0%*
Good	15.2*	22.8	9.9*	19.0*	22.8	35.3*	32.6*	20.1*
Fair or poor	2.1*	3.9	1.0*	2.0*	3.9	22.7*	13.8*	0.9*
Impairments								
Impairment requiring special equipment	1.2%*	1.6%	1.1%*	0.7%*	1.6%	11.2%*	5.0%*	0.4%*
Impairment limits ability to crawl, walk, run, play[7]	2.0*	3.1	1.5*	1.3*	3.1	19.9*	10.8*	0.5*
Impairment lasted, or expected to last 12+ months[8]	1.8*	2.8	1.3*	1.1*	2.8	19.9*	9.9*	0.4*
Specific health conditions								
Ever told child has:								
ADHD/ADD[8]	7.9%*	10.7%	6.8%*	5.2%*	10.7%	38.8%*	38.2%*	2.1%*
Asthma	13.9*	17.0	12.4*	11.0*	17.0	32.3*	40.2*	11.1*
Autism[7]	1.0*	1.3	0.9*	0.5*	1.3	14.0*	4.0*	0.0*
Cerebral palsy[7]	0.3*	0.4	0.2*	†	0.4	6.2*	1.3*	†
Congenital heart disease	1.3*	1.7	1.1*	0.8*	1.7	7.1*	5.0*	0.8*
Diabetes	0.2	0.3	0.2	†	0.3	†	1.4*	†
Down syndrome[7]	0.1*	0.2	0.1*	†	0.2	3.6*	0.6*	†
Intellectual disability (mental retardation)[7]	0.8*	1.4	0.5*	†	1.4	16.2*	4.6*	0.0*
Other developmental delay[7]	4.3*	5.8	3.8*	3.1*	5.8	43.1*	19.9*	0.9*
Sickle cell anemia[7]	0.1*	0.3	0.0*	†	0.3	1.6	0.8*	0.1*

See Table 5 for notes.
Source: MACPAC analysis of the 2009-2011 National Health Interview Survey (NHIS).

TABLE 5. Use of Care by Non-Institutionalized Individuals Aged 0–18 by Source of Health Insurance, 2009–2011

	All Children	Selected Sources of Insurance[1]				Medicaid/CHIP[2]		
		Medicaid/ CHIP[2]	Private[3]	Uninsured[4]	Medicaid/ CHIP children	SSI	Non-SSI CSHCN[5]	Neither SSI nor CSHCN
Received well-child check-up in past 12 months[7]	79.4%*	81.1%	82.1%	51.6%*	81.1%	81.6%	85.1%*	80.2%
Regularly taking prescription drug(s) for 3+ months[8]	13.4*	15.7	13.3*	5.7*	15.7	45.0*	54.3*	5.3*
Number of times saw a doctor or other health professional in past 12 months (categories sum to 100%)								
None	10.1%*	8.8%	7.4%*	32.9%*	8.8%	5.6%*	3.4%*	10.2%*
1	20.5*	18.8	20.8*	24.9*	18.8	11.6*	10.1*	21.1*
2–3	36.7	35.5	38.8*	27.5*	35.5	24.7*	26.8*	38.0*
4+	32.7*	36.8	33.0*	14.7*	36.8	58.2*	59.7*	30.8*
Number of emergency room visits in past 12 months (categories sum to 100%)								
None	79.4%*	72.1%	83.7%*	83.4%*	72.1%	67.8%	57.6%*	75.6%*
1	13.5*	16.5	11.9*	10.5*	16.5	16.8	18.7*	16.0
2–3	5.7*	8.6	3.8*	4.8*	8.6	8.5	16.3*	6.9*
4+	1.5*	2.8	0.6*	1.3*	2.8	7.0*	7.4*	1.6*

Notes: CHIP is State Children's Health Insurance Program. SSI is Supplemental Security Income. CSHCN is children with special health care needs. ADHD is attention deficit hyperactivity disorder. ADD is attention deficit disorder.

† Estimate has a relative standard error of greater than 50 percent.

* Statistically different from Medicaid/CHIP at the (.05) level, two-tailed test.

– Quantity zero; amounts shown as 0.0 round to less than 0.1.

[1] Health insurance coverage is defined at the time of the survey. Totals of health insurance coverage may sum to more than 100 percent because individuals may have multiple sources of coverage. Responses to recent-care questions are based on the previous 12 months, during which time the individual may have had different coverage than that shown in the table. Not separately shown are the estimates of children covered by Medicare (generally children with end-stage renal disease), any type of military health plan (VA, TRICARE, and CHAMP-VA), or other government-sponsored programs.

[2] Medicaid/CHIP also includes persons covered by other state-sponsored health plans.

[3] Private health insurance coverage excludes plans that paid for only one type of service, such as accidents or dental care.

[4] Individuals were defined as uninsured if they did not have any private health insurance, Medicaid, CHIP, Medicare, state-sponsored or other government-sponsored health plan, or military plan. Individuals were also defined as uninsured if they had only Indian Health Service coverage or had only a private plan that paid for one type of service, such as accidents or dental care.

[5] Due in part to changes in the 2011 National Health Interview Survey (NHIS) questionnaire, the CSHCN definition differs slightly from the definition used in prior MACPAC reports using earlier NHIS data. The CSHCN definition applied here is based on an approach developed by the Child and Adolescent Health Measurement Initiative (CAHMI) to identify "children with chronic conditions and elevated service use or need" in the 2007 NHIS and other prior research. (See CAMHI, *Identifying children with chronic conditions and elevated service use or need (CCCESUN) in the National Health Interview Survey (NHIS)*, Portland, OR: Oregon Health and Science University, 2012; A.J. Davidoff, Identifying children with special health care needs in the National Health Interview Survey: a new resource for policy analysis, *Health Services Research* 39 (1): 53-71, 2004). CSHCN in this analysis must have at least one diagnosed or parent-reported condition expected to be an ongoing health condition, and also meet at least one of five criteria related to elevated service use or elevated need, including reported unmet need for care. For more information on the methods used to identify CSHCN, see text and endnotes in Section 5 of MACStats.

[6] For a child to be eligible for SSI, one of the criteria is that the child has a medically determinable physical or mental impairment(s) that results in marked and severe functional limitations and generally is expected to last at least 12 months or result in death. Thus, children who are eligible for SSI should meet the criteria for being a CSHCN; however, some do not. While we do not have enough information to assess the reasons that these Medicaid/CHIP children who are reported to have SSI did not meet the criteria for CSHCN, it could be because: (1) the parents erroneously reported in the survey that the children received SSI, or (2) the parents neglected to report in the survey the children's health information related to their eligibility for SSI and thus as CSHCN.

[7] Question only asked for children aged 0 to 17.

[8] Question only asked for children aged 2 to 17.

Source: MACPAC analysis of the 2009–2011 National Health Interview Survey (NHIS).

TABLE 6. Health Insurance and Demographic Characteristics of Non-Institutionalized Individuals Aged 19–64 by Source of Health Insurance, 2009–2011

	Adults Aged 19–64	Selected Sources of Insurance[1]				Medicaid[2]			
		Medicaid[2]	Private[3]	Medicare	Uninsured[4]	Medicaid adults aged 19–64	Medicare (dual eligibles)	Non-dual SSI	Neither SSI nor Medicare
Health Insurance Coverage		9.5%	65.2%	3.5%	21.3%	100.0%	11.4%	15.0%	73.6%
Age (categories sum to 100%)									
19–24	13.6%*	19.7%	11.0%*	1.8%*	19.7%	19.7%	2.6%*	11.5%*	23.9%*
25–44	43.5*	46.8	42.2*	20.8*	49.9*	46.8	30.8*	36.1*	51.6*
45–54	23.7*	19.2	25.6*	28.6*	19.2	19.2	33.6*	27.9*	15.2*
55–64	19.2*	14.4	21.2*	48.8*	11.3*	14.4	33.0*	24.5*	9.4*
Gender (categories sum to 100%)									
Male	49.2%*	35.5%	49.0%*	49.0%*	54.6%*	35.5%	43.1%*	42.4%*	32.9%*
Female	50.8*	64.5	51.0*	51.0*	45.4*	64.5	56.9*	57.6*	67.1*
Race (categories sum to 100%)									
Hispanic	15.3%*	21.1%	9.7%*	8.7%*	30.1%*	21.1%	9.0%*	13.5%*	24.7%*
White, non-Hispanic	66.3*	49.5	74.4*	69.4*	49.5	49.5	64.3*	54.0	46.4*
Black, non-Hispanic	12.5*	24.0	9.6*	19.5*	14.9*	24.0	24.7	28.0	23.0
Other and multiple races, non-Hispanic	5.9	5.3	6.3*	2.4*	5.5	5.3	2.0*	4.6	6.0
Family characteristics									
Parent of a dependent child[5]	38.0%*	49.2%	38.0%*	13.3%*	35.7%*	49.2%	13.7%*	16.5%*	61.5%*
Health insurance									
Medicaid/CHIP	9.5%*	100.0%	0.4%*	30.3%*	–	100.0%	100.0%	100.0%	100.0%
Medicare	3.5*	11.3	1.1*	100.0*	–	11.3	100.0*	–	–
Private	65.2*	2.6	100.0*	21.2*	–	2.6	2.2	2.7	2.7

See Table 8 for notes.
Source: MACPAC analysis of the 2009–2011 National Health Interview Survey (NHIS).

SECTION 2

MACStats

TABLE 7. Health Characteristics of Non-Institutionalized Individuals Aged 19–64 by Source of Health Insurance, 2009–2011

	Adults Aged 19–64	Selected Sources of Insurance[1]				Medicaid adults aged 19–64	Medicaid Medicare (dual eligibles)	Medicaid[2] Non-dual SSI	Neither SSI nor Medicare
		Medicaid[2]	Private[3]	Medicare	Uninsured[4]				
Disability and work status									
Receives Supplemental Security Income (SSI)	2.4%*	19.9%	0.3%*	21.1%	0.4%*	19.9%	42.7%*	100.0%*	—
Receives Social Security Disability Insurance (SSDI)	3.5*	14.4	1.4*	63.9*	0.5*	14.4	67.2*	18.2*	5.5%*
Working	70.3*	33.5	81.2*	10.9*	59.8*	33.5	8.2*	7.2*	42.8*
Current health status (categories sum to 100%)									
Excellent or very good	63.6%*	40.5%	71.3%*	12.9%*	55.5%*	40.5%	10.8%*	16.4%*	50.1%*
Good	25.3*	29.4	22.5*	27.9	31.7*	29.4	28.0	27.1	30.0
Fair or poor	11.1*	30.1	6.3*	59.2*	12.8*	30.1	61.2*	56.5*	19.9*
Health compared to 12 months ago (categories sum to 100%)									
Better	19.2%*	20.6%	19.5%	16.8%*	18.0%*	20.6%	20.0%	19.5%	21.0%
Worse	8.1*	15.2	5.9*	26.0*	9.6*	15.2	26.4*	21.4*	12.2*
Same	72.7*	64.2	74.6*	57.2*	72.3*	64.2	53.6*	59.1*	66.9*
Activities of daily living (ADLs)									
Help with any personal care needs[6]	1.3%*	6.3%	0.5%*	13.1%*	0.6%*	6.3%	19.6%*	17.0%*	2.2%*
Help with bathing/showering	0.7*	4.3	0.2*	7.7*	0.3*	4.3	12.5*	12.8*	1.3*
Help with dressing	0.7*	3.7	0.3*	7.5*	0.3*	3.7	11.4*	10.9*	1.1*
Help with eating	0.3*	1.7	0.1*	3.0*	0.1*	1.7	5.7*	5.3*	0.4*
Help with transferring (in/out of bed or chairs)	0.6*	3.1	0.2*	6.6*	0.3*	3.1	10.2*	7.9*	1.1*
Help with toileting	0.4*	2.5	0.2*	4.5*	0.1*	2.5	7.7*	7.2*	0.7*
Help getting around in home	0.5*	2.8	0.2*	5.7*	0.2*	2.8	9.3*	6.6*	1.0*
Number of above ADLs reported (categories sum to 100%)									
0	98.7%*	93.7%	99.5%*	86.9%*	99.4%*	93.7%	80.4%*	83.0%*	97.9%*
1	0.2*	0.8	0.1*	2.1*	0.2*	0.8	3.0*	1.7	0.3*
2	0.2*	1.0	0.1*	1.8*	0.1*	1.0	2.2*	3.1*	0.3*
3	0.3*	1.2	0.1*	3.1*	0.1*	1.2	4.3*	2.7*	0.4*
4+	0.6*	3.3	0.2*	6.0*	0.2*	3.3	10.0*	9.4*	1.1*

TABLE 7, Continued

	Adults Aged 19–64	Selected Sources of Insurance[1]				Medicaid[2]			
		Medicaid[2]	Private[3]	Medicare	Uninsured[4]	Medicaid adults aged 19–64	Medicare (dual eligibles)	Non-dual SSI	Neither SSI nor Medicare
Specific health conditions									
Currently pregnant[7]	3.5%*	9.7%	2.8%*	†	1.6%*	9.7%	†	3.1%*	11.2%
Functional limitation[8]	29.7*	47.7	26.1*	84.5%*	27.6*	47.7	84.9%*	76.8*	36.0*
Difficulty walking without equipment	3.2*	11.5	1.7*	31.3*	2.0*	11.5	32.6*	24.6*	5.6*
Health condition that requires special equipment (e.g., cane, wheelchair)	4.1*	11.8	2.7*	32.8*	2.4*	11.8	32.8*	24.7*	6.0*
Lost all natural teeth	4.5*	8.8	3.3*	18.5*	5.0*	8.8	20.7*	16.7*	5.4*
Depressed/anxious feelings[9]	13.1*	27.9	8.6*	37.9*	18.0*	27.9	44.5*	41.1*	22.8*
Ever told had hypertension	23.5*	30.9	23.1*	57.0*	18.0*	30.9	53.8*	47.2*	24.1*
Ever told had coronary heart disease	2.5*	4.4	2.3*	14.0*	1.4*	4.4	11.7*	7.9*	2.6*
Ever told had heart attack	1.8*	3.8	1.4*	11.6*	1.4*	3.8	9.9*	6.5*	2.3*
Ever told had stroke	1.5*	4.2	1.0*	11.1*	1.1*	4.2	11.6*	8.6*	2.2*
Ever told had cancer	5.2	5.8	5.6	13.1*	2.8*	5.8	11.3*	9.5*	4.2*
Ever told had diabetes	6.8*	12.5	6.1*	25.2*	5.0*	12.5	27.2*	21.6*	8.5*
Ever told had arthritis	17.7*	24.5	17.6*	53.5*	11.3*	24.5	53.2*	39.5*	17.0*
Ever told had asthma	13.1*	20.0	12.2*	23.5*	12.1*	20.0	28.9*	27.2*	17.1*
Past 12 months, told had chronic bronchitis	4.0*	8.2	3.1*	15.0*	3.5*	8.2	17.4*	14.2*	5.6*
Past 12 months, told had liver condition	1.4*	3.4	1.0*	6.1*	1.2*	3.4	7.2*	7.3*	2.1*
Past 12 months, told had weak/failing kidneys	1.3*	4.1	0.8*	8.8*	1.3*	4.1	11.6*	6.3*	2.5*

See Table 8 for notes.
Source: MACPAC analysis of the 2009–2011 National Health Interview Survey (NHIS).

TABLE 8. Use of Care by Non-Institutionalized Individuals Aged 19–64 by Source of Health Insurance, 2009–2011

	Adults Aged 19–64	Selected Sources of Insurance[1]				Medicaid[2]			
		Medicaid[2]	Private[3]	Medicare	Uninsured[4]	Medicaid adults aged 19–64	Medicare (dual eligibles)	Non-dual SSI	Neither SSI nor Medicare
Received at-home care in past 12 months	1.2%*	4.7%	0.9%*	9.1%*	0.4%*	4.7%	15.4%*	8.2%*	2.3%*
Number of times saw a doctor or other health professional in past 12 months (categories sum to 100%)									
None	21.9%*	14.0%	15.3%*	6.0%*	47.6%*	14.0%	4.9%*	8.9%*	16.3%*
1	17.8*	12.6	19.0*	4.9*	17.7*	12.6	4.2*	8.7*	14.7*
2–3	26.1*	20.6	29.9*	17.0*	17.1*	20.6	17.2	15.0*	22.2
4+	34.2*	52.9	35.8*	72.1*	17.5*	52.9	73.7*	67.4*	46.8*
Number of emergency room visits in past 12 months (categories sum to 100%)									
None	79.8%*	60.3%	83.6%*	59.6%	78.5%*	60.3%	53.2%*	54.5%*	62.5%*
1	12.7*	18.6	11.6*	17.8	12.5*	18.6	17.7	19.3	18.6
2–3	5.3*	13.0	3.7*	13.4	6.2*	13.0	17.3*	14.5	12.0
4+	2.3*	8.1	1.0*	9.1	2.8*	8.1	11.9*	11.7*	6.8*

Notes: SSI is Supplemental Security Income.

† Estimate has a relative standard error of greater than 50 percent.

* Statistically different from Medicaid at the (.05) level, two-tailed test.

– Quantity zero; amounts shown as 0.0 round to less than 0.1 in this table.

[1] Health insurance coverage is defined as coverage at the time of the survey. Totals of health insurance coverage may sum to more than 100 percent because individuals may have multiple sources of coverage. Responses to recent-care questions are based on the previous 12 months, during which time the individual may have had different coverage than that shown in the table. Not separately shown are the estimates of individuals covered by any type of military health plan (VA, TRICARE, and CHAMP-VA) or other government-sponsored programs.

[2] Medicaid also includes adults reporting coverage through the CHIP program or other state-sponsored health plans. Medicaid and CHIP cannot be distinguished from each other in the National Health Interview Survey. CHIP enrollment of adults is small, totaling approximately 218,000 ever enrolled during FY 2012. (See March 2013 MACStats Table 3.)

[3] Private health insurance coverage excludes plans that paid for only one type of service, such as accidents or dental care.

[4] Individuals were defined as uninsured if they did not have any private health insurance, Medicaid, CHIP, Medicare, state-sponsored or other government-sponsored health plan, or military plan. Individuals were also defined as uninsured if they had only Indian Health Service coverage or had only a private plan that paid for one type of service, such as accidents or dental care.

[5] Parent of a dependent child is defined as an adult with at least one dependent child (biological, adopted, step, or foster) in the household; a dependent child is defined as a child age 18 and under or a child age 23 and under who is not working because of going to school.

[6] Only adults who report needing assistance with personal care needs are asked about each of the specific personal care needs. Each specific personal care need is reported as the overall population prevalence (rather than the prevalence among those needing help with any personal care needs).

[7] Question only asked for females aged 18 to 49.

[8] Individuals with a functional limitation are those who reported any degree of difficulty—ranging from "only a little difficult" to "can't do at all"—doing any of a dozen activities (e.g., walking a quarter of a mile, stooping or kneeling) by themselves and without special equipment.

[9] Reports feeling sad, hopeless, worthless, nervous, restless, or that everything was an effort all or most of the time.

Source: MACPAC analysis of the 2009–2011 National Health Interview Survey (NHIS).

TABLE 9. Health Insurance and Demographic Characteristics of Non-Institutionalized Individuals Aged 65 and Older by Source of Health Insurance, 2009–2011

	Adults Aged 65+	Selected Sources of Insurance[1]			Medicaid[2]		
		Medicaid[2]	Private[3]	Medicare	All Medicaid adults aged 65+	Functional limitation[4]	No functional limitation
Health Insurance Coverage		7.5%	54.4%	94.9%	100.0%	80.0%	20.0%
Age (categories sum to 100%)							
65–74	54.9%	54.1%	54.3%	53.9%	54.1%	52.4%	60.9%*
75–84	33.3	34.9	33.9	34.0	34.9	35.2	33.9
85+	11.8	11.0	11.8	12.1	11.0	12.4	5.1*
Gender (categories sum to 100%)							
Male	43.6%*	33.3%	43.4%*	43.0%*	33.3%	30.8%	42.9%*
Female	56.4*	66.7	56.6*	57.0*	66.7	69.2	57.1*
Race (categories sum to 100%)							
Hispanic	7.2%*	22.1%	3.1%*	6.6%*	22.1%	21.0%	26.4%
White, non-Hispanic	80.0*	49.6	88.3*	81.3*	49.6	51.0	44.3
Black, non-Hispanic	8.6*	18.4	5.9*	8.2*	18.4	19.3	14.7
Other and multiple races, non-Hispanic	4.2*	9.8	2.8*	3.9*	9.8	8.6	14.5
Health insurance							
Medicaid/CHIP	7.5%*	100.0%	0.7%*	7.2%*	100.0%	100.0%	100.0%
Medicare	94.9*	90.8	94.1*	100.0*	90.8	91.7	87.5
Private	54.4*	5.3	100.0*	53.9*	5.3	4.7	7.8

See Table 11 for notes.
Source: MACPAC analysis of the 2009–2011 National Health Interview Survey (NHIS).

TABLE 10. Health Characteristics of Non-Institutionalized Individuals Aged 65 and Older by Source of Health Insurance, 2009–2011

	Adults Aged 65+	Selected Sources of Insurance[1]			All Medicaid adults aged 65+	Medicaid[2]	
		Medicaid[2]	Private[3]	Medicare		Functional limitation[4]	No functional limitation
Disability and work status							
Receives Supplemental Security Income (SSI)	3.9%*	32.5%	0.7%*	3.8%*	32.5%	35.3%	20.5%*
Working	15.7*	3.5	19.2*	14.3*	3.5	2.5	7.6*
Current health status (categories sum to 100%)							
Excellent or very good	42.6%*	19.4%	47.4%*	42.5%*	19.4%	13.4%*	43.8%*
Good	33.9*	29.9	34.5*	33.9*	29.9	28.8	35.0
Fair or poor	23.4*	50.7	18.1*	23.6*	50.7	57.9*	21.1*
Health compared to 12 months ago (categories sum to 100%)							
Better	13.4%	13.2%	12.9%	13.3%	13.2%	13.6%	11.9%
Worse	12.5*	21.5	11.2*	12.6*	21.5	25.3*	6.1*
Same	74.1*	65.3	75.9*	74.0*	65.3	61.1*	82.0*
Activities of daily living (ADLs)							
Help with any personal care needs[5]	6.7%*	20.2%	4.8%*	6.7%*	20.2%	24.5%*	2.9%*
Help with bathing/showering	4.9*	15.9	3.5*	5.0*	15.9	19.2*	2.5*
Help with dressing	3.9*	13.2	2.6*	3.9*	13.2	16.0	2.2*
Help with eating	1.4*	5.0	0.8*	1.4*	5.0	5.9	1.7*
Help with transferring (in/out of bed or chairs)	2.9*	9.2	2.1*	2.9*	9.2	11.0	2.2*
Help with toileting	2.1*	6.8	1.6*	2.2*	6.8	8.0	2.0*
Help getting around in home	2.7*	8.5	1.9*	2.7*	8.5	10.0	2.0*
Number of above ADLs reported (categories sum to 100%)							
0	93.4%*	79.8%	95.2%*	93.3%*	79.8%	75.5%*	97.1%*
1	0.7*	2.3	0.6*	0.7*	2.3	2.8	†
2	1.4*	2.7	1.1*	1.5*	2.7	3.3	†
3	1.5*	4.9	1.1*	1.5*	4.9	6.1	0.0*
4+	2.9*	10.3	2.0*	3.0*	10.3	12.3	2.2*

TABLE 10, Continued

	Adults Aged 65+	Selected Sources of Insurance[1]			All Medicaid adults aged 65+	Medicaid[2]	
		Medicaid[2]	Private[3]	Medicare		Functional limitation[4]	No functional limitation
Specific health conditions							
Functional limitation[4]	65.3%*	80.0%	63.8%*	66.0%*	80.0%	100.0%*	0.0%*
Difficulty walking without equipment	18.7*	37.5	16.1*	19.1*	37.5	45.0*	6.5*
Health condition that requires special equipment (e.g., cane, wheelchair)	20.7*	37.8	18.1*	21.2*	37.8	45.3*	7.8*
Lost all natural teeth	23.8*	42.3	19.9*	23.9*	42.3	45.5	29.0*
Depressed/anxious feelings[6]	9.9*	22.0	8.1*	9.8*	22.0	26.1*	5.9*
Ever told had hypertension	62.2*	70.0	61.5*	62.5*	70.0	73.5	55.4*
Ever told had coronary heart disease	15.8*	18.8	15.9*	16.1*	18.8	20.9	10.2*
Ever told had heart attack	10.6*	14.1	10.1*	10.8*	14.1	15.6	8.2*
Ever told had stroke	8.5*	13.8	7.6*	8.6*	13.8	16.4	3.2*
Ever told had cancer	24.3*	17.4	26.9*	24.7*	17.4	18.8	10.7*
Ever told had diabetes	20.5*	30.1	18.7*	20.6*	30.1	33.7	16.4*
Ever told had arthritis	50.8*	57.0	51.6*	51.5*	57.0	65.1*	23.7*
Ever told had asthma	10.9*	15.8	10.2*	11.1*	15.8	17.1	10.2*
Past 12 months, told had chronic bronchitis	6.3*	10.3	5.8*	6.4*	10.3	11.8	4.1*
Past 12 months, told had liver condition	1.3*	2.9	1.1*	1.3*	2.9	3.3	†
Past 12 months, told had weak/failing kidneys	4.6*	9.9	3.8*	4.7*	9.9	11.8	2.5*

See Table 11 for notes.
Source: MACPAC analysis of the 2009–2011 National Health Interview Survey (NHIS).

MACStats

SECTION 2

TABLE 11. Use of Care by Non-Institutionalized Individuals Aged 65 and Older by Source of Health Insurance, 2009–2011

	Adults Aged 65+	Selected Sources of Insurance[1]			Medicaid[2]		
		Medicaid[2]	Private[3]	Medicare	All Medicaid adults aged 65+	Functional limitation[4]	No functional limitation
Received at-home care in past 12 months	8.1%*	19.1%	7.3%*	8.3%*	19.1%	22.8%	4.1%*
Number of times saw a doctor or other health professional in past 12 months (categories sum to 100%)							
None	5.9%	7.2%	4.5%*	5.5%*	7.2%	4.8%*	16.5%*
1	10.2*	7.0	9.8*	9.9*	7.0	5.3	13.8*
2–3	25.3*	17.8	26.2*	25.1*	17.8	16.3	23.5
4+	58.7*	68.1	59.5*	59.5*	68.1	73.6*	46.3*
Number of emergency room visits in past 12 months (categories sum to 100%)							
None	76.1%*	67.4%	77.1%*	75.7%*	67.4%	63.8%	81.7%*
1	16.0	17.5	15.8	16.2	17.5	18.8	12.3*
2–3	6.0*	10.4	5.4*	6.0*	10.4	11.8	4.6*
4+	2.0*	4.7	1.7*	2.0*	4.7	5.5	1.4*

Notes:
† Estimate has a relative standard error of greater than 50 percent.
* Statistically different from Medicaid at the (.05) level, two-tailed test.
– Quantity zero; amounts shown as 0.0 round to less than 0.1 in this table.

[1] Health insurance coverage is defined as coverage at the time of the survey. Totals of health insurance coverage may sum to more than 100 percent because individuals may have multiple sources of coverage. Responses to recent-care questions are based on the previous 12 months, during which time the individual may have had different coverage than that shown in the table. Not separately shown are the estimates of individuals covered by any type of military health plan (VA, TRICARE, and CHAMP-VA) or other government-sponsored programs.
[2] Medicaid also includes adults reporting coverage through CHIP or other state-sponsored health plans.
[3] Private health insurance coverage excludes plans that paid for only one type of service, such as accidents or dental care.
[4] Individuals with a functional limitation are those who reported any degree of difficulty—ranging from "only a little difficult" to "can't do at all"—doing any of a dozen activities (e.g., walking a quarter of a mile, stooping or kneeling) by themselves and without special equipment.
[5] Only adults who report needing assistance with personal care needs are asked about each of the following specific personal care needs. Each need is reported as the overall population prevalence (rather than the prevalence among those needing help with any personal care needs).
[6] Reports feeling sad, hopeless, worthless, nervous, restless, or that everything was an effort all or most of the time.

Source: MACPAC analysis of the 2009–2011 National Health Interview Survey (NHIS).

MACStats

MAC Stats

SECTION 3

Key Points

Medicaid Enrollment and Benefit Spending

- Individuals eligible on the basis of a disability and those aged 65 and older account for about a quarter of Medicaid enrollees, but about two-thirds of program spending (Tables 12 and 13).

- Medicaid spending per enrollee is affected by large numbers of individuals with limited benefits in some states (Table 14).

- Among individuals dually enrolled in Medicaid and Medicare, those aged 65 and older account for about 60 percent of enrollment and Medicaid benefit spending (Tables 12 and 13).

- A large share of Medicaid spending for enrollees eligible on the basis of a disability and enrollees aged 65 and older is for long-term services and supports (LTSS), while a substantial portion of spending for non-disabled children and adults is for capitation payments to managed care plans (Figures 3 and 4).

- Long-term services and supports (LTSS) users account for only about 6 percent of Medicaid enrollees, but nearly half of all Medicaid spending (Figure 5). Acute care represents a minority of Medicaid spending for most LTSS users (Figure 6), and average Medicaid benefit spending for these individuals is more than 10 times that of enrollees who are not using LTSS (Figure 7).

- Medicaid benefit spending per enrollee varies substantially across states (Table 14). Reasons for this variation may include the breadth of benefits that states choose to cover; the proportion of enrollees receiving the full benefit package or a more limited version; enrollee case mix (based on health status and other characteristics); the underlying costs of delivering health care services in specific geographic areas; and state policies regarding provider payments, care management, and other program features.

SECTION 3

MACStats

TABLE 12. Medicaid Enrollment by State, Eligibility Group, and Dual Eligible Status, FY 2010 (thousands)

State	Total	Percentage of Enrollees in Eligibility Group[1]				Dual Eligible Status[2]					
						All dual eligibles		Dual eligibles with full benefits		Dual eligibles with limited benefits	
		Children	Adults	Disabled	Aged	Total	Percentage age 65+	Total	Percentage age 65+	Total	Percentage age 65+
Total	**66,024**	**48.1%**	**27.8%**	**14.5%**	**9.5%**	**9,755**	**59.6%**	**7,366**	**59.8%**	**2,389**	**58.9%**
Alabama	1,016	50.1	17.3	20.9	11.6	206	56.3	97	52.7	109	59.5
Alaska	126	55.4	24.4	13.2	7.0	14	53.8	14	53.4	0	67.2
Arizona	1,531	44.5	40.3	8.9	6.2	153	58.4	119	54.6	34	71.7
Arkansas	699	52.1	17.0	20.9	10.0	125	53.9	70	59.6	55	46.7
California	11,335	38.3	43.7	9.1	9.0	1,262	70.3	1,231	70.2	31	76.2
Colorado	700	58.3	19.7	13.7	8.3	89	58.8	66	61.1	23	52.2
Connecticut	712	44.4	32.5	10.2	12.9	133	65.3	79	58.3	54	75.6
Delaware	225	40.8	41.6	11.1	6.4	26	53.6	12	54.4	14	52.9
District of Columbia	213	37.9	36.6	17.4	8.1	26	60.2	20	59.4	6	63.2
Florida	3,703	51.1	20.8	15.4	12.7	676	65.2	369	69.1	307	60.5
Georgia	1,870	59.2	16.3	15.2	9.3	272	58.9	138	59.1	135	58.6
Hawaii	261	41.5	38.7	10.4	9.4	35	68.2	31	68.7	4	63.9
Idaho[3]	223	61.4	13.5	17.5	7.6	32	49.7	22	49.3	10	50.6
Illinois	2,780	53.6	27.7	11.0	7.6	346	56.3	307	55.5	39	62.5
Indiana	1,174	55.2	22.3	14.8	7.6	166	48.9	106	53.8	60	40.4
Iowa	555	47.2	30.5	14.5	7.8	86	50.2	71	47.4	15	63.3
Kansas	394	56.4	14.4	19.6	9.6	68	50.8	48	52.9	20	45.8
Kentucky	907	47.8	15.9	25.7	10.6	185	50.8	110	51.7	75	49.4
Louisiana	1,177	52.0	19.4	18.9	9.7	191	58.3	109	56.2	81	61.0
Maine	411	30.7	27.3	25.8	16.3	105	60.2	57	46.0	48	76.9
Maryland	952	47.7	29.1	15.2	8.0	120	56.8	80	56.7	40	57.1
Massachusetts	1,654	29.2	44.4	16.2	10.2	270	53.0	248	49.1	22	96.8
Michigan	2,257	52.0	26.0	15.6	6.3	275	47.6	240	47.1	35	50.9
Minnesota	936	47.4	28.3	14.0	10.4	143	54.1	129	53.1	14	63.3
Mississippi	772	51.8	15.0	21.7	11.6	158	56.2	83	58.6	74	53.5
Missouri[3]	1,033	52.8	18.4	19.6	9.1	181	49.7	164	49.5	17	51.8
Montana	133	56.8	16.4	17.3	9.6	24	53.2	16	53.7	8	52.4
Nebraska	250	57.5	18.1	15.3	9.1	41	51.4	38	50.5	3	62.2
Nevada	340	59.5	19.6	12.8	8.0	45	59.4	23	65.4	22	53.1
New Hampshire	167	59.2	14.1	17.3	9.4	33	45.6	22	45.8	10	45.1

TABLE 12, Continued

State	Total	Percentage of Enrollees in Eligibility Group[1]				Dual Eligible Status[2]					
		Children	Adults	Disabled	Aged	All dual eligibles		Dual eligibles with full benefits		Dual eligibles with limited benefits	
						Total	Percentage age 65+	Total	Percentage age 65+	Total	Percentage age 65+
New Jersey	1,026	55.3%	12.9%	17.1%	14.8%	210	66.1%	183	65.5%	27	69.8%
New Mexico	576	60.4	20.1	12.1	7.5	70	59.9	39	60.2	30	59.6
New York	5,570	37.6	39.1	12.2	11.1	797	67.9	694	66.6	103	76.9
North Carolina	1,876	52.3	20.8	17.0	9.8	324	55.6	253	55.2	71	57.2
North Dakota	82	52.9	21.5	14.1	11.5	16	58.0	13	57.4	3	60.4
Ohio	2,246	49.6	25.0	17.3	8.1	326	50.4	222	52.9	104	45.0
Oklahoma	829	55.5	21.9	14.6	8.0	120	53.7	99	53.6	21	54.2
Oregon	644	50.1	25.9	15.0	9.0	100	56.3	65	58.1	35	52.8
Pennsylvania	2,417	44.6	20.8	24.6	10.0	415	54.5	348	53.3	68	60.8
Rhode Island	205	44.8	20.9	20.1	14.1	42	58.3	36	57.0	6	66.3
South Carolina	909	51.0	22.9	16.9	9.2	155	53.9	135	53.3	20	58.0
South Dakota	131	58.6	17.1	14.5	9.8	22	59.1	14	60.8	8	55.8
Tennessee	1,502	51.9	20.7	17.9	9.5	269	52.1	157	50.0	111	55.2
Texas	4,844	63.9	13.7	13.1	9.2	666	65.5	421	67.0	245	63.0
Utah	352	58.0	25.3	12.1	4.7	32	45.1	29	44.3	4	51.2
Vermont	196	34.8	41.6	12.2	11.4	36	60.1	28	55.9	8	75.5
Virginia	1,007	54.7	16.8	17.6	10.9	184	56.6	124	59.4	60	50.7
Washington	1,353	56.1	21.5	15.3	7.1	172	54.3	129	57.4	43	45.3
West Virginia	430	47.5	15.0	27.7	9.8	84	49.6	51	50.6	33	48.1
Wisconsin	1,232	39.1	36.1	13.1	11.8	222	64.3	202	64.2	20	64.7
Wyoming	87	64.9	15.6	12.8	6.8	11	52.3	7	51.8	4	53.5

Notes: Enrollment numbers generally include individuals ever enrolled in Medicaid-financed coverage during the year, even if for a single month; however, in the event individuals were also enrolled in CHIP-financed Medicaid coverage (i.e., Medicaid-expansion CHIP) during the year, they are excluded if their most recent enrollment month was in Medicaid-expansion CHIP. Numbers exclude individuals enrolled only in Medicaid-expansion CHIP during the year and enrollees in the territories.

Although state-level information is not yet available, the estimated number of individuals ever enrolled in Medicaid (excluding Medicaid-expansion CHIP) is 70.7 million for fiscal year (FY) 2011 and 71.6 million for FY 2012. These FY 2011–FY 2012 figures exclude about 1 million enrollees in the territories (MACPAC communication with Centers for Medicare & Medicaid Services Office of the Actuary, February 2013).

[1] Children and adults under age 65 who qualify for Medicaid on the basis of a disability are included in the disabled category. About 690,000 enrollees aged 65 and older are identified in the data as disabled; given that disability is not an eligibility pathway for individuals aged 65 and older, MACPAC recodes these enrollees as aged.

[2] Dual eligibles are individuals who are enrolled in both Medicare and Medicaid; those with limited benefits only receive Medicaid assistance with Medicare premiums and cost sharing. Zeroes indicate enrollment counts less than 500 that round to zero.

[3] FY 2010 data unavailable for Idaho and Missouri; FY 2009 values shown instead.

Source: MACPAC analysis of Medicaid Statistical Information System (MSIS) annual person summary (APS) data from CMS as of May 2013.

SECTION 3

TABLE 13. Medicaid Benefit Spending by State, Eligibility Group, and Dual Eligible Status, FY 2010 (millions)

State	Total	Percentage of Benefit Spending Attributable to Eligibility Group[1]				All dual eligibles		Dual Eligible Status[2]		Dual eligibles with limited benefits	
		Children	Adults	Disabled	Aged	Total	Percentage attributable to age 65+	Dual eligibles with full benefits Total	Percentage attributable to age 65+	Total	Percentage attributable to age 65+
Total	$388,611	19.1%	14.7%	42.8%	23.3%	$140,573	60.5%	$135,406	60.8%	$5,166	52.5%
Alabama	4,749	27.2	9.1	38.6	25.1	1,757	65.9	1,516	67.7	242	55.2
Alaska	1,207	28.2	15.9	38.0	17.8	335	54.2	334	54.2	1	70.5
Arizona	9,384	20.9	36.9	29.0	13.3	1,913	59.3	1,852	59.1	61	64.4
Arkansas	3,940	21.2	4.8	46.5	27.5	1,736	59.8	1,510	63.3	226	37.0
California	42,142	15.9	15.2	41.5	27.4	15,358	67.9	15,272	67.9	87	69.9
Colorado	4,052	22.6	12.8	42.3	22.3	1,371	60.8	1,337	61.2	34	45.4
Connecticut	5,744	15.3	12.6	36.4	35.6	3,091	62.7	2,994	62.8	96	60.4
Delaware	1,289	19.0	30.6	33.2	17.2	369	57.8	340	58.9	29	45.8
District of Columbia	1,792	11.9	12.6	54.2	21.3	544	60.8	523	61.2	21	49.4
Florida	17,390	17.9	13.4	42.2	26.6	6,894	62.9	6,168	64.2	726	51.5
Georgia	7,785	22.3	14.1	43.1	20.6	2,228	62.7	1,998	64.0	230	51.7
Hawaii	1,428	15.9	26.5	29.7	27.8	536	72.4	528	72.6	8	61.1
Idaho[3]	1,277	20.7	10.3	51.0	18.0	408	52.0	392	52.4	16	42.5
Illinois	15,336	24.8	18.5	40.1	16.6	3,992	55.5	3,904	55.8	88	45.1
Indiana	5,921	18.1	11.7	45.2	25.1	2,581	55.9	2,454	57.1	127	33.2
Iowa	3,119	17.3	12.1	48.0	22.6	1,385	50.4	1,355	50.3	30	55.6
Kansas	2,438	19.5	8.5	48.6	23.4	1,020	53.2	986	53.7	34	38.9
Kentucky	5,606	23.4	12.4	45.7	18.5	1,781	57.1	1,644	58.1	137	45.3
Louisiana	6,964	19.7	12.4	50.5	17.5	2,044	56.5	1,882	56.7	162	54.3
Maine	2,296	16.2	10.4	47.6	25.8	1,062	54.6	988	53.1	74	74.3
Maryland	7,082	18.9	16.8	44.6	19.7	2,127	59.1	2,016	59.5	111	50.1
Massachusetts	11,781	13.6	19.3	42.4	24.6	4,864	55.9	4,826	55.6	38	95.9
Michigan	11,655	19.0	15.7	45.1	20.2	3,822	58.7	3,741	59.0	81	43.0
Minnesota	7,589	17.5	12.2	47.5	22.8	3,278	50.5	3,255	50.5	23	52.3
Mississippi	4,146	21.7	11.5	42.9	23.8	1,484	65.5	1,308	67.9	176	47.4
Missouri[3]	7,748	23.4	9.4	48.1	19.1	2,603	52.9	2,568	53.1	35	40.9
Montana	936	23.7	11.9	39.1	25.4	375	63.8	356	64.8	20	46.7
Nebraska	1,730	23.6	10.0	42.8	23.6	697	53.9	693	53.9	4	60.4

TABLE 13, Continued

State	Total	Percentage of Benefit Spending Attributable to Eligibility Group[1]				All dual eligibles		Dual Eligible Status[2]			
		Children	Adults	Disabled	Aged	Total	Percentage attributable to age 65+	Dual eligibles with full benefits		Dual eligibles with limited benefits	
								Total	Percentage attributable to age 65+	Total	Percentage attributable to age 65+
Nevada	1,509	28.5%	12.8%	41.9%	16.9%	383	62.1%	340	64.1%	43	46.6%
New Hampshire	1,332	24.8	8.4	38.1	28.7	622	58.4	598	58.8	24	49.1
New Jersey	10,224	16.2	7.1	44.6	32.0	4,770	63.8	4,727	63.7	43	69.4
New Mexico	3,443	45.7	19.3	31.6	3.4	339	30.4	286	25.5	53	56.7
New York	52,122	10.5	18.8	42.2	28.5	22,770	60.9	22,517	60.8	253	72.5
North Carolina	10,907	21.8	14.2	45.0	19.1	3,518	58.6	3,397	59.0	121	48.0
North Dakota	688	15.4	9.9	42.5	32.2	382	57.0	378	57.1	5	52.6
Ohio	15,262	13.6	13.6	47.2	25.6	6,051	58.7	5,801	59.7	250	36.6
Oklahoma	4,119	26.9	12.3	42.0	18.8	1,366	53.7	1,338	53.7	28	50.8
Oregon	4,007	17.5	17.7	40.6	24.2	1,457	64.7	1,399	65.5	58	45.7
Pennsylvania	18,766	16.7	9.0	49.5	24.8	7,122	62.0	7,018	62.0	104	56.7
Rhode Island	1,926	22.2	12.1	46.4	19.2	695	51.4	688	51.4	8	53.3
South Carolina	5,173	20.5	15.7	43.9	20.0	1,743	59.3	1,719	59.4	24	53.4
South Dakota	784	24.9	11.8	41.2	22.1	294	58.3	276	59.0	18	48.8
Tennessee	8,518	24.6	17.3	40.9	17.2	2,503	56.5	2,286	57.9	217	41.4
Texas	27,200	32.2	9.5	40.3	18.0	7,213	64.8	6,542	64.7	671	65.2
Utah	1,716	25.9	14.3	48.8	11.1	470	37.5	462	37.5	8	40.9
Vermont	1,250	[4]	[4]	[4]	[4]	[4]	[4]	[4]	[4]	[4]	[4]
Virginia	6,467	23.3	10.3	45.0	21.3	2,274	55.6	2,158	56.3	116	43.1
Washington	7,063	22.7	15.3	40.8	21.3	2,319	62.8	2,220	63.7	99	41.1
West Virginia	2,553	16.2	7.6	47.7	28.5	1,076	66.7	1,018	67.8	59	47.7
Wisconsin	6,521	11.9	17.9	41.1	29.1	3,163	58.5	3,133	58.6	30	53.8
Wyoming	538	22.9	10.5	43.1	23.6	240	52.6	224	53.1	16	45.3

Notes: Includes federal and state funds. Excludes administrative spending, the territories, and Medicaid-expansion CHIP enrollees. Benefit spending from Medicaid Statistical Information System (MSIS) data has been adjusted to reflect CMS-64 totals; see Section 5 of MACStats for methodology.

[1] Children and adults under age 65 who qualify for Medicaid on the basis of a disability are included in the disabled category. About 690,000 enrollees aged 65 and older are identified in the data as disabled; given that disability is not an eligibility pathway for individuals aged 65 and older, MACPAC recodes these enrollees as aged.

[2] Dual eligibles are individuals who are enrolled in both Medicaid and Medicare; those with limited benefits only receive Medicaid assistance with Medicare premiums and cost sharing.

[3] Fiscal year (FY) 2010 data unavailable for Idaho and Missouri; FY 2009 values shown instead.

[4] Due to large differences in the way managed care spending is reported by Vermont in Medicaid Statistical Information System (MSIS) annual person summary (APS) data and CMS-64 Financial Management Report (FMR) net expenditure data from CMS as of May 2013.

Sources: MACPAC analysis of Medicaid Statistical Information System (MSIS) annual person summary (APS) data and CMS-64 Financial Management Report (FMR) net expenditure data from CMS as of May 2013.

SECTION 3

MACStats

TABLE 14. Medicaid Benefit Spending Per Full-Year Equivalent (FYE) Enrollee by State and Eligibility Group, FY 2010

State	Total - Percentage of FYEs with limited benefits[1]	Total - Benefit spending per FYE - All enrollees	Total - Benefit spending per FYE - Excluding those with limited benefits[2]	Children - Percentage of FYEs with limited benefits[1]	Children - Benefit spending per FYE - All enrollees	Children - Benefit spending per FYE - Excluding those with limited benefits[2]	Children - Percentage of FYEs with limited benefits[1]	Adults - Benefit spending per FYE - All enrollees	Adults - Benefit spending per FYE - Excluding those with limited benefits[2]	Adults - Percentage of FYEs with limited benefits[1]	Disabled - Benefit spending per FYE - All enrollees	Disabled - Benefit spending per FYE - Excluding those with limited benefits[2]	Disabled - Percentage of FYEs with limited benefits[1]	Aged - Benefit spending per FYE - All enrollees	Aged - Benefit spending per FYE - Excluding those with limited benefits[2]
Total	**11.5%**	**$7,264**	**$7,915**	**1.5%**	**$2,848**	**$2,871**	**27.7%**	**$4,343**	**$5,259**	**9.9%**	**$19,166**	**$20,889**	**23.0%**	**$16,430**	**$20,549**
Alabama	22.8	5,613	6,572	0.1	3,071	3,070	74.3	3,355	6,747	19.9	9,637	11,316	55.0	11,216	22,140
Alaska	0.3	12,016	12,041	0.0	5,954	5,953	0.0	9,350	9,348	0.6	30,857	31,027	2.5	27,651	28,271
Arizona	7.9	7,161	7,436	2.5	3,320	3,358	11.1	6,913	7,381	7.0	20,851	21,317	26.7	13,937	17,921
Arkansas	19.9	6,697	7,736	2.4	2,680	2,709	71.5	2,186	5,391	19.7	14,196	16,284	36.9	17,700	25,896
California	29.0	4,773	6,256	7.2	1,937	2,032	64.8	1,828	3,162	0.8	18,399	18,465	3.9	12,550	12,859
Colorado	4.3	7,584	7,687	0.2	2,942	2,910	3.8	5,804	5,330	10.8	20,567	22,635	19.9	17,886	21,861
Connecticut	6.8	10,010	10,559	—	3,222	3,222	0.0	4,467	4,467	16.3	32,003	37,552	38.6	27,982	44,274
Delaware	14.8	7,129	7,999	2.1	3,280	3,333	17.7	5,626	6,385	26.0	18,514	24,093	52.3	17,199	33,871
District of Columbia	3.0	10,969	11,074	—	3,013	3,013	0.6	5,099	4,773	5.0	29,002	30,195	19.9	25,645	31,107
Florida	10.3	6,164	6,453	0.2	2,079	2,062	5.9	5,543	5,308	20.9	14,650	17,531	39.1	11,362	17,006
Georgia	8.3	5,345	5,593	0.0	1,991	1,988	0.8	6,191	5,838	19.2	13,126	15,689	45.6	10,443	17,709
Hawaii	1.4	6,423	6,476	0.0	2,365	2,365	0.0	4,761	4,755	4.6	17,027	17,723	9.1	18,259	19,825
Idaho[3]	5.0	7,425	7,715	—	2,531	2,531	0.0	7,576	7,576	11.8	18,366	20,531	30.0	15,685	21,727
Illinois	5.2	6,295	6,501	0.1	2,882	2,881	13.9	4,369	4,684	4.8	21,931	22,824	11.5	13,581	15,103
Indiana	5.4	6,158	6,371	—	1,955	1,955	0.0	3,764	3,764	19.9	17,194	20,775	28.1	19,755	26,705
Iowa	10.5	7,037	7,576	1.1	2,532	2,546	26.3	3,172	3,397	6.3	20,137	21,294	22.3	19,196	24,112
Kansas	5.7	7,884	8,210	0.0	2,712	2,708	0.6	5,953	5,737	14.0	17,530	20,031	24.7	18,015	23,380
Kentucky	9.0	7,500	8,024	0.0	3,660	3,657	0.4	7,473	7,422	15.8	12,146	13,991	39.2	12,176	18,838
Louisiana	15.3	6,738	7,552	0.0	2,478	2,477	47.5	4,918	7,381	14.3	17,407	19,851	44.4	11,805	19,705
Maine	12.9	6,927	7,700	0.1	3,409	3,412	0.4	2,605	2,610	13.1	14,974	16,945	57.1	10,291	21,768
Maryland	7.9	8,987	9,301	0.9	3,471	3,464	12.0	5,775	5,422	11.0	24,115	26,642	29.9	21,103	28,865
Massachusetts	6.6	8,527	9,026	3.4	4,054	4,169	9.0	3,898	4,167	0.3	19,717	19,762	16.6	19,590	23,007
Michigan	6.1	6,247	6,538	1.0	2,203	2,216	17.2	4,307	4,944	4.6	16,547	17,161	13.2	19,677	22,258
Minnesota	5.2	10,395	10,841	0.9	3,737	3,752	11.7	4,967	5,473	3.9	30,498	31,526	11.8	24,671	27,493
Mississippi	15.3	6,517	7,104	0.0	2,783	2,782	36.3	5,771	6,439	21.0	11,912	14,280	44.3	12,295	20,223
Missouri[3]	5.3	9,305	9,633	0.1	3,991	3,991	23.1	5,657	6,181	4.1	21,770	22,579	9.2	18,890	20,614
Montana	6.5	9,037	9,461	—	3,763	3,763	—	7,845	7,845	15.9	18,403	21,246	33.5	22,308	32,229
Nebraska	1.1	8,740	8,807	0.0	3,362	3,362	0.2	6,665	6,620	2.2	21,791	22,242	7.8	24,653	26,602
Nevada	7.4	5,922	6,077	0.1	2,816	2,802	2.0	4,642	4,253	22.3	16,905	20,738	41.3	10,930	16,867
New Hampshire	6.3	9,924	10,405	—	4,073	4,073	—	7,379	7,379	18.8	20,515	24,661	29.6	29,207	40,177

TABLE 14, Continued

State	Percentage of FYEs with limited benefits[1]	Total Benefit spending per FYE – All enrollees	Total Benefit spending per FYE – Excluding those with limited benefits[2]	Children Percentage of FYEs with limited benefits[1]	Children Benefit spending per FYE – All enrollees	Children Benefit spending per FYE – Excluding those with limited benefits[2]	Adults Percentage of FYEs with limited benefits[1]	Adults Benefit spending per FYE – All enrollees	Adults Benefit spending per FYE – Excluding those with limited benefits[2]	Disabled Percentage of FYEs with limited benefits[1]	Disabled Benefit spending per FYE – All enrollees	Disabled Benefit spending per FYE – Excluding those with limited benefits[2]	Aged Percentage of FYEs with limited benefits[1]	Aged Benefit spending per FYE – All enrollees	Aged Benefit spending per FYE – Excluding those with limited benefits[2]
New Jersey	3.2%	$11,645	$11,866	0.0%	$3,374	$3,373	1.8%	$8,081	$7,376	5.0%	$28,228	$29,570	13.7%	$24,188	$27,639
New Mexico	12.3	7,055	7,549	0.0	5,247	5,239	38.8	7,641	9,548	17.0	17,266	20,329	40.9	3,092	3,908
New York	5.5	11,139	11,500	2.2	3,136	3,184	6.5	5,647	5,616	3.5	34,495	35,508	15.0	26,814	30,703
North Carolina	8.9	7,197	7,676	0.1	2,941	2,938	28.0	6,072	7,494	9.3	16,887	18,350	21.9	12,763	15,879
North Dakota	4.6	10,821	11,262	—	3,084	3,084	0.0	6,125	6,124	11.1	28,518	31,806	22.8	28,228	36,153
Ohio	4.7	7,987	8,248	—	2,138	2,138	0.0	4,707	4,707	14.5	20,853	23,859	26.3	25,418	33,672
Oklahoma	7.5	6,227	6,575	0.1	2,889	2,889	28.0	4,531	5,484	7.6	16,034	17,199	17.1	13,346	15,795
Oregon	10.7	8,083	8,807	3.0	2,796	2,868	14.3	6,621	7,213	16.4	18,572	21,785	31.9	19,346	27,597
Pennsylvania	7.5	9,267	9,866	0.2	3,486	3,481	24.3	4,494	5,390	4.5	17,185	17,881	17.1	22,357	26,574
Rhode Island	3.4	11,126	11,356	0.0	5,519	5,490	3.9	7,120	7,121	3.3	23,427	24,005	13.8	15,061	17,085
South Carolina	8.7	6,822	7,249	0.1	2,705	2,702	32.4	5,334	6,669	5.0	16,169	16,898	12.8	13,856	15,683
South Dakota	6.3	7,512	7,829	0.0	3,141	3,141	0.1	6,424	6,401	17.0	19,231	22,505	33.7	15,759	22,563
Tennessee	7.6	6,639	6,975	0.0	3,099	3,094	0.1	6,019	5,916	18.1	14,711	17,304	43.1	11,752	19,399
Texas	9.6	7,365	7,663	0.0	3,698	3,670	38.0	7,524	9,120	14.0	18,937	21,311	34.9	12,199	16,676
Utah	1.6	6,941	6,918	0.0	3,075	3,069	1.1	4,674	4,333	4.4	22,763	23,615	12.7	13,980	15,610
Vermont	4.4	7,792	[4]	—	[4]	[4]	—	[4]	[4]	7.4	[4]	[4]	26.7	[4]	[4]
Virginia	7.2	7,842	8,225	0.0	3,289	3,288	6.6	5,903	5,956	16.1	18,421	21,390	27.6	14,475	19,169
Washington	11.1	6,426	6,781	0.2	2,500	2,486	43.4	5,527	7,051	11.2	16,028	17,572	19.7	18,208	21,905
West Virginia	8.1	7,319	7,785	0.0	2,488	2,488	0.0	4,824	4,823	13.8	11,432	12,922	37.9	20,052	31,036
Wisconsin	9.2	6,289	6,754	4.7	1,944	1,986	16.5	3,228	3,510	4.3	18,060	18,721	8.7	14,858	16,130
Wyoming	6.7	7,971	8,200	0.8	2,776	2,794	12.2	6,576	6,700	14.6	23,778	26,833	35.0	25,971	37,698

Notes: Includes federal and state funds. Excludes administrative spending, the territories, and Medicaid-expansion CHIP Children and adults under age 65 who qualify for Medicaid on the basis of a disability are included in the disabled category. About 690,000 enrollees aged 65 and older are identified in the data as disabled; given that disability is not an eligibility pathway for individuals aged 65 and older, MACPAC recodes these enrollees as aged. Benefit spending from Medicaid Statistical Information System (MSIS) data has been adjusted to reflect CMS-64 totals; see Section 5 of MACStats for methodology.

In this table, enrollees with limited benefits are defined as those reported by states in MSIS as receiving coverage of only family planning services, assistance with Medicare premiums and cost sharing, or emergency services. Additional individuals may receive limited benefits for other reasons, but are not broken out here.

Zeroes indicate amounts less than 0.05 percent that round to zero. Dashes indicate amounts that are true zeroes.

[1] These percentages are likely to be underestimated because comparisons with other data sources indicate that some states do not identify all of their limited-benefit enrollees in MSIS.
[2] Calculated by removing limited-benefit enrollees and their spending.
[3] Fiscal year (FY) 2010 data unavailable for Idaho and Missouri; FY 2009 values shown instead.
[4] Due to large differences in the way managed care spending is reported by Vermont in CMS-64 and MSIS data, MACPAC's adjustment methodology is only applied to total Medicaid spending.

Sources: MACPAC analysis of Medicaid Statistical Information System (MSIS) annual person summary (APS) data and CMS-64 Financial Management Report (FMR) net expenditure data from CMS as of May 2013.

FIGURE 3. Distribution of Medicaid Benefit Spending by Eligibility Group and Service Category, FY 2010

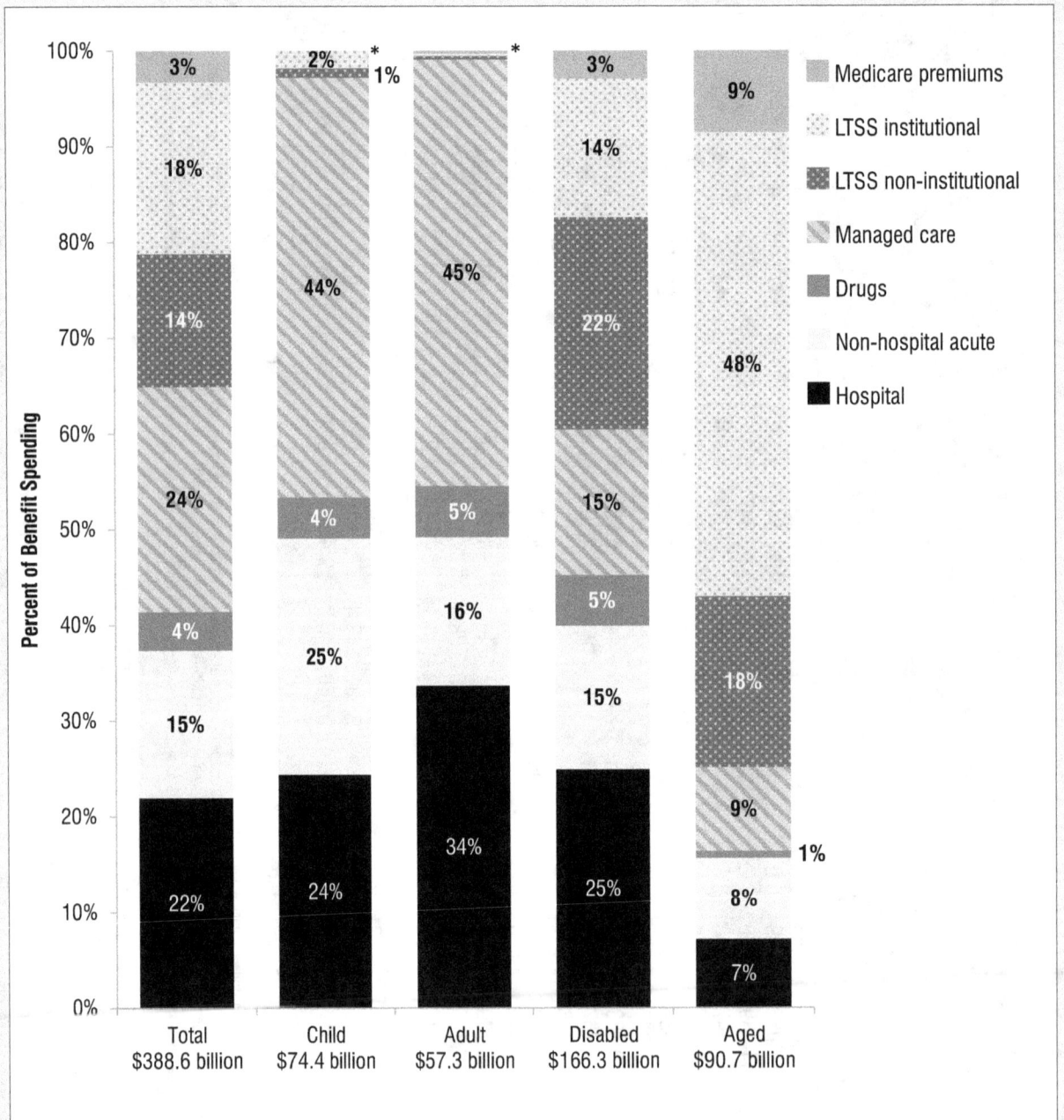

Notes: LTSS is long-term services and supports. Includes federal and state funds. Excludes spending for administration, the territories, and Medicaid-expansion CHIP enrollees. Children and non-aged adults who qualify for Medicaid on the basis of a disability are included in the disabled category. About 690,000 enrollees aged 65 and older are identified in the data as disabled; given that disability is not an eligibility pathway for individuals aged 65 and older, MACPAC recodes these enrollees as aged. Amounts are fee for service unless otherwise noted. Benefit spending from Medicaid Statistical Information System (MSIS) data has been adjusted to reflect CMS-64 totals; see Section 5 of MACStats for methodology, including a list of services in each category. Fiscal year (FY) 2010 data unavailable for Idaho and Missouri; FY 2009 values used instead.

* Values less than 1 percent are not shown.

Sources: MACPAC analysis of Medicaid Statistical Information System (MSIS) annual person summary (APS) data and CMS-64 Financial Management Report (FMR) net expenditure data from CMS as of May 2013.

FIGURE 4. Medicaid Benefit Spending Per Full-Year Equivalent (FYE) Enrollee by Eligibility Group and Service Category, FY 2010

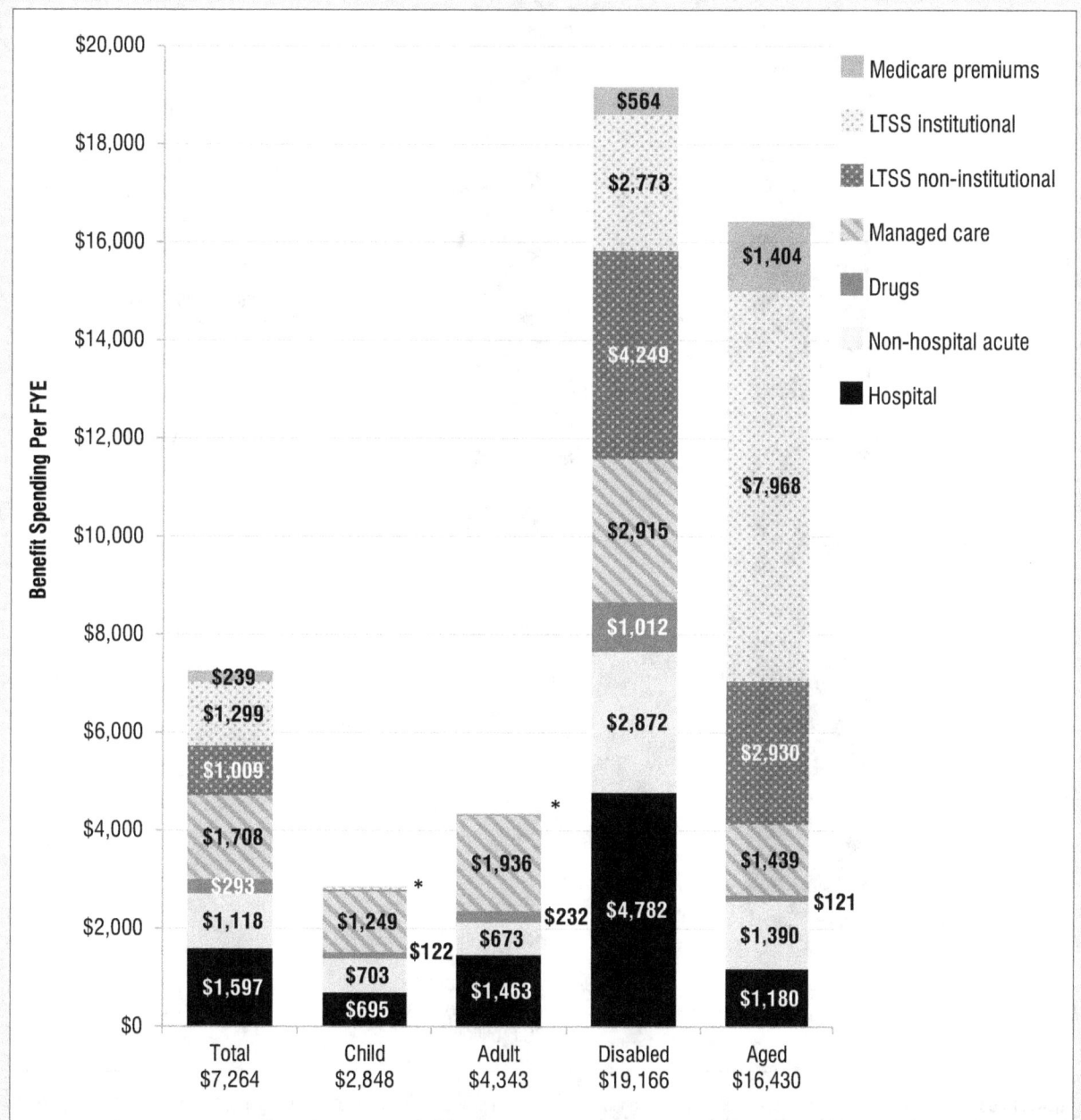

Notes: LTSS is long-term services and supports. Includes federal and state funds. Excludes spending for administration, the territories, and Medicaid-expansion CHIP enrollees. Children and non-aged adults who qualify for Medicaid on the basis of a disability are included in the disabled category. About 690,000 enrollees aged 65 and older are identified in the data as disabled; given that disability is not an eligibility pathway for individuals aged 65 and older, MACPAC recodes these enrollees as aged. Amounts are fee for service unless otherwise noted. Benefit spending from Medicaid Statistical Information System (MSIS) data has been adjusted to reflect CMS-64 totals; see Section 5 of MACStats for methodology, including a list of services in each category. Amounts reflect all enrollees, including those with limited benefits; see Table 14 notes for more information. Fiscal year (FY) 2010 data unavailable for Idaho and Missouri; FY 2009 values used instead.

* Values less than $100 not shown.

Sources: MACPAC analysis of Medicaid Statistical Information System (MSIS) annual person summary (APS) data and CMS-64 Financial Management Report (FMR) net expenditure data from CMS as of May 2013.

FIGURE 5. Distribution of Medicaid Enrollment and Benefit Spending by Users and Non-Users of Long-Term Services and Supports, FY 2010

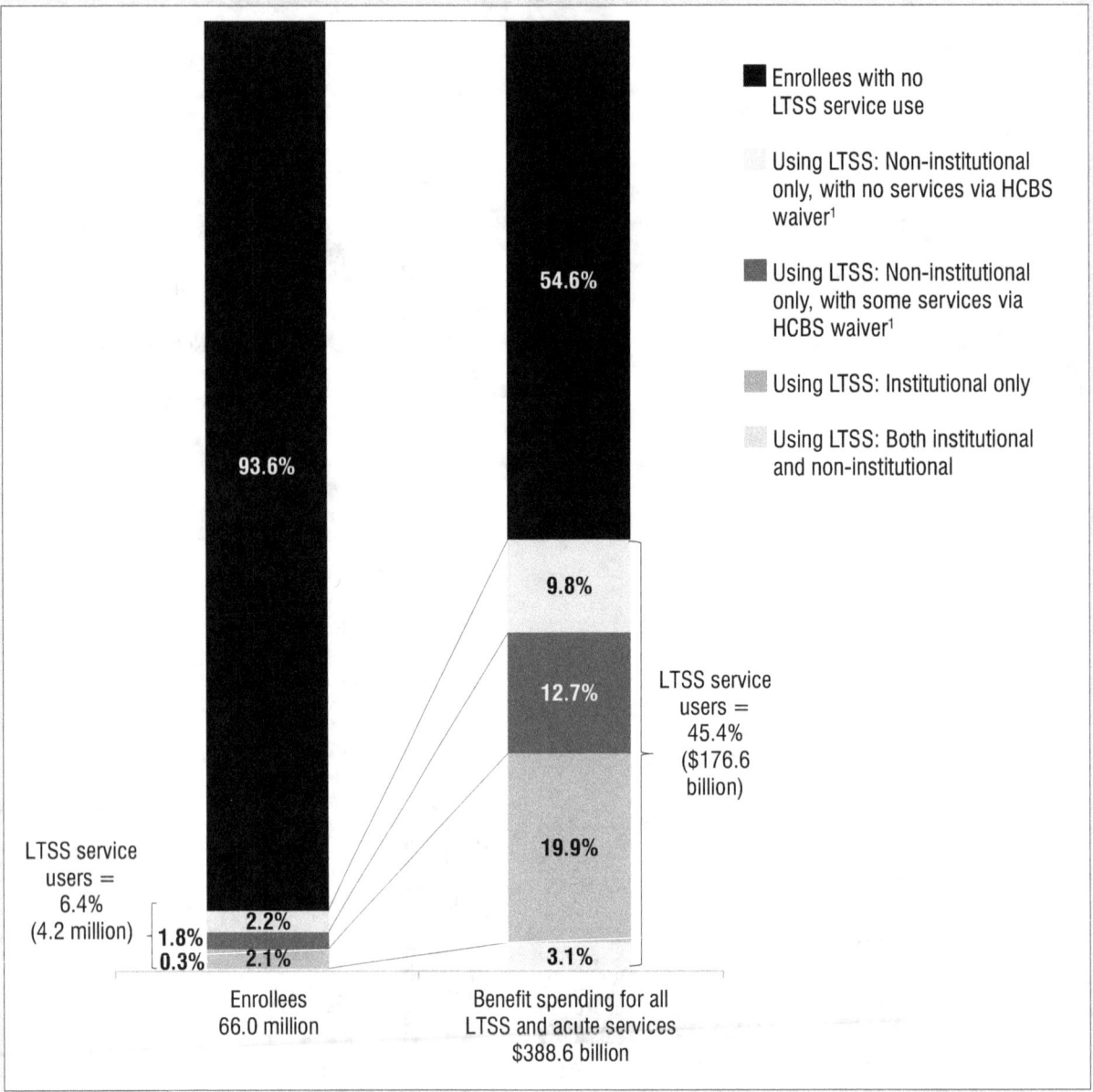

Notes: HCBS is home and community-based services; LTSS is long-term services and supports. Includes federal and state funds. Excludes administrative spending and spending and enrollees in the territories and in Medicaid-expansion CHIP. Benefit spending from Medicaid Statistical Information System (MSIS) data has been adjusted to match CMS-64 totals; see Section 5 of MACStats for methodology, including a list of services in each category. Fiscal year (FY) 2010 data unavailable for Idaho and Missouri; FY 2009 values used instead. LTSS users are defined here as enrollees using at least one LTSS service during the year under a fee-for-service arrangement, regardless of the amount. (The data do not allow a breakout of LTSS services delivered through managed care.) For example, an enrollee with a short stay in a nursing facility for rehabilitation following a hospital discharge and an enrollee with permanent residence in a nursing facility would both be counted as LTSS users. More refined definitions that take these and other factors into account would produce different results and will be considered in future Commission work.

[1] All states have HCBS waivers that provide a range of LTSS for targeted populations of enrollees who require institutional levels of care. Based on a comparison with CMS-372 data (a state-reported source containing aggregate spending and enrollment for HCBS waivers), the number of HCBS waiver enrollees may be underreported in MSIS.

Sources: MACPAC analysis of Medicaid Statistical Information System (MSIS) annual person summary (APS) data and CMS-64 Financial Management Report (FMR) net expenditure data from CMS as of May 2013.

FIGURE 6. Distribution of Medicaid Benefit Spending by Long-Term Services and Supports Use and Service Category, FY 2010

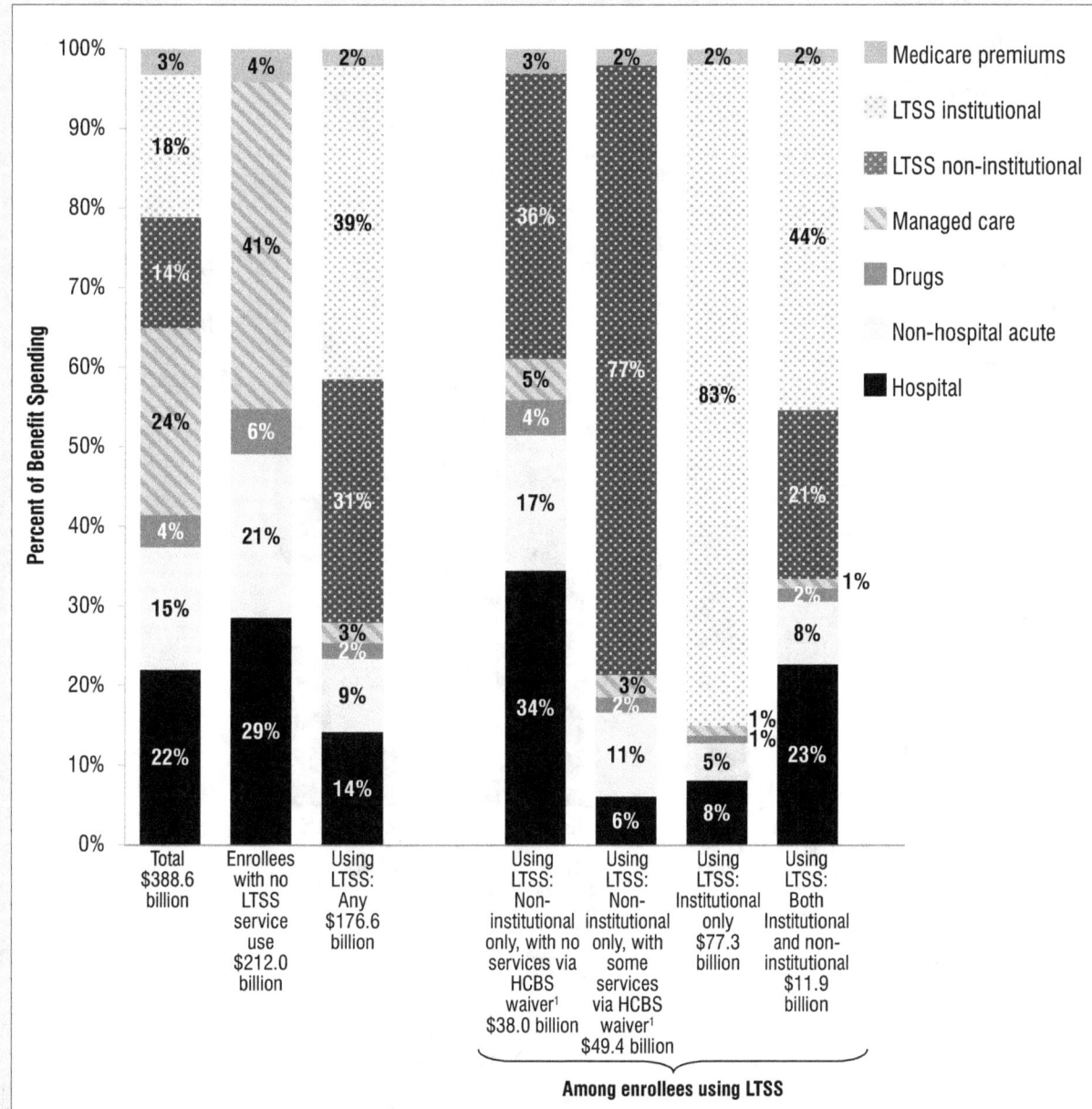

Notes: HCBS is home and community-based services, LTSS is long-term services and supports. Includes federal and state funds. Excludes administrative spending and spending and enrollees in the territories and in Medicaid-expansion CHIP. Benefit spending from Medicaid Statistical Information System (MSIS) data has been adjusted to match CMS-64 totals; see Section 5 of MACStats for methodology, including a list of services in each category. Fiscal year (FY) 2010 data unavailable for Idaho and Missouri; FY 2009 values used instead. LTSS users are defined here as enrollees using at least one LTSS service during the year under a fee-for-service arrangement, regardless of the amount. (The data do not allow a breakout of LTSS services delivered through managed care.) For example, an enrollee with a short stay in a nursing facility for rehabilitation following a hospital discharge and an enrollee with permanent residence in a nursing facility would both be counted as LTSS users. More refined definitions that take these and other factors into account would produce different results and will be considered in future Commission work.

[1] All states have HCBS waivers that provide a range of LTSS for targeted populations of enrollees who require institutional levels of care. Based on a comparison with CMS-372 data (a state-reported source containing aggregate spending and enrollment for HCBS waivers), the number of HCBS waiver enrollees may be underreported in MSIS.

Sources: MACPAC analysis of Medicaid Statistical Information System (MSIS) annual person summary (APS) data and CMS-64 Financial Management Report (FMR) net expenditure data from CMS as of May 2013.

FIGURE 7. Medicaid Benefit Spending Per Full-Year Equivalent (FYE) Enrollee by Long-Term Services and Supports Use and Service Category, FY 2010

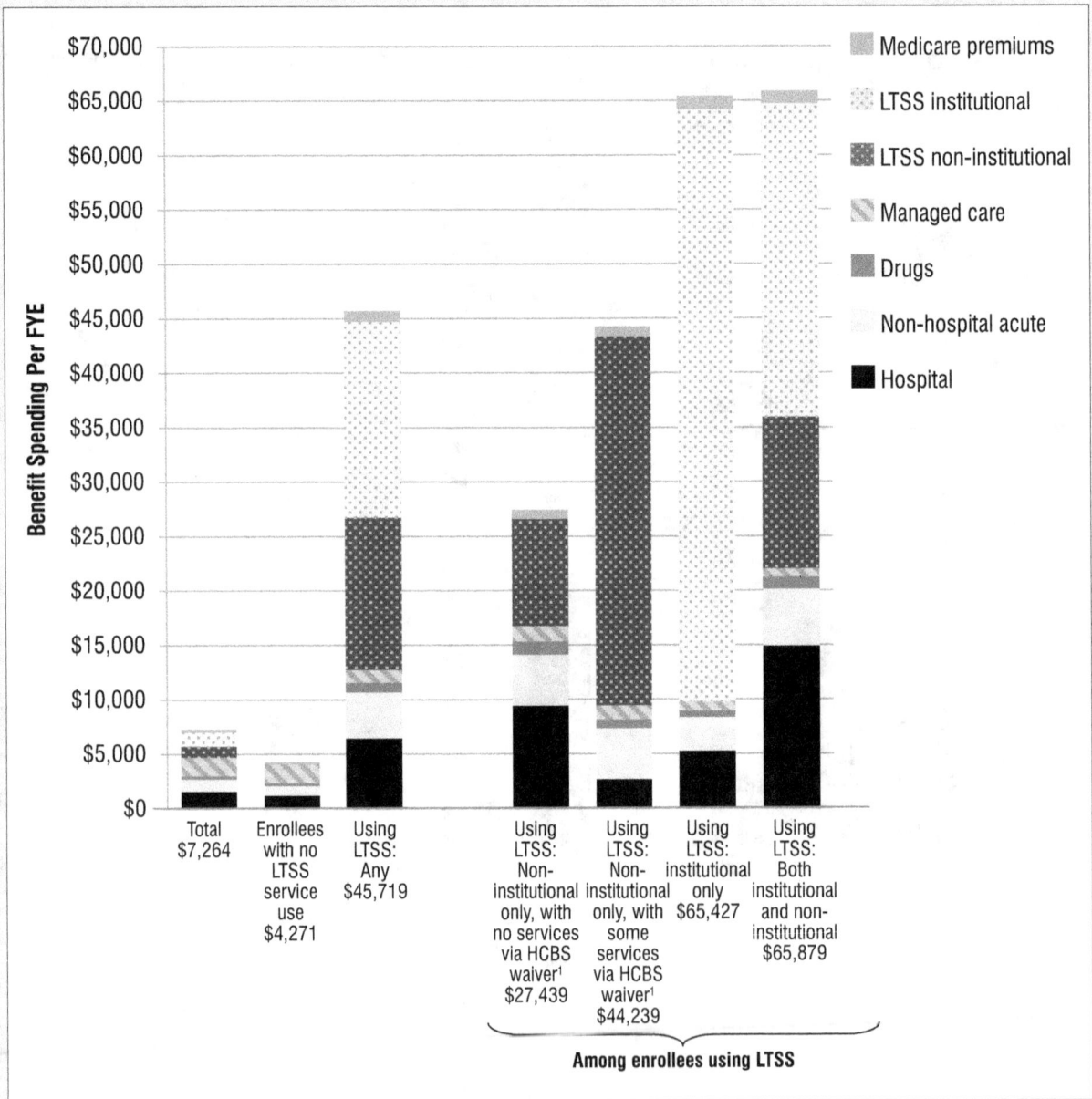

Notes: HCBS is home and community-based services, LTSS is long-term services and supports. Includes federal and state funds. Excludes administrative spending and spending and enrollees in the territories and in Medicaid-expansion CHIP. Benefit spending from Medicaid Statistical Information System (MSIS) data has been adjusted to match CMS-64 totals; see Section 5 of MACStats for methodology, including a list of services in each category. Fiscal year (FY) 2010 data unavailable for Idaho and Missouri; FY 2009 values used instead. LTSS users are defined here as enrollees using at least one LTSS service during the year under a fee-for-service arrangement, regardless of the amount. The data do not allow a breakout of LTSS services delivered through managed care. For example, an enrollee with a short stay in a nursing facility for rehabilitation following a hospital discharge and an enrollee with permanent residence in a nursing facility would both be counted as LTSS users. More refined definitions that take these and other factors into account would produce different results and will be considered in future Commission work.

[1] All states have HCBS waivers that provide a range of LTSS for targeted populations of enrollees who require institutional levels of care. Based on a comparison with CMS-372 data (a state-reported source containing aggregate spending and enrollment for HCBS waivers), the number of HCBS waiver enrollees may be underreported in MSIS.

Sources: MACPAC analysis of Medicaid Statistical Information System (MSIS) annual person summary (APS) data and CMS-64 Financial Management Report (FMR) net expenditure data from CMS as of May 2013.

MAC Stats

MACStats

SECTION 4

Key Points
Medicaid Managed Care

- The term managed care may refer to several different arrangements, including comprehensive risk-based and limited-benefit plans that provide a contracted set of services in exchange for a capitated (per member per month) payment, as well as primary care case management (PCCM) programs that typically pay primary care providers a small monthly fee to coordinate enrollees' care. Depending on the definition that is used, the national percentage of Medicaid enrollees in managed care ranges from about half (reflecting individuals in comprehensive risk-based plans) to more than 70 percent (Tables 15 and 17).

- The use of managed care varies widely by state, both in the arrangements used and the populations served. In 2011, all but three states reported using some form of managed care, including comprehensive risk-based plans, limited-benefit plans, or PCCM programs (Tables 15 and 16).

- The national percentage of Medicaid enrollees in any form of managed care ranged from 41 percent among enrollees aged 65 and older to 87 percent among non-disabled child enrollees in fiscal year (FY) 2010 (Table 17). Participation in comprehensive risk-based managed care plans was lowest among the aged and disabled eligibility groups (12 and 29 percent, respectively) and highest among non-disabled adults and children (47 and 62 percent).

- For individuals dually enrolled in Medicaid and Medicare, enrollment in Medicaid limited-benefit plans (which typically cover only behavioral health, transportation, or dental services) is more common than enrollment in Medicaid comprehensive risk-based plans or PCCM programs. Forty-one percent of individuals dually enrolled in Medicaid and Medicare were enrolled in some form of Medicaid managed care in FY 2010 (Table 17).

- The national percentage of Medicaid benefit spending on any form of managed care ranges from about 9 percent among enrollees aged 65 and older to more than 40 percent among non-disabled child and adult enrollees (Table 18). In states with comprehensive risk-based managed care, these plans account for the majority of managed care spending.

TABLE 15. Medicaid Enrollees in Managed Care by State, July 1, 2011

State	Number	All Medicaid Enrollees Percentage in managed care			Individuals Dually Enrolled in Medicaid and Medicare	
		Any managed care[1]	Comprehensive risk-based or PCCM[2,3]	Comprehensive risk-based[2]	PCCM	Number	Percentage in comprehensive risk-based managed care[2]

State	Number	Any managed care[1]	Comprehensive risk-based or PCCM[2,3]	Comprehensive risk-based[2]	PCCM	Number	Percentage in comprehensive risk-based managed care[2]
Total	56,006,959	74.1%	65.9%	50.2%	15.8%	8,922,794	10.5%
Alabama	930,736	61.1	58.7	–	58.7	196,313	–
Alaska	120,611	–	–	–	–	13,879	–
Arizona	1,351,988	88.7	88.7	88.7	–	153,637	69.9
Arkansas	608,332	78.4	61.8	–	61.8	116,855	0.1
California	7,580,978	60.1	59.7	59.7	–	1,188,551	23.3
Colorado	583,618	94.6	16.7	8.3	8.3	82,104	5.5
Connecticut	578,620	68.6	68.6	68.5	0.1	121,149	–
Delaware	200,810	80.5	77.1	77.1	–	24,403	–
District of Columbia[4]	201,777	67.4	68.1	68.1	–	14,458	0.6
Florida	3,069,456	63.8	60.5	40.7	19.8	637,738	4.7
Georgia	1,548,090	91.3	71.9	61.5	10.5	233,374	–
Hawaii	272,218	98.7	98.0	98.0	–	30,839	87.8
Idaho	230,725	100.0	91.1	–	91.1	19,054	–
Illinois[4]	2,787,200	67.8	67.8	7.7	60.1	327,851	–
Indiana	1,055,779	70.3	70.1	66.8	3.3	145,859	–
Iowa	440,993	91.1	44.6	–	44.5	77,874	–
Kansas	354,664	87.4	58.8	51.3	7.5	72,505	0.3
Kentucky	823,133	89.4	64.7	20.8	43.9	174,351	7.9
Louisiana	1,208,859	65.3	63.4	–	63.4	181,277	0.1
Maine	357,706	49.3	49.3	–	49.3	93,914	–
Maryland	986,304	74.6	74.6	74.6	–	110,648	0.1
Massachusetts[4]	1,566,222	53.1	53.4	32.8	20.7	254,449	7.2
Michigan	1,818,312	88.4	66.7	66.7	–	263,576	0.2
Minnesota	847,638	65.7	65.7	65.7	–	127,651	41.0
Mississippi	621,607	87.2	8.3	8.3	–	144,764	–
Missouri	895,998	97.7	45.4	45.4	–	168,335	0.1
Montana[5]	106,493	76.1	76.1	–	76.1	21,314	–
Nebraska	237,484	85.1	45.6	42.5	3.1	33,994	–
Nevada	297,640	83.6	56.7	56.7	–	43,522	–
New Hampshire	135,092	–	–	–	–	28,153	–

TABLE 15, Continued

State	All Medicaid Enrollees					Individuals Dually Enrolled in Medicaid and Medicare	
	Number	Percentage in managed care				Number	Percentage in comprehensive risk-based managed care[2]
		Any managed care[1]	Comprehensive risk-based or PCCM[2,3]	Comprehensive risk-based[2]	PCCM		
New Jersey	1,098,608	77.7%	77.7%	77.7%	—	195,802	14.1%
New Mexico[4]	551,017	72.8	72.9	72.9	—	65,637	50.5
New York	4,925,236	76.7	76.0	75.7	0.3%	706,454	1.3
North Carolina	1,488,263	83.2	77.2	—	77.2	301,493	0.1
North Dakota[4]	66,698	63.6	63.7	0.1	63.6	14,226	0.4
Ohio	2,129,706	75.4	75.4	75.4	—	301,063	0.2
Oklahoma	684,387	86.5	64.2	—	64.2	105,532	0.1
Oregon	652,846	98.2	76.7	76.3	0.5	96,210	37.5
Pennsylvania	2,134,956	81.5	68.2	54.1	14.2	322,835	1.6
Rhode Island[4]	197,248	68.6	69.5	68.6	1.0	37,280	0.5
South Carolina	862,145	100.0	66.3	49.8	16.5	143,325	0.2
South Dakota	120,474	75.8	75.8	—	75.8	17,846	—
Tennessee	1,218,676	100.0	96.4	96.4	—	236,408	57.9
Texas	3,943,189	70.7	70.7	47.5	23.2	615,435	22.0
Utah	269,643	99.8	45.7	19.1	26.6	33,767	0.6
Vermont	177,108	58.5	58.5	58.5	—	33,453	1.1
Virginia[4]	915,038	58.2	64.2	58.2	5.9	168,354	0.4
Washington	1,182,587	88.1	61.8	61.8	—	158,096	1.2
West Virginia[4]	326,749	51.0	52.6	51.0	1.6	74,765	—
Wisconsin	1,173,355	63.7	60.7	60.7	—	182,499	7.2
Wyoming	69,947	—	—	—	—	9,923	—

Notes: PCCM is primary care case management. Excludes the territories. Unlike most other tables and figures in the June 2013 MACStats (with the exception of those in Section 2), this table includes Medicaid-expansion CHIP enrollees.

— Quantity zero.

[1] Any managed care includes comprehensive risk-based plans, limited-benefit plans, and PCCM programs.

[2] Comprehensive risk-based managed care includes plans categorized by the Centers for Medicare & Medicaid Services (CMS) and states as commercial, Medicaid-only, Health Insuring Organizations (HIOs), and Programs of All-Inclusive Care for the Elderly (PACE). HIOs exist only in California where selected county-organized health systems serve Medicaid enrollees. PACE combines Medicare and Medicaid financing for qualifying frail elderly individuals who are dually eligible for Medicare and Medicaid.

[3] Figure is based on the sum of enrollees reported in comprehensive risk-based plans and PCCM programs.

[4] The number of enrollees reported by the state for the managed care types shown exceeds the unduplicated number of enrollees in any form of managed care. It is unclear whether this is a reporting error or whether there were some enrollees participating in more than one of the plan types shown (e.g., both comprehensive risk-based and PCCM) as of the reporting date.

[5] Montana reported 153,588 PCCM enrollees, which exceeds the total Medicaid enrollment reported by the state (106,493) and the unduplicated enrollees in any form of managed care (81,085). PCCM figure shown here was capped at 81,085.

Source: Source: MACPAC analysis of data from CMS, *Medicaid Managed Care Enrollment Report: Summary Statistics as of July 1, 2011*, 2011, http://www.medicaid.gov/Medicaid-CHIP-Program-Information/By-Topics/Data-and-Systems/Downloads/2011-Medicaid-MC-Enrollment-Report.pdf.

TABLE 16. Number of Managed Care Entities by State and Type, July 1, 2011

	Comprehensive Risk-based Plans				Limited-benefit Plans			
State	Commercial MCO	Medicaid-only MCO	HIO	PACE	PIHP	PAHP	PCCM	Other
Total	148	175	5	79	162	63	40	11
Alabama	–	–	–	–	–	1	1	–
Alaska	–	–	–	–	–	–	–	–
Arizona	–	29	–	1	1	–	1	–
Arkansas	–	–	–	1	–	–	1	–
California	21	3	5	5	10	13	–	2
Colorado	–	1	–	3	6	–	3	1
Connecticut	1	2	–	–	–	–	1	–
Delaware	–	2	–	–	1	1	–	–
District of Columbia	–	2	–	–	–	–	–	–
Florida	22	6	–	3	27	6	1	2
Georgia	–	3	–	–	–	1	1	–
Hawaii	4	1	–	–	–	–	–	–
Idaho	–	–	–	–	–	3	1	–
Illinois	2	3	–	–	–	–	1	–
Indiana	6	–	–	–	–	–	2	1
Iowa	–	–	–	1	1	1	1	–
Kansas	–	2	–	2	1	2	1	–
Kentucky	–	1	–	–	–	1	1	1
Louisiana	–	–	–	2	–	–	1	–
Maine	–	–	–	–	1	–	1	–
Maryland	–	7	–	1	–	5	–	1
Massachusetts	3	6	–	6	1	–	1	–
Michigan	–	14	–	4	18	1	1	1
Minnesota	5	3	–	–	–	–	–	–
Mississippi	–	2	–	–	–	1	1	–
Missouri	–	12	–	1	–	1	–	–
Montana	–	–	–	–	–	–	2	1
Nebraska	2	–	–	–	–	–	1	1

TABLE 16, Continued

State	Comprehensive Risk-based Plans				Limited-benefit Plans				
	Commercial MCO	Medicaid-only MCO	HIO	PACE	PIHP	PAHP	PCCM	Other	
Nevada	1	1	–	–	–	1	–	–	
New Hampshire	–	–	–	–	–	–	–	–	
New Jersey	–	4	–	3	–	1	–	–	
New Mexico	6	–	–	1	1	–	–	–	
New York	20	13	–	7	22	–	3	–	
North Carolina	–	–	–	4	1	–	2	–	
North Dakota	–	–	–	1	–	1	1	–	
Ohio	–	7	–	2	–	–	–	–	
Oklahoma	–	–	–	1	–	1	2	–	
Oregon	2	13	–	1	10	8	1	–	
Pennsylvania	12	–	–	15	37	2	1	–	
Rhode Island	1	1	–	–	–	1	1	–	
South Carolina	–	4	–	2	–	2	3	–	
South Dakota	–	–	–	–	–	–	1	–	
Tennessee	–	6	–	1	1	2	1	–	
Texas	6	14	–	3	1	1	1	–	
Utah	1	1	–	–	10	2	1	–	
Vermont	–	1	–	–	–	–	–	–	
Virginia	3	2	–	5	–	1	1	–	
Washington	8	–	–	1	2	2	–	–	
West Virginia	3	–	–	–	–	–	1	–	
Wisconsin	19	9	–	1	11	–	–	1	
Wyoming	–	–	–	–	–	–	–	–	

Notes: HIO is Health Insuring Organization; MCO is managed care organization; PACE is Program of All-Inclusive Care for the Elderly; PAHP is prepaid ambulatory health plan; PIHP is prepaid inpatient health plan; PCCM is primary care case management. Excludes the territories.

Comprehensive risk-based managed care includes plans categorized by the Centers for Medicare & Medicaid Services (CMS) and states as commercial, Medicaid-only, Health Insuring Organizations (HIOs), and Programs of All-Inclusive Care for the Elderly (PACE). HIOs exist only in California where selected county-organized health systems serve Medicaid enrollees. PACE combines Medicare and Medicaid financing for qualifying frail elderly individuals who are dually eligible for Medicare and Medicaid. In the data reporting instructions provided by CMS to states, commercial plans are those that provide comprehensive services to both Medicaid and commercial and/or Medicare enrollees; Medicaid-only plans are those that provide comprehensive services to only Medicaid enrollees, not to commercial or Medicare enrollees.

Source: MACPAC analysis of data from CMS, *Medicaid Managed Care Enrollment Report: Summary Statistics as of July 1, 2011*, http://www.medicaid.gov/Medicaid-CHIP-Program-Information/By-Topics/Data-and-Systems/Downloads/2011-Medicaid-MC-Enrollment-Report.pdf.

MACStats

SECTION 4

TABLE 17. Percentage of Medicaid Enrollees in Managed Care by State and Eligibility Group, FY 2010

	Percentage of Enrollees						Comprehensive risk-based managed care					
	Any managed care											
State	Total	Children	Adults	Disabled	Aged	Dual eligibles[1]	Total	Children	Adults	Disabled	Aged	Dual eligibles[1]
Total	**71.7%**	**87.0%**	**60.5%**	**63.1%**	**40.6%**	**40.7%**	**48.3%**	**62.2%**	**46.8%**	**28.7%**	**12.4%**	**11.9%**
Alabama	72.8	97.2	44.0	66.1	23.0	22.2	3.0	—	0.0	6.5	14.3	14.9
Alaska	—	—	—	—	—	—	—	—	—	—	—	—
Arizona	91.3	96.8	87.5	93.8	73.5	79.0	85.1	90.9	80.5	88.3	68.0	74.1
Arkansas	79.8	97.1	47.9	78.5	47.3	47.9	—	—	—	—	—	—
California	58.8	79.0	28.1	92.3	89.0	92.4	38.5	64.3	22.9	26.9	15.9	17.7
Colorado	90.8	95.0	87.6	85.7	78.0	73.2	13.3	14.1	11.7	13.6	10.8	8.9
Connecticut	62.3	94.8	61.7	1.0	0.0	0.6	62.3	94.8	61.7	1.0	0.0	0.6
Delaware	88.0	96.8	88.6	75.9	49.1	49.0	76.5	88.5	82.8	49.1	6.3	5.6
District of Columbia	90.7	95.1	88.6	92.5	76.3	76.5	68.2	88.8	87.2	14.9	0.2	1.8
Florida	71.7	90.3	71.6	55.8	16.0	11.3	71.7	90.3	71.6	55.8	16.0	11.3
Georgia	88.9	97.1	89.8	77.5	53.6	51.5	69.4	93.1	84.9	3.2	0.1	0.4
Hawaii	95.8	97.6	95.7	94.8	89.6	89.4	95.8	97.6	95.7	94.8	89.6	89.4
Idaho[2]	90.8	98.2	93.6	80.5	49.8	57.3	—	—	—	—	—	—
Illinois	71.7	84.4	78.1	37.6	9.1	3.7	7.2	9.6	7.3	0.1	0.1	0.1
Indiana	77.7	93.1	88.0	43.1	3.3	4.2	70.7	89.3	87.2	13.1	0.3	1.9
Iowa	78.1	94.9	49.6	90.8	64.7	74.7	0.0	—	—	0.1	0.1	0.1
Kansas	84.0	92.1	85.5	78.1	46.1	55.9	53.6	75.8	72.0	2.1	0.6	0.9
Kentucky	90.2	98.4	96.8	83.0	61.1	60.5	20.1	25.2	20.8	15.7	6.5	8.1
Louisiana	62.1	88.4	41.1	42.1	1.7	3.3	0.0	0.0	—	0.0	0.2	0.1
Maine	—	—	—	—	—	—	—	—	—	—	—	—
Maryland	72.9	95.6	63.7	56.9	1.4	4.1	72.9	95.6	63.7	56.9	1.4	4.1
Massachusetts	72.6	89.2	81.6	54.7	14.2	13.1	48.5	60.6	58.4	22.2	12.6	9.6
Michigan	88.9	95.9	75.6	90.7	81.6	85.0	70.9	85.5	68.8	53.2	3.4	7.1
Minnesota	67.6	84.4	70.5	11.4	58.8	43.6	67.6	84.4	70.5	11.4	58.8	43.6
Mississippi	—	—	—	—	—	—	—	—	—	—	—	—

TABLE 17, Continued

State	Total	Any managed care					Comprehensive risk-based managed care					
		Children	Adults	Disabled	Aged	Dual eligibles[1]	Total	Children	Adults	Disabled	Aged	Dual eligibles[1]
Missouri[2]	72.4%	66.7%	60.0%	91.6%	89.4%	89.9%	46.6%	66.7%	59.7%	2.0%	0.0%	0.4%
Montana	66.0	82.4	69.9	44.6	1.1	2.4	–	–	–	–	–	–
Nebraska	42.3	51.8	46.9	23.9	3.8	1.6	38.1	47.4	39.4	21.9	3.5	0.9
Nevada	89.2	96.5	89.6	75.1	56.6	51.5	60.8	77.8	72.6	2.0	0.0	0.4
New Hampshire	–	–	–	–	–	–	–	–	–	–	–	–
New Jersey	93.4	96.1	90.0	93.9	85.3	85.8	72.8	93.0	81.0	52.5	13.4	12.4
New Mexico	67.3	82.4	58.3	46.3	3.5	4.0	67.3	82.4	58.3	46.2	3.5	4.0
New York	65.9	78.9	73.1	48.8	15.0	12.8	65.9	78.9	73.1	48.8	15.0	12.8
North Carolina	80.9	96.4	72.8	72.7	30.2	37.6	0.0	–	–	0.0	0.1	0.0
North Dakota	56.1	75.1	75.1	1.8	–	0.3	–	–	–	–	–	–
Ohio	75.7	91.2	92.2	40.3	4.9	3.6	75.7	91.2	92.2	40.3	4.9	3.6
Oklahoma	81.1	94.6	46.0	83.6	79.8	77.7	0.0	–	–	0.0	0.1	0.0
Oregon	87.0	95.1	80.3	83.2	67.5	66.1	74.6	86.0	73.2	62.0	36.3	38.4
Pennsylvania	86.8	95.5	78.9	92.1	51.1	65.4	59.7	74.2	60.5	53.7	8.2	7.6
Rhode Island	59.2	88.0	78.2	16.7	0.1	1.1	59.2	88.0	78.2	16.7	0.1	1.1
South Carolina	91.9	99.1	77.0	93.7	86.0	87.0	53.3	69.4	54.3	32.3	0.6	2.5
South Dakota	92.1	93.3	88.4	91.7	91.5	92.5	–	–	–	–	–	–
Tennessee	92.7	97.4	97.7	89.5	62.0	70.8	92.7	97.4	97.7	89.5	62.0	70.8
Texas	74.1	92.4	52.0	46.7	19.5	21.1	48.1	61.4	32.8	22.1	14.9	15.5
Utah	89.6	98.6	67.5	94.2	85.4	88.6	0.3	0.1	–	1.8	0.1	1.0
Vermont	[3]	[3]	[3]	[3]	[3]	[3]	[3]	[3]	[3]	[3]	[3]	[3]
Virginia	66.5	83.1	71.1	42.4	15.1	9.7	60.8	78.4	66.7	35.7	4.0	2.0
Washington	68.7	90.5	61.8	24.7	12.1	12.1	67.5	89.9	61.1	20.8	11.5	11.7
West Virginia	54.5	90.0	73.4	2.6	0.0	0.4	51.8	85.7	70.8	1.8	0.0	0.4
Wisconsin	64.5	82.5	71.0	36.0	16.1	20.5	58.7	82.4	71.0	4.8	2.3	3.5
Wyoming	–	–	–	–	–	–	–	–	–	–	–	–

SECTION 4

TABLE 17, Continued. Percentage of Medicaid Enrollees in Managed Care by State and Eligibility Group, FY 2010

	Percentage of Enrollees										
	Limited-benefit plan						Primary care case management				
State	Total	Children	Adults	Disabled	Aged	Dual eligibles[1]	Total	Children	Adults	Disabled	Aged	Dual eligibles[1]
Total	**36.4%**	**41.6%**	**26.1%**	**42.1%**	**31.2%**	**32.0%**	**12.5%**	**17.3%**	**8.3%**	**11.5%**	**2.0%**	**2.4%**
Alabama	69.9	97.1	44.0	59.8	9.0	7.7	46.4	71.5	14.0	38.2	1.4	1.4
Alaska	–	–	–	–	–	–	–	–	–	–	–	–
Arizona	87.8	96.5	87.1	71.6	53.3	60.4	–	–	–	–	–	–
Arkansas	78.7	95.3	47.0	78.4	47.3	47.7	60.7	85.9	24.6	54.7	3.9	5.2
California	55.2	72.4	25.8	91.9	88.2	91.8	–	–	–	–	–	–
Colorado	90.6	95.0	87.6	85.5	76.1	71.8	–	–	–	–	–	–
Connecticut	–	–	–	–	–	–	–	–	–	–	–	–
Delaware	87.1	95.9	87.4	75.5	49.0	48.8	–	–	–	–	–	–
District of Columbia	24.0	7.0	2.0	83.1	76.3	75.3	–	–	–	–	–	–
Florida	–	–	–	–	–	–	–	–	–	–	–	–
Georgia	88.5	96.5	89.4	77.4	53.6	51.5	8.7	0.4	0.1	50.1	8.2	6.7
Hawaii	0.5	1.1	–	0.6	–	–	–	–	–	–	–	–
Idaho[2]	70.6	93.2	92.7	3.7	3.6	4.3	86.0	93.4	83.2	79.2	46.8	54.1
Illinois	2.7	3.7	2.6	0.0	0.0	0.0	65.4	75.8	72.0	37.5	9.0	3.6
Indiana	–	–	–	–	–	–	11.8	4.9	18.8	31.8	3.1	3.1
Iowa	78.0	94.9	49.2	90.8	64.7	74.6	38.9	62.3	30.5	1.5	0.0	0.3
Kansas	83.9	92.1	85.5	78.0	45.6	55.6	5.2	3.0	1.1	16.6	1.6	1.2
Kentucky	89.9	98.1	96.4	82.8	61.0	60.3	46.2	68.6	67.6	9.8	0.8	0.9
Louisiana	–	–	–	–	–	–	62.0	88.4	41.1	42.0	1.5	3.1
Maine	–	–	–	–	–	–	–	–	–	–	–	–
Maryland	29.6	35.4	29.8	36.1	1.8	3.8	–	–	–	–	–	–
Massachusetts	88.7	95.6	75.4	90.6	81.3	84.8	–	–	–	–	–	–
Michigan	–	–	–	–	–	–	0.0	–	–	0.0	0.0	0.0
Minnesota	–	–	–	–	–	–	–	–	–	–	–	–
Mississippi	26.2	0.1	0.4	91.2	89.4	89.7	–	–	–	–	–	–
Missouri[2]	–	–	–	–	–	–	66.0	82.4	69.9	44.6	1.1	2.4
Montana	–	–	–	–	–	–	21.7	27.3	22.2	11.8	2.0	0.8
Nebraska	89.2	96.5	89.6	75.1	56.6	51.5	–	–	–	–	–	–
Nevada	–	–	–	–	–	–	–	–	–	–	–	–
New Hampshire	–	–	–	–	–	–	–	–	–	–	–	–
New Jersey	70.7	66.6	62.7	81.2	81.3	82.2	–	–	–	–	–	–
New Mexico	67.0	82.4	58.1	44.7	1.9	2.3	–	–	–	–	–	–
New York	–	–	–	–	–	–	–	–	–	–	–	–

TABLE 17, Continued

State	Limited-benefit plan						Primary care case management				
	Total	Children	Adults	Disabled	Aged	Dual eligibles[1]	Total	Children	Adults	Disabled	Aged	Dual eligibles[1]
North Carolina	69.8%	88.6%	65.4%	54.4%	5.8%	8.4%	74.8%	93.6%	60.1%	62.9%	26.7%	34.2%
North Dakota	—	—	—	—	—	—	56.1	75.1	75.1	1.8	—	0.3
Ohio	—	—	—	—	—	—	—	—	—	—	—	—
Oklahoma	81.1	94.6	46.0	83.6	79.7	77.7	2.0	2.9	1.0	1.4	0.1	0.1
Oregon	86.9	94.9	80.3	83.2	67.5	66.1	0.6	0.6	0.2	0.9	1.1	1.0
Pennsylvania	86.2	95.1	77.8	91.9	50.2	64.8	17.0	21.2	17.0	16.1	1.0	1.7
Rhode Island	—	—	—	—	—	—	—	—	—	—	—	—
South Carolina	91.7	98.8	76.9	93.6	86.0	87.0	14.8	18.6	9.7	14.4	7.2	9.4
South Dakota	87.3	88.0	79.3	91.0	91.5	92.4	44.8	56.7	55.3	14.3	0.4	0.8
Tennessee	8.5	5.2	9.9	19.4	2.5	10.8	—	—	—	—	—	—
Texas	10.8	13.1	5.4	9.7	4.3	4.8	25.2	31.9	19.6	16.0	0.3	1.0
Utah	89.6	98.6	67.5	94.2	85.4	88.6	—	—	—	—	—	—
Vermont	[3]	[3]	[3]	[3]	[3]	[3]	[3]	[3]	[3]	[3]	[3]	[3]
Virginia	—	—	—	—	—	—	5.9	4.9	4.6	7.0	11.2	7.7
Washington	—	—	—	—	—	—	1.6	1.1	1.1	4.7	0.8	0.6
West Virginia	—	—	—	—	—	—	3.5	5.7	3.5	0.9	0.0	0.0
Wisconsin	5.9	0.2	0.1	32.1	13.8	17.1	—	—	—	—	—	—
Wyoming	—	—	—	—	—	—	—	—	—	—	—	—

Notes: Excludes the territories and Medicaid-expansion CHIP enrollees. Children and adults under age 65 who qualify for Medicaid on the basis of a disability are included in the disabled category. About 690,000 enrollees aged 65 and older are identified in the data as disabled; given that disability is not an eligibility pathway for individuals aged 65 and older, MACPAC recodes these enrollees as aged. Any managed care includes comprehensive risk-based plans, limited-benefit plans, and primary care case management programs. Enrollees are counted as participating in managed care if they were enrolled during the fiscal year and at least one managed care payment was made on their behalf during the fiscal year; this method underestimates participation somewhat because it does not capture enrollees who entered managed care late in the year but for whom a payment was not made until the following fiscal year. Managed care types do not sum to total because individuals are counted in every category for which a payment was made on their behalf during the year.

Figures shown here may differ from Table 9, which uses Medicaid managed care enrollment report data. Reasons for differences include differing time periods (the Medicaid Statistical Information System (MSIS) data used here include those ever enrolled in fiscal year (FY) 2010), state reporting anomalies (e.g., some states report a very small number of comprehensive risk-based enrollees in MSIS who may be miscategorized), and Medicaid-expansion CHIP enrollees (excluded here but included in Table 15). Although the enrollment report used for Table 9 is a commonly cited source, it does not provide information on the characteristics of enrollees in managed care (e.g., eligibility group) or their spending and non-managed care service use. MSIS data are used here to provide this additional level of detail.

Zeroes indicate amounts less than 0.05 percent that round to zero. Dashes indicate amounts that are true zeroes.

[1] Dual eligibles are individuals who are enrolled in both Medicaid and Medicare; these figures include those with full Medicaid benefits and those with limited benefits who only receive Medicaid assistance with Medicare premiums and cost sharing. For dual eligibles enrolled in a comprehensive Medicaid managed care plan, Medicare is still the primary payer of most acute care services; as a result, the Medicaid plan may only provide a subset of the comprehensive services normally covered under its contract with the state.

[2] FY 2010 data unavailable for Idaho and Missouri; FY 2009 values shown instead.

[3] Due to large differences in the way managed care spending is reported by Vermont in CMS-64 and MSIS data, managed care enrollment (which, for this table, is based on the presence of managed care spending in MSIS for a given enrollee) is not reported here.

Source: MACPAC analysis of Medicaid Statistical Information System (MSIS) annual person summary (APS) data from CMS as of May 2013.

MACStats

SECTION 4

TABLE 18. Percentage of Medicaid Benefit Spending on Managed Care by State and Eligibility Group, FY 2010

	Percentage of Benefit Spending										
	Any managed care						Comprehensive risk-based managed care				
State	Total	Children	Adults	Disabled	Aged	Dual eligibles[1]	Total	Children	Adults	Disabled	Aged	Dual eligibles[1]
Total	**23.5%**	**43.9%**	**44.6%**	**15.2%**	**8.8%**	**8.0%**	**21.6%**	**41.1%**	**42.7%**	**13.3%**	**7.5%**	**6.1%**
Alabama	15.8	38.3	24.0	7.6	1.0	0.9	0.2	–	0.0	0.2	0.3	0.4
Alaska	–	–	–	–	–	–	–	–	–	–	–	–
Arizona	87.0	88.7	90.1	84.4	81.3	82.5	86.0	87.6	88.5	84.1	80.7	82.0
Arkansas	0.4	1.3	0.6	0.2	0.1	0.1	–	–	–	–	–	–
California	15.5	42.3	16.8	8.8	9.4	10.0	14.8	41.8	16.6	8.5	7.7	8.6
Colorado	11.4	16.5	8.5	10.4	9.8	9.6	5.9	5.4	4.6	4.9	9.0	6.6
Connecticut	12.7	47.2	43.2	0.1	0.0	0.0	12.7	47.2	43.2	0.1	0.0	0.0
Delaware	46.6	63.0	80.4	28.7	2.7	2.1	46.5	62.8	80.3	28.6	2.5	1.9
District of Columbia	22.8	62.8	78.6	9.6	0.8	1.6	21.8	62.3	78.6	8.4	0.0	0.3
Florida	17.0	33.1	18.5	13.9	10.4	5.9	17.0	33.1	18.5	13.9	10.4	5.9
Georgia	28.7	77.5	75.8	1.2	1.2	1.3	28.0	77.4	75.8	0.3	0.0	0.1
Hawaii	76.0	74.4	81.2	62.2	86.6	75.4	76.0	74.4	81.2	62.2	86.6	75.4
Idaho[2]	3.1	11.3	3.8	0.4	0.6	0.8	–	–	–	–	–	–
Illinois	2.2	4.8	5.2	0.1	0.3	0.2	1.6	3.3	3.9	0.0	0.2	0.2
Indiana	21.5	63.0	73.2	3.5	0.1	0.2	21.0	62.2	73.0	2.8	0.0	0.2
Iowa	4.3	8.2	5.8	4.2	0.5	2.1	0.1	–	–	0.1	0.1	0.1
Kansas	23.3	60.2	72.3	9.8	3.0	4.3	16.8	52.8	71.5	0.6	0.7	0.6
Kentucky	13.4	22.1	19.8	11.9	2.0	2.4	12.5	19.8	18.7	11.4	1.7	2.0
Louisiana	0.1	0.4	0.1	0.0	0.2	0.1	0.0	0.0	–	0.0	0.2	0.1
Maine	–	–	–	–	–	–	–	–	–	–	–	–
Maryland	35.7	55.4	76.5	27.5	0.6	1.5	35.7	55.4	76.5	27.5	0.6	1.5
Massachusetts	27.2	51.1	55.9	14.5	13.4	8.0	24.1	45.8	50.8	11.3	13.3	7.9
Michigan	49.5	65.7	73.2	53.1	7.5	25.7	41.2	63.8	66.7	40.4	1.7	4.1
Minnesota	34.5	77.1	80.2	5.3	38.3	21.5	34.5	77.1	80.2	5.3	38.3	21.5
Mississippi	–	–	–	–	–	–	–	–	–	–	–	–
Missouri[2]	15.4	47.3	40.3	0.7	1.0	0.9	14.9	47.3	40.3	0.2	0.0	0.1
Montana	0.7	2.2	0.9	0.3	0.0	0.0	–	–	–	–	–	–
Nebraska	6.2	11.3	16.2	4.0	0.9	0.2	6.2	11.3	16.2	4.0	0.9	0.2
Nevada	19.2	44.2	49.8	0.4	0.3	0.4	18.9	43.9	49.6	0.2	0.0	0.1
New Hampshire	–	–	–	–	–	–	–	–	–	–	–	–

TABLE 18, Continued

State	Percentage of Benefit Spending									
	Any managed care						Comprehensive risk-based managed care			
	Total	Children	Adults	Disabled	Aged	Dual eligibles[1]	Total	Children	Adults	Disabled	Aged	Dual eligibles[1]
New Jersey	18.7%	48.6%	61.4%	12.1%	3.4%	2.3%	18.3%	48.4%	61.3%	11.7%	2.6%	1.4%
New Mexico	64.8	76.3	68.8	49.6	28.1	8.9	64.7	76.3	68.8	49.6	28.1	8.9
New York	18.7	44.3	42.9	8.3	8.7	5.8	18.7	44.3	42.9	8.3	8.7	5.8
North Carolina	2.5	3.8	2.2	2.7	0.6	1.5	0.0	–	–	0.0	0.1	0.1
North Dakota	0.5	2.3	1.2	0.0	–	0.0	–	–	–	–	–	–
Ohio	29.7	71.3	79.3	18.4	2.1	0.8	29.7	71.3	79.3	18.4	2.1	0.8
Oklahoma	4.2	6.5	1.5	3.5	4.4	3.8	0.2	–	–	0.0	0.8	0.2
Oregon	42.4	76.5	75.7	34.7	6.0	8.2	40.7	73.6	74.6	32.7	5.4	7.1
Pennsylvania	45.5	82.4	71.5	47.4	7.3	6.5	41.5	76.4	69.1	42.9	5.1	3.4
Rhode Island	29.2	63.7	83.5	10.5	0.0	0.2	29.2	63.7	83.5	10.5	0.0	0.2
South Carolina	24.9	44.8	43.3	19.6	1.9	2.6	24.0	43.3	42.8	19.2	0.3	1.3
South Dakota	0.2	0.6	0.2	0.1	0.1	0.1	–	–	–	–	–	–
Tennessee	57.9	70.6	89.9	47.1	33.3	32.9	57.9	70.6	89.9	47.1	33.3	32.9
Texas	18.1	34.9	21.7	8.6	7.7	7.6	17.8	34.4	21.5	8.2	7.6	7.5
Utah	20.7	19.4	10.5	26.8	10.4	24.2	0.5	0.2	–	0.9	0.1	0.7
Vermont	81.2	[3]	[3]	[3]	[3]	[3]	[3]	[3]	[3]	[3]	[3]	[3]
Virginia	25.9	43.0	60.9	19.4	3.8	0.9	25.8	42.9	60.9	19.4	3.8	0.9
Washington	25.8	71.5	53.0	3.0	1.4	1.3	25.8	71.5	53.0	2.9	1.4	1.3
West Virginia	12.7	53.1	52.3	0.2	0.0	0.1	12.6	53.1	52.3	0.2	0.0	0.1
Wisconsin	39.6	53.4	55.0	33.0	33.9	34.9	19.2	52.1	54.8	3.4	6.3	5.6
Wyoming	–	–	–	–	–	–	–	–	–	–	–	–

Notes: Includes federal and state funds. Excludes administrative spending, the territories, and Medicaid-expansion CHIP enrollees. Children and non-aged adults who qualify for Medicaid on the basis of a disability are included in the disabled category. About 690,000 enrollees aged 65 and older are identified in the data as disabled; given that disability is not an eligibility pathway for individuals aged 65 and older, MACPAC recodes these enrollees as aged. Benefit spending from Medicaid Statistical Information System (MSIS) data has been adjusted to match CMS-64 totals; see Section 5 of MACStats for methodology. Any managed care includes comprehensive risk-based plans, limited-benefit plans, and primary care case management programs.

Zeroes indicate amounts less than 0.05 percent that round to zero. Dashes indicate amounts that are true zeroes.

[1] Dual eligibles are individuals who are enrolled in both Medicaid and Medicare; these figures include those with full Medicaid benefits and those with limited benefits who only receive Medicaid assistance with Medicare premiums and cost sharing. For dual eligibles enrolled in a comprehensive Medicaid managed care plan, Medicare is still the primary payer of most acute care services; as a result, the Medicaid plan may only provide a subset of the comprehensive services normally covered under its contract with the state.

[2] Fiscal year (FY) 2010 data unavailable for Idaho and Missouri; FY 2009 values shown instead.

[3] Due to large differences in the way managed care spending is reported by Vermont in CMS-64 and MSIS data, benefit spending based on MACPAC's adjustment methodology is not reported at a level lower than total Medicaid managed care.

Source: MACPAC analysis of Medicaid Statistical Information System (MSIS) annual person summary (APS) data and CMS-64 Financial Management Report (FMR) net expenditure data from CMS as of May 2013.

MAC Stats

SECTION 5

Technical Guide to the June 2013 MACStats

This section provides supplemental information to accompany the tables and figures in Sections 1–4 of MACStats. It describes some of the data sources used in MACStats, the methods that MACPAC uses to analyze these data, and reasons why numbers in MACStats tables and figures—such as those on enrollment and spending—may differ from each other or from those published elsewhere.

Interpreting Medicaid and CHIP Enrollment and Spending Numbers

Previous MACPAC reports have discussed reasons why estimates of Medicaid and State Children's Health Insurance Program (CHIP) enrollment and spending may vary.[1] Here, Tables 19–22 are used to illustrate how various factors can affect enrollment numbers. Table 19 shows enrollment numbers for the entire U.S. population in 2010.[2] Tables 20–22 divide the U.S. population into the three age groups that are commonly used in MACPAC analyses because they correspond to some of the key eligibility pathways in Medicaid and CHIP: children aged 0 to 18; adults aged 19 to 64; and adults aged 65 and older.

Data sources

Medicaid and CHIP enrollment and spending numbers are available from administrative data, which states and the federal government compile in the course of administering these programs. The latest year of available data may differ, depending on the source. The administrative data used in this edition of MACStats include the following, which are submitted by the states to the Centers for Medicare & Medicaid Services (CMS):

▶ Form CMS-64 data for state-level Medicaid spending, which is used throughout MACStats;

TABLE 19. Medicaid and CHIP Enrollment by Data Source and Enrollment Period, 2010

Medicaid and CHIP Enrollment (All Ages)	Administrative Data		Survey Data (NHIS)
	Ever enrolled during the year	Point in time	Point in time
Medicaid	66.0 million	53.5 million	Not available
CHIP	7.9 million	5.3 million	Not available
Totals for Medicaid and CHIP	74.0 million	58.8 million	47.7 million
U.S. Population	**Census Bureau**		**Survey Data (NHIS)**
	310.3 million	308.8 million	304.1 million, excluding active-duty military and individuals in institutions
Medicaid and CHIP Enrollment as a Percentage of U.S. Population			
	23.8%	19.1%	15.7%

See Table 22 for notes.

Sources: MACPAC analysis of Medicaid Statistical Information System (MSIS) annual person summary (APS) data from CMS as of May 2013, CHIP Statistical Enrollment Data System (SEDS) data from CMS as of May 2013, data from the National Health Interview Survey (NHIS), and U.S. Census Bureau data on the monthly postcensal resident population, by single year of age, sex, race, and Hispanic origin.

TABLE 20. Medicaid and CHIP Enrollment by Data Source and Enrollment Period Among Children Under Age 19, 2010

Medicaid and CHIP Enrollment Among Children Under Age 19	Administrative Data		Survey Data (NHIS)
	Ever enrolled during the year	Point in time	Point in time
Medicaid	32.1 million	26.7 million	Not available
CHIP	7.7 million	5.1 million	Not available
Totals for Medicaid and CHIP	39.8 million	31.8 million	28.2 million
Children Under Age 19	**Census Bureau**		**Survey Data (NHIS)**
	79.1 million	78.8 million	79.0 million, excluding active-duty military and individuals in institutions
Medicaid and CHIP Enrollment as a Percentage of All Children Under 19			
	50.3%	40.4%	35.7%

See Table 22 for notes.

Sources: MACPAC analysis of Medicaid Statistical Information System (MSIS) annual person summary (APS) data from CMS as of May 2013, CHIP Statistical Enrollment Data System (SEDS) data from CMS as of May 2013, data from the National Health Interview Survey (NHIS), and U.S. Census Bureau data on the monthly postcensal resident population, by single year of age, sex, race, and Hispanic origin.

TABLE 21. Medicaid and CHIP Enrollment by Data Source and Enrollment Period Among Adults Aged 19-64, 2010

Medicaid and CHIP Enrollment Among Adults Age 19–64	Administrative Data		Survey Data (NHIS)
	Ever enrolled during the year	Point in time	Point in time
Medicaid	27.7 million	21.2 million	Not available
CHIP	0.2 million	0.2 million	Not available
Totals for Medicaid and CHIP	27.9 million	21.4 million	16.5 million
Adults Age 19–64	**Census Bureau**		**Survey Data (NHIS)**
	190.6 million	189.7 million	186.4 million, excluding active-duty military and individuals in institutions
Medicaid and CHIP Enrollment as a Percentage of All Adults Age 19–64			
	14.6%	11.3%	8.9%

See Table 22 for notes.

Sources: MACPAC analysis of Medicaid Statistical Information System (MSIS) annual person summary (APS) data from CMS as of May 2013, CHIP Statistical Enrollment Data System (SEDS) data from CMS as of May 2013, data from the National Health Interview Survey (NHIS), and U.S. Census Bureau data on the monthly postcensal resident population, by single year of age, sex, race, and Hispanic origin.

TABLE 22. Medicaid and CHIP Enrollment by Data Source and Enrollment Period Among Adults Aged 65 and Older, 2010

Medicaid and CHIP Enrollment Among Adults Age 65 and Older	Administrative Data		Survey Data (NHIS)
	Ever enrolled during the year	Point in time	Point in time
Medicaid	6.3 million	5.5 million	Not available
CHIP	–	–	Not available
Totals for Medicaid and CHIP	6.3 million	5.5 million	3.0 million
Adults Age 65 and Older	**Census Bureau**		**Survey Data (NHIS)**
	40.7 million	40.2 million	38.7 million, excluding active-duty military and individuals in institutions
Medicaid and CHIP Enrollment as a Percentage of All Adults Age 65 and Older			
	15.5%	13.8%	7.7%

Notes: Excludes U.S. territories. Medicaid enrollment numbers obtained from administrative data include 8.5 million individuals ever enrolled during the year who received limited benefits (e.g., emergency services only, Medicaid payment only for Medicare enrollees' cost sharing), of whom 0.6 million were under age 19, 6.4 million were aged 19 to 64, and 1.5 million were aged 65 or older. In the event individuals were reported to be in both Medicaid and CHIP during the year, individuals were counted only once in the administrative data, based on their most recent source of coverage. Overcounting of enrollees in the administrative data may occur because individuals may move and be enrolled in two states' Medicaid programs during the year. The National Health Interview Survey (NHIS) excludes individuals in institutions (such as nursing homes) and active-duty military; in addition, surveys such as NHIS generally do not count limited benefits as Medicaid/CHIP coverage. Administrative data (with the exception of Idaho and Missouri, for which fiscal year (FY) 2009 values were used) and Census Bureau data are for FY 2010 (October 2009 through September 2010); the NHIS data are for sources of insurance at the time of the survey in calendar year 2010. The Census Bureau number in the ever-enrolled column was the estimated U.S. resident population in the month in FY 2010 with the largest count; the number of residents ever living in the United States during the year is not available. The Census Bureau point-in-time number is the average estimated monthly number of U.S. residents for FY 2010.

Sources: MACPAC analysis of Medicaid Statistical Information System (MSIS) annual person summary (APS) data from CMS as of May 2013, CHIP Statistical Enrollment Data System (SEDS) data from CMS as of May 2013, data from the National Health Interview Survey (NHIS), and U.S. Census Bureau data on the monthly postcensal resident population, by single year of age, sex, race, and Hispanic origin.

- Medicaid Statistical Information System (MSIS) data for person-level detail, which is used throughout MACStats;
- Medicaid managed care enrollment reports, which are used in Tables 15 and 16;[3] and
- Statistical Enrollment Data System (SEDS) data for CHIP enrollment, used in Tables 19–22.

Additional information is available from nationally representative surveys based on interviews of individuals. The survey data used in Tables 3–11 are from the federal National Health Interview Survey (NHIS), which is described below in more detail.

Tables 19–22 show 2010 survey-based estimates of Medicaid/CHIP enrollment as well as comparable (point-in-time) estimates from the administrative data. Estimates of Medicaid/CHIP enrollment from survey data tend to be lower than numbers from administrative data because survey respondents tend to underreport Medicaid and CHIP, among other reasons described later in this section.

Enrollment period examined

The number of individuals enrolled at a particular point during the year will be lower than the total number enrolled at any point during an entire year. For example, the administrative data in Table 20 show that 50.3 percent of children (39.8 million) were enrolled in Medicaid or CHIP at some time during fiscal year (FY) 2010. However, numbers from the same data source illustrate that the number of children enrolled at a particular point in time (31.8 million, or approximately 40.4 percent of children) is much smaller than the number ever enrolled during the year.

Point-in-time data may also be referred to as average monthly enrollment or full-year equivalent enrollment.[4] Full-year equivalent enrollment is often used for budget analyses (such as those by the CMS Office of the Actuary) and when comparing enrollment and expenditure numbers (such as in Figure 1). Per enrollee spending levels based on full-year equivalents (Table 14) ensure that amounts are not biased by individuals' transitions in and out of Medicaid coverage during the year.

Enrollees versus beneficiaries

Depending on the source and the year in question, data may include slightly different numbers of individuals in Medicaid. Certain terms commonly used to refer to people with Medicaid have very specific definitions in administrative data sources provided by CMS:[5]

- Enrollees (less commonly referred to as eligibles) are individuals who are eligible for and enrolled in Medicaid or CHIP. Prior to FY 1990, CMS did not track the number of Medicaid enrollees, only beneficiaries. For some historical numbers, CMS has estimated the number of enrollees prior to 1990 (Figure 1).

- Beneficiaries or persons served (less commonly referred to as recipients) are enrollees who receive covered services or for whom Medicaid or CHIP payments are made. Prior to FY 1998, individuals were not counted as beneficiaries if managed care payments were the only Medicaid payments made on their behalf. Beginning in FY 1998, however, Medicaid managed care enrollees with no fee-for-service (FFS) spending were also counted as beneficiaries, which had a large impact on the numbers (Table 1).[6]

The following example illustrates the difference in these terms. In FY 2010, there were 31.8 million non-disabled child Medicaid enrollees (Table 12). However, there were 30 million beneficiaries in this eligibility group—that is, during FY 2010, a

Medicaid FFS or managed care capitation payment was made on their behalf (Table 1).[7] Generally, the number of beneficiaries will approach the number of enrollees as more of these individuals use Medicaid-covered services or are enrolled in managed care.[8]

Institutionalized and limited-benefit enrollees

Administrative Medicaid data include enrollees who were in institutions such as nursing homes, as well as individuals who received only limited benefits (for example, only coverage for emergency services). Survey data tend to exclude such individuals from counts of coverage; the NHIS estimates in Tables 3–11 do not include the institutionalized.

Table 22 shows point-in-time enrollment among those aged 65 and older—5.5 million from the administrative data and 3.0 million from the survey data (NHIS). In percentage terms, the difference between the administrative data and the survey data is largest for this age group. This is primarily because the NHIS excludes the institutionalized and because, when Medicaid pays only for Medicare enrollees' cost sharing, the NHIS generally does not count it as Medicaid coverage. Based on administrative data, 1.5 million Medicaid enrollees aged 65 and older received only limited benefits from Medicaid.

State Children's Health Insurance Program Enrollees

Medicaid-expansion CHIP enrollees are children who are entitled to the covered services of a state's Medicaid program, but whose Medicaid coverage is generally funded with CHIP dollars. Depending on the data source, Medicaid enrollment and spending figures may include both Medicaid enrollees funded with Medicaid dollars and Medicaid-expansion CHIP enrollees funded with CHIP dollars. We generally exclude Medicaid-expansion CHIP enrollees from Medicaid analyses where possible in MACStats, but in some cases data sources do not allow these children to be broken out separately.

Methodology for Adjusting Benefit Spending Data

The FY 2010 Medicaid benefit spending amounts shown in the June 2013 MACStats were calculated based on MSIS data that have been adjusted to match total benefit spending reported by states in CMS-64 data.[9] Although the CMS-64 provides a more complete accounting of spending and is preferred when examining state or federal spending totals, MSIS is the only data source that allows for analysis of benefit spending by eligibility group and other enrollee characteristics.[10] We adjust the MSIS amounts for several reasons:

- CMS-64 data provide an official accounting of state spending on Medicaid for purposes of receiving federal matching dollars; in contrast, MSIS data are used primarily for statistical purposes.
- MSIS generally understates total Medicaid benefit spending because it excludes disproportionate share hospital payments and additional types of supplemental payments made to hospitals and other providers, Medicare premium payments, and certain other amounts.[11]
- MSIS generally overstates net spending on prescribed drugs, because it excludes rebates from drug manufacturers.
- Even after accounting for differences in their scope and design, MSIS still tends to produce lower total benefit spending than the CMS-64.[12]

- The extent to which MSIS differs from the CMS-64 varies by state, meaning that a cross-state comparison of unadjusted MSIS amounts may not reflect true differences in benefit spending. See Table 23 for unadjusted benefit spending amounts in MSIS as a percentage of benefit spending in the CMS-64.

The methodology MACPAC uses for adjusting the MSIS benefit spending data involves the following steps:

- We aggregate the service types into broad categories that are comparable between the two sources. This is necessary because there is not a one-to-one correspondence of service types in the MSIS and CMS-64 data. Even service types that have identical names may still be reported differently in the two sources due to differences in the instructions given to states. Table 24 provides additional detail on the categories used.

- We calculate state-specific adjustment factors for each of the service categories by dividing CMS-64 benefit spending by MSIS benefit spending.

- We then multiply MSIS dollar amounts in each service category by the state-specific factors to obtain adjusted MSIS spending. For example, in a state with a FFS hospital factor of 1.2, each Medicaid enrollee with hospital spending in MSIS would have that spending multiplied by 1.2; doing so makes the sum of adjusted hospital spending amounts among individual Medicaid enrollees in MSIS total the aggregate hospital spending reported by states in the CMS-64.[13]

By making these adjustments to the MSIS data, we are attempting to provide more complete estimates of Medicaid benefit spending across states that can be analyzed by eligibility group and other enrollee characteristics. Other organizations, including the Office of the Actuary at CMS, the Kaiser Commission on Medicaid and the Uninsured, and the Urban Institute use methodologies that are similar to MACPAC's but may differ in various ways—for example, by using different service categories or producing estimates for future years based on actual data for earlier years.

Understanding Data on Health and Other Characteristics of Medicaid/CHIP Populations

Section 2 of MACStats, which encompasses Tables 3–11, uses data from the federal National Health Interview Survey to describe Medicaid and CHIP enrollees in terms of their self-reported demographic, socioeconomic, and health characteristics as well as their use of care. Background information on the NHIS is provided here, along with information on how children with special health care needs are identified in Tables 3–5 using this data source.

National Health Interview Survey data

Every year, thousands of non-institutionalized Americans are interviewed about their health insurance and health status for the NHIS.[14] Individuals' responses to the NHIS questions are the basis for the results in Tables 3–11.

The NHIS is an annual face-to-face household survey of civilian non-institutionalized persons designed to monitor the health of the U.S. population through the collection of information on a broad range of health topics.[15] Administered by the National Center for Health Statistics within the Centers for Disease Control and Prevention, the NHIS consists of a nationally representative sample from approximately 35,000 households containing about 87,500 people.[16] Tables 3–11

TABLE 23. Medicaid Benefit Spending in MSIS and CMS-64 Data by State, FY 2010 (billions)

State	MSIS	CMS-64	MSIS as a Percentage of CMS-64
Total	$339.9	$388.6	87.5%
Alabama	4.0	4.7	85.1
Alaska	1.2	1.2	96.8
Arizona	9.5	9.4	101.4
Arkansas	3.7	3.9	93.7
California	34.4	42.1	81.7
Colorado	3.3	4.1	81.4
Connecticut	5.4	5.7	93.8
Delaware	1.3	1.3	104.1
District of Columbia	1.8	1.8	100.1
Florida	16.1	17.4	92.7
Georgia	7.0	7.8	89.5
Hawaii	1.3	1.4	92.3
Idaho[1]	1.3	1.3	104.1
Illinois	11.5	15.3	75.1
Indiana	5.7	5.9	95.6
Iowa	3.0	3.1	96.0
Kansas	2.3	2.4	94.1
Kentucky	5.2	5.6	92.5
Louisiana	5.3	7.0	75.9
Maine	1.5	2.3	63.8
Maryland	6.6	7.1	93.6
Massachusetts	10.8	11.8	92.0
Michigan	11.4	11.7	97.5
Minnesota	7.1	7.6	94.0
Mississippi	3.4	4.1	81.1
Missouri[1]	5.7	7.7	73.2
Montana	0.8	0.9	81.4
Nebraska	1.5	1.7	88.5
Nevada	1.3	1.5	86.2
New Hampshire	1.0	1.3	75.7
New Jersey	8.0	10.2	78.7
New Mexico	2.4	3.4	70.6
New York	47.4	52.1	90.9
North Carolina	9.5	10.9	87.2
North Dakota	0.7	0.7	97.9
Ohio	14.1	15.3	92.5
Oklahoma	3.6	4.1	86.6
Oregon	3.2	4.0	79.5
Pennsylvania	15.9	18.8	84.7
Rhode Island	1.5	1.9	77.3
South Carolina	5.0	5.2	96.7
South Dakota	0.8	0.8	96.5
Tennessee	9.0	8.5	105.5
Texas	20.7	27.2	76.2
Utah	2.0	1.7	116.3
Vermont	1.0	1.3	79.9
Virginia	5.8	6.5	89.9
Washington	6.3	7.1	89.4
West Virginia	2.7	2.6	105.4
Wisconsin	5.4	6.5	82.2
Wyoming	0.6	0.5	106.3

Note: See text for a discussion of differences between Medicaid Statistical Information System (MSIS) and CMS-64 data. Both sources reflect unadjusted amounts as reported by states. Includes federal and state funds. Both sources exclude spending on administration, the territories, and Medicaid-expansion CHIP enrollees; in addition, the CMS-64 amounts exclude $6.7 billion in offsetting collections from third-party liability, estate, and other recoveries.

[1] Fiscal year (FY) 2010 data unavailable for Idaho and Missouri; FY 2009 values shown instead.

Sources: MACPAC analysis of Medicaid Statistical Information System (MSIS) annual person summary (APS) data and CMS-64 Financial Management Report (FMR) net expenditure data from CMS as of May 2013.

TABLE 24. Service Categories Used to Adjust FY 2010 Medicaid Benefit Spending in MSIS to Match CMS-64 Totals

Service Category	MSIS Service Types	CMS-64 Service Types
Hospital	- Inpatient hospital - Outpatient hospital	- Inpatient hospital non-DSH - Inpatient hospital DSH - Inpatient hospital non-DSH supplemental payments - Inpatient hospital GME payments - Outpatient hospital non-DSH - Outpatient hospital non-DSH supplemental payments - Emergency services for aliens[1] - Emergency hospital services - Critical access hospitals
Non-hospital acute care	- Physician - Dental - Nurse midwife - Nurse practitioner - Other practitioner - Non-hospital outpatient clinic - Lab and X-ray - Sterilizations - Abortions - Hospice - Targeted case management - Physical, occupational, speech, and hearing therapy - Non-emergency transportation - Private duty nursing - Rehabilitative services - Other care, excluding HCBS waiver	- Physician - Physician services supplemental payments - Dental - Nurse midwife - Nurse practitioner - Other practitioner - Other practitioner supplemental payments - Non-hospital clinic - Rural health clinic - Federally qualified health center - Lab and X-ray - Sterilizations - Abortions - Hospice - Targeted case management - Statewide case management - Physical therapy - Occupational therapy - Services for speech, hearing, and language - Non-emergency transportation - Private duty nursing - Rehabilitative services (non-school-based) - School-based services - EPSDT screenings - Diagnostic screening and preventive services - Prosthetic devices, dentures, eyeglasses - Care not otherwise categorized

TABLE 24, Continued

Service Category	MSIS Service Types	CMS-64 Service Types
Drugs	▸ Drugs (gross spending)	▸ Drugs (gross spending) ▸ Drug rebates
Managed care and premium assistance	▸ HMO (i.e., comprehensive risk-based managed care; includes PACE) ▸ PHP ▸ PCCM	▸ MCO (i.e., comprehensive risk-based managed care) ▸ MCO drug rebates ▸ PACE ▸ PAHP ▸ PIHP ▸ PCCM ▸ Premium assistance for private coverage
LTSS non-institutional	▸ Home health ▸ Personal care ▸ HCBS waiver	▸ Home health ▸ Personal care ▸ Personal care – 1915(j) ▸ HCBS waiver ▸ HCBS – 1915(i) ▸ HCBS – 1915(j)
LTSS institutional	▸ Nursing facility ▸ ICF/ID ▸ Inpatient psychiatric for individuals under age 21 ▸ Mental health facility for individuals aged 65 and older	▸ Nursing facility ▸ Nursing facility supplemental payments ▸ ICF/ID ▸ ICF/ID supplemental payments ▸ Mental health facility for under age 21 or aged 65+ non-DSH ▸ Mental health facility for under age 21 or aged 65+ DSH
Medicare[2,3]		▸ Medicare Part A and Part B premiums ▸ Medicare coinsurance and deductibles for QMBs

Notes: DSH is disproportionate share hospital; EPSDT is Early and Periodic Screening, Diagnostic, and Treatment; GME is graduate medical education; HCBS is home and community-based services; HMO is health maintenance organization; ICF/ID is intermediate care facility for persons with intellectual disabilities; LTSS is long-term services and supports; MCO is managed care organization; MSIS is Medicaid Statistical Information System; PACE is Program of All-inclusive Care for the Elderly; PAHP is prepaid ambulatory health plan; PIHP is prepaid inpatient health plan; PHP is prepaid health plan, either a PAHP or a PIHP; PCCM is primary care case management; QMB is qualified Medicare beneficiary.

Service categories and types reflect fee-for-service spending unless noted otherwise. Service types with identical names in MSIS and CMS-64 data may still be reported differently in the two sources due to differences in the instructions given to states; amounts for those that appear only in the CMS-64 (e.g., DSH) are distributed across Medicaid enrollees with MSIS spending in the relevant service categories (e.g., hospital).

[1] Emergency services for aliens are reported under individual service types throughout MSIS, but primarily inpatient and outpatient hospital. As a result, we include this CMS-64 amount in the hospital category.

[2] Medicare premiums are not reported in MSIS. We distribute CMS-64 amounts across dual-eligible enrollees in MSIS.

[3] Medicare coinsurance and deductibles are reported under individual service types throughout MSIS. We distribute the CMS-64 amount for QMBs across CMS-64 spending in the hospital and non-hospital acute categories prior to calculating adjustment factors, based on the distribution of spending for these categories among QMBs in MSIS.

Sources: MACPAC analysis of MSIS Annual Person Summary (APS) data and CMS-64 Financial Management Report (FMR) net expenditure data from CMS.

are based on NHIS data, pooling the years 2009 through 2011.[17] Although there are other federal surveys, the NHIS is used here because it is generally considered to be one of the best surveys for health insurance coverage estimates, and it captures detailed information on individuals' health status.[18]

As with most surveys, information about participation in programs such as Medicaid, CHIP, Medicare, Supplemental Security Income (SSI), and Social Security Disability Insurance (SSDI) may not be accurately reported by respondents in the NHIS. As a result, they may not match estimates of program participation computed from the programs' administrative data. In addition, although the NHIS asks separately about participation in Medicaid and CHIP, estimates for the programs are not produced separately from the survey data for several reasons. For example, many states' CHIP and Medicaid programs use the same name, so respondents would not necessarily know whether their children's coverage was funded by Medicaid or CHIP. The separate survey questions are used to reduce surveys' undercount of Medicaid and CHIP enrollees, not to produce valid estimates separately for each program. Thus, survey estimates generally combine Medicaid and CHIP into a single category, as is done in Section 2 of MACStats.

Children with special health care needs

Tables 3–5 in MACStats present figures for children with special health care needs (CSHCN) who are enrolled in Medicaid or CHIP. As described here, MACPAC uses NHIS data to construct a CSHCN indicator based on responses to a number of questions contained in the survey.

CSHCN are defined by the Maternal and Child Health Bureau (MCHB) within the Health Resources and Services Administration as a group of children who "have or are at increased risk for a chronic physical, developmental, behavioral, or emotional condition and who also require health and related services of a type or amount beyond that required by children generally."[19] This definition is used by all states for policy and program planning purposes for CSHCN and encompasses children with disabilities and also children with chronic conditions (e.g., asthma, juvenile diabetes, sickle cell anemia) that range from mild to severe. Children with special health care needs are a broader group than children with conditions severe enough and family incomes so low as to qualify for SSI.[20] Table 3 shows that only 3.3 percent of children with Medicaid or CHIP receive SSI.

To operationalize the MCHB definition of CSHCN, researchers developed a set of survey questions referred to as the CSHCN Screener.[21] The CSHCN Screener is currently used in several national surveys, but not the NHIS. It incorporates four components of the definition of CSHCN considered by researchers as essential: functional limitations, need for health-related services, presence of a health condition, and minimum expected duration of health condition (e.g., 12 months).[22]

It should be noted that CSHCN can vary substantially in their health status and use of health care services. A CSHCN could be a child with intensive health care needs and high health care expenses who has severe functional limitations (e.g., spina bifida, paralysis) and would qualify for SSI if his or her family income were low enough.[23] On the other hand, a CSHCN could also be a child who has asthma, attention deficit disorder, or depression that is well managed through the use of prescription medications. Regardless of whether functional limitations are mild, moderate, or severe, however, CSHCN share a heightened need for health care services in order to maintain their health and to be able to function appropriately for their age.

Since the NHIS does not include the validated CSHCN Screener, MACPAC's analysis is based on an alternative approach developed by the Child and Adolescent Health Measurement Initiative (CAHMI 2012), specifically for use in the 2007 NHIS, and on other prior research.[24] The CAHMI definition of CSHCN (CAHMI uses the term "children with chronic conditions and elevated service use or need–CCCESUN") includes children with at least one diagnosed or parent-reported condition expected to be an ongoing health condition, and who also meet at least one of five criteria related to elevated service use or elevated need:

- is limited or prevented in his or her ability to do things most children of the same age can do;
- needs or uses medications prescribed by a doctor (other than vitamins);
- needs or uses specialized therapies such as physical, occupational, or speech therapy;
- has above-routine need or use of medical, mental health, home care, or education services; or
- needs or receives treatment or counseling for an emotional, behavioral, or developmental problem.[25]

The NHIS varies from year to year in the diagnoses and health conditions that parents are asked about, so establishing a consistent definition across the 2009–2011 NHIS data in this analysis required modifying the survey items used in the CAHMI construct of CSHCN. Estimates for CSHCN in this analysis are not directly comparable to those in prior MACPAC reports because the definition of CSHCN used here differs slightly from the one used previously.[26]

Understanding Managed Care Enrollment and Spending Data

There are four main sources of data on Medicaid managed care available from CMS.

- **Medicaid Managed Care Data Collection System (MMCDCS).** The MMCDCS provides state-reported aggregate enrollment statistics and other basic information for each managed care plan within a state. CMS uses the MMCDCS to create an annual Medicaid managed care enrollment report, which is the source of information on Medicaid managed care most commonly cited by CMS, as well as by outside analysts and researchers.[27] CMS also uses the MMCDCS to produce an annual summary of state Medicaid managed care programs that describes the managed care programs within a state (generally defined by the statutory authority under which they operate), each of which may include several managed care plans.[28]

- **Medicaid Statistical Information System (MSIS).** The MSIS provides person-level and claims-level information for all Medicaid enrollees.[29] With regard to managed care, the information collected for each enrollee includes: (1) plan ID numbers and types for up to four managed care plans (including comprehensive risk-based plans, primary care case management programs, and limited-benefit plans) under which the enrollee is covered, (2) the waiver ID number, if enrolled in a 1915(b) or other waiver, (3) claims that provide a record of each capitated payment made on behalf of the enrollee to a managed care plan (generally referred to as capitated claims), and (4) in some states, a record of each service received by the enrollee from a provider under contract with a managed care plan (which generally do not include a payment amount and are referred to as encounter or "dummy" claims). As discussed in Chapter 4, all states collect encounter data from their Medicaid managed care plans, but some do not report them in MSIS. Managed care enrollees may also have FFS claims in MSIS if they used services that were not included in their managed care plan's contract with the state.

- **CMS-64.** The CMS-64 provides aggregate spending information for Medicaid by major benefit categories, including managed care. The spending amounts reported by states on the CMS-64 are used to calculate their federal matching dollars.

- **Statistical Enrollment Data System (SEDS).** The SEDS provides aggregate statistics on CHIP enrollment and child Medicaid enrollment that include the number covered under FFS and managed care systems. SEDS is the only comprehensive source of information on managed care participation among separate CHIP enrollees across states.

In Tables 15 and 16, the statistics cited on managed care are from CMS's annual Medicaid managed care enrollment report. However, this enrollment report does not provide information on characteristics of enrollees in managed care aside from dual eligibility for Medicare (e.g., basis of eligibility and demographics such as age, sex, race, and ethnicity). It also does not include information on their spending and service use outside of managed care. As a result, we supplement statistics from the enrollment report with MSIS and CMS-64 data; for example, Tables 17 and 18 use MSIS data to show the percentage of various populations in managed care and the percentage of their Medicaid benefit spending accounted for by managed care.

When examining managed care statistics from various sources, the following issues should be noted:

- Figures in the annual Medicaid managed care enrollment report published by CMS include Medicaid-expansion CHIP enrollees. Although we generally exclude these children (about 2 million, depending on the time period) from Medicaid analyses, it is not possible to do so with the enrollment report data cited for Tables 15 and 16. Tables 17 and 18—which show the percentage of child, adult, disabled, aged, and dual-eligible enrollees who are enrolled in Medicaid managed care and the percentage of their Medicaid benefit spending that was for managed care—are based on MSIS data and exclude Medicaid-expansion CHIP enrollees.[30]

- The types of managed care reported by states may differ somewhat between the Medicaid managed care enrollment report and the MSIS. For example, some states report a small number of enrollees in comprehensive risk-based managed care in one data source but not the other (Tables 15 and 17). Anomalies in the MSIS data are documented by CMS as it reviews each state's quarterly submission, but not all issues may be identified in this process.[31]

- The Medicaid managed care enrollment report provides point-in-time figures (e.g., as of July 1, 2011). In contrast, CMS generally uses MSIS to report on the number of enrollees ever in managed care during a fiscal year (although point-in-time enrollment can also be calculated from MSIS based on the monthly data it contains).

Endnotes

[1] Medicaid and CHIP Payment and Access Commission (MACPAC), *Report to the Congress on Medicaid and CHIP,* March 2012 (Washington, DC: MACPAC, 2012): 87–89. http://www.macpac.gov/reports/.

[2] Table 19 is modeled after Table 1 in the March 2013 edition of MACStats (Medicaid and CHIP Payment and Access Commission (MACPAC), *Report to the Congress on Medicaid and CHIP,* March 2013 (Washington, DC: MACPAC, 2013): 75. http://www.macpac.gov/reports/). Table 1 of the March 2013 MACStats shows estimates for 2012 and is partly based on projections by the CMS Office of the Actuary. To produce the age breaks used in Tables 19–22, however, numbers were calculated by MACPAC directly from the MSIS. FY 2010 is the latest year for which data are available in MSIS for all but two states.

[3] MACPAC has adjusted benefit spending from MSIS to match CMS-64 totals; see the discussion later in Section 5 for details.

[4] Because administrative data are grouped by month, the point-in-time number from administrative data generally appears under a few different titles—average monthly enrollment, full-year equivalent enrollment, or person-years. Average monthly enrollment takes the state-submitted monthly enrollment numbers and averages them over the 12-month period. It produces the same result as full-year equivalent enrollment or person-years, which is the sum of the monthly enrollment totals divided by 12.

[5] See, for example, Centers for Medicare & Medicaid Services (CMS), Brief summaries and glossary in *Health care financing review 2010 statistical supplement* (Baltimore, MD: CMS, 2010). http://www.cms.gov/Research-Statistics-Data-and-Systems/Statistics-Trends-and-Reports/MedicareMedicaidStatSupp/Medicare-and-Medicaid-Statistical-Supplement-List.html.

[6] States make capitated payments for all individuals enrolled in managed care plans, even if no health care services are used. Therefore, all managed care enrollees are currently counted as beneficiaries, regardless of whether or not they have any health service use.

[7] Some individuals who are counted as beneficiaries in CMS data for a particular fiscal year were not enrolled in Medicaid during that year; they are individuals who were enrolled and received services in a prior year, but for whom a lagged payment was made in the following year. These individuals usually have an "unknown" basis of eligibility in CMS data.

[8] Analyses of growth in the number of Medicaid beneficiaries will sometimes refer to "enrollment growth" in a generic sense.

[9] Medicaid benefit spending reported here excludes amounts for Medicaid-expansion CHIP enrollees, the territories, administrative activities, the Vaccines for Children program (which is authorized by the Medicaid statute but operates as a separate program), and offsetting collections from third-party liability, estate, and other recoveries.

[10] For a discussion of these data sources, see Chapter 4 and Medicaid and CHIP Payment and Access Commission (MACPAC), Improving Medicaid and CHIP data for policy analysis and program accountability, in *Report to the Congress on Medicaid and CHIP,* March 2011 (Washington, DC: MACPAC, 2011). http://www.macpac.gov/reports/MACPAC_March2011_web.pdf.

[11] Some of these amounts, including disproportionate share hospital (DSH) and other supplemental payments, are lump sums not related to service use by an individual Medicaid enrollee. Nonetheless, we refer to these CMS-64 amounts as benefit spending, and the adjustment methodology described here distributes them across Medicaid enrollees with MSIS spending in the relevant service categories (e.g., hospital).

[12] Government Accountability Office (GAO), *Medicaid: Data sets provide inconsistent picture of expenditures* (Washington, DC: 2012). http://www.gao.gov/assets/650/649733.pdf; Administrative databases, in *Databases for estimating health insurance coverage for children: A workshop summary,* edited by T. Plewes (Washington, DC: The National Academies Press, 2010): 72. http://www.nap.edu/catalog/13024.html.

[13] The sum of adjusted MSIS benefit spending amounts for all service categories totals CMS-64 benefit spending, exclusive of offsetting collections from third-party liability, estate, and other recoveries. These collections, $6.8 billion in FY 2010, are not reported by type of service in the CMS-64 and are not reported at all in MSIS.

[14] Although the discussion in this section generally omits the term non-institutionalized for brevity, all estimates exclude individuals living in nursing homes and other institutional settings.

[15] Centers for Disease Control and Prevention (CDC), *About the National Health Interview Survey* (Atlanta, GA: CDC, 2012). http://www.cdc.gov/nchs/nhis/about_nhis.htm.

[16] The annual NHIS questionnaire consists of three major components—the Family Core, the Sample Adult Core, and the Sample Child Core. The Family Core collects information for all family members regarding household composition and socioeconomic and demographic characteristics, along with basic indicators of health status, activity limitation, and health insurance. The Sample Adult and Sample Child Cores obtain additional information on the health of one randomly selected adult and child in the family.

[17] Data were pooled to yield sufficiently large samples to produce reliable subgroup estimates and to increase the capacity to detect meaningful differences between subgroups and insurance categories.

[18] G. Kenney and V. Lynch, Monitoring children's health insurance coverage under CHIPRA using federal surveys, in *Databases for estimating health insurance coverage for children: A workshop summary,* edited by T. Plewes (Washington, DC: The National Academies Press, 2010): 72. http://www.nap.edu/catalog/13024.html.

[19] M. McPherson, et al., A new definition of children with special health care needs, *Pediatrics* 102 (1998): 137–140.

[20] For children under age 18 to be determined disabled under SSI rules, the child must have a medically determinable physical or mental impairment(s) that causes marked and severe functional limitations and that can be expected to cause death or last at least 12 months (§1614(a)(3)(C)(i) of the Social Security Act). For additional discussion of disability as determined under the SSI program and its interaction with Medicaid eligibility, see Chapter 1 in MACPAC's March 2012 report to the Congress.

[21] The CSHCN Screener was developed by CAHMI and is currently used in the National Survey of Children with Special Health Care Needs, the Medical Expenditure Panel Survey, and other federal surveys. For more information on the CSHCN Screener, see C.D. Bethell, D. Read, R.E. Stein, et al., Identifying children with special health care needs: Development and evaluation of a short screening instrument. *Ambulatory Pediatrics* 2 (2002): 38–48.

[22] Child and Adolescent Health Measurement Initiative (CAHMI), *Approaches to identifying children and adults with special health care needs: A resource manual for state Medicaid agencies and managed care organizations* (Baltimore, MD: Centers for Medicare and Medicaid Services, 2002).

[23] Children who are receiving SSI should meet the criteria for being a CSHCN; however, some do not. While we do not have enough information to assess the reasons that children who are reported to have SSI did not meet the criteria for CSHCN, it could be because: (1) the parent erroneously reported in the survey that the child received SSI, or (2) the NHIS condition list did not capture, or the parent did not recognize, any of the NHIS conditions as reflecting the child's health circumstances.

[24] Child and Adolescent Health Measurement Initiative (CAHMI), *Identifying children with chronic conditions and elevated service use or need (CCCESUN) in the National Health Interview Survey (NHIS)* (Portland, OR: Oregon Health and Science University, 2012); Davidoff, A.J., Identifying children with special health care needs in the National Health Interview Survey: A new resource for policy analysis. *Health Services Research* 39 (2004): 53–71.

[25] The CAHMI algorithm differs from the CSHCN Screener in three main respects (CAHMI 2012—see endnote 24 for source). First, the CSHCN Screener uses a non-condition specific approach, which identifies a broader range of children with chronic childhood conditions who have special needs. The CAHMI algorithm limits CSHCN to children identified by parents as having a specific diagnosis in a condition set collected in the NHIS. Second, the CSHCN Screener captures children with above routine use of medical and health services that is the result of an ongoing condition, based on brief follow-up questions. The NHIS does not include the duration of conditions or identify elevated service use or need directly related to each condition. Thus, the CAHMI algorithm collects data on elevated service use and need independent from the condition set. Third, the CAHMI algorithm identifies a small number of additional children as having elevated need when parents report an unmet need due to cost through one of three survey items. As a result of these differences, the children identified from the CAHMI algorithm in the NHIS are not equivalent in health and function characteristics to children identified by the CSHCN Screener in other surveys. The CAHMI criteria differ from criteria developed by Davidoff (2004—see endnote 24 for source) in that Davidoff does not recognize unmet need due to cost as part of the definition of elevated need.

[26] The algorithm in this analysis begins with the NHIS conditions referred to as the limited condition set by CAHMI (2012—see endnote 24 for source), then excludes seven conditions that were dropped in the 2011 NHIS (depression, learning disability, cancer, neurological problem, phobia or fears, gum disease, lung or breathing problem). To capture CSHCN potentially lost from this change and other children with a broader range of chronic conditions, affirmative responses to three other survey items were treated as qualifying conditions (has difficulties with emotions/concentration/behavior or getting along in last four weeks, has chronic condition that limits activity, and fair or poor health). These items were also added to better align the CSHCN definition with the 18-year-olds, whom the NHIS treats as adults. The NHIS Sample Adult Core contains slightly different condition items. In order to align the CSHCN definitions more closely, the condition set for 18-year-olds was expanded to add mental retardation or developmental problems that cause difficulty with activity, cancer, symptoms of depression in the past 30 days, fair or poor health, and any unspecified condition that causes functional limitation and is chronic. In the MACPAC analysis, two or more emergency department visits reported in the last 12 months was added as another measure of elevated service use.

[27] Centers for Medicare & Medicaid Services (CMS), *Medicaid managed care enrollment report* (Baltimore, MD: CMS). http://www.medicaid.gov/Medicaid-CHIP-Program-Information/By-Topics/Data-and-Systems/Medicaid-Managed-Care/Medicaid-Managed-Care-Enrollment-Report.html.

[28] Centers for Medicare & Medicaid Services (CMS), *National summary of state Medicaid managed care programs as of July 1, 2011* (Baltimore, MD: CMS). http://www.medicaid.gov/Medicaid-CHIP-Program-Information/By-Topics/Data-and-Systems/Medicaid-Managed-Care/State-Program-Descriptions.html.

[29] For enrollees with no paid claims during a given period (e.g., fiscal year), their MSIS data are limited to person-level information (e.g., basis of eligibility, age, sex, etc.).

[30] We generally exclude Medicaid-expansion CHIP children from Medicaid analyses because their funding stream (CHIP, under Title XXI of the Social Security Act) differs from that of other Medicaid enrollees (Medicaid, under Title XIX). In addition, spending (and often enrollment) for the Medicaid-expansion CHIP population is reported by CMS in CHIP statistics, along with information on separate CHIP enrollees.

[31] See Centers for Medicare & Medicaid Services (CMS), *MSIS state data characteristics/anomalies report,* January 7, 2013 (Baltimore, MD: CMS, 2013). http://www.cms.gov/Research-Statistics-Data-and-Systems/Computer-Data-and-Systems/MedicaidDataSourcesGenInfo/downloads/anomalies1.pdf.

CHAPTER 3

Access to Care for Persons with Disabilities

Key Points

Access to Care for Persons with Disabilities

- This chapter summarizes a literature review on access to care for non-institutionalized adults with disabilities under age 65 who are Medicaid-only enrollees, a group with a wide range of health care needs and functional limitations. We found little research directly examining access to acute care for our study population and therefore reviewed a wider range of studies based on large-scale population surveys, provider and stakeholder data, consumer interviews and other qualitative data, and state Medicaid program data.

- Access to health care among Medicaid-only enrollees with disabilities is comparable to that of other insured persons with disabilities, based on large-scale population survey data.

- Unmet need among Medicaid-only enrollees with disabilities is lower compared to individuals with disabilities covered by private insurance or Medicare-only, based on survey data. Preventive services are potentially underused among Medicaid enrollees with disabilities, though findings vary by service.

- Interviews with providers, plans, and other stakeholders share three areas of concern: 1) disability competency training in medical schools for non-pediatric specialists; 2) accessibility of equipment and services; and 3) access to dental services. However, studies specific to Medicaid are rare and leave an unclear picture of access for our study population.

- Several access barriers figure prominently in qualitative studies of adults with disabilities: 1) scheduling appointments and receiving timely primary care; 2) communication with providers and staff; 3) accessibility of health care facilities and services; 4) finding a doctor who understands their disability; and 5) transportation. However, these experiences may not be representative of experiences among Medicaid enrollees with disabilities.

- Studies using state Medicaid program data provide little information on access to care for Medicaid enrollees with disabilities. Studies do not have comparison groups with other forms of coverage and include no data on service use prior to enrollment.

- Further research is needed on: 1) the impact of enabling services on access to care; 2) disability competency and accessibility in Medicaid provider networks; and 3) evaluation and best practices in risk-based managed care. Additional areas of research are the role of non-physician practitioners in access to care for subpopulations with disabilities, and best practices in service delivery.

CHAPTER 3

Access to Care for Persons with Disabilities

Medicaid enrollees under age 65 with disabilities are a heterogeneous population with a wide range of health care needs and functional limitations, including mobility and cognitive limitations, difficulty with self-care, and difficulty participating in everyday activities (KCMU 2011, Allen et al. 2000). They include persons with genetic disorders, such as Down syndrome; persons with traumatic brain injury and spinal cord injury; and persons with disabilities stemming from degenerative diseases, chronic diseases, and serious mental illnesses.

This chapter presents information from a literature review on access to care for adults with disabilities under age 65, with a specific focus on non-institutionalized individuals enrolled in Medicaid and not dually enrolled in Medicare. Medicaid-only enrollees constitute over 60 percent of individuals under age 65 who are eligible for Medicaid on the basis of disability (MACPAC 2012).[1]

Persons with disabilities require a wide range of services to address the underlying causes of disabilities as well as co-occurring conditions prevalent in this population, especially mental illness.[2] Nearly half of Medicaid-only enrollees qualifying on the basis of disability have a mental illness such as depression, schizophrenia, or bipolar disorder (Kronick et al. 2009). The prevalence of mental illness is even higher among enrollees with physical health conditions (Kronick et al. 2007). Among enrollees who have one of the five most common physical conditions, approximately two-thirds also have a mental illness (Boyd et al. 2010).[3]

Providing appropriate access to care for this population is relatively challenging because a broad range of services may be needed, and each provider must accommodate the unique needs related to an individual's disability and consider the cause and nature of the disability in treatment plans.

Scope of Literature Review

Study population. In our review, we found little research directly examining persons with disabilities enrolled only in Medicaid and therefore we reviewed a wider range of studies to learn about access in selected care settings or among persons with a common disability (e.g., intellectual disabilities). Throughout this chapter, we note which studies provide evidence specifically for our study population—persons with disabilities under age 65 enrolled in Medicaid only—and which provide evidence for a more general population.

Services. The health services we examined are broadly defined as acute care services and included acute care hospital services, physician and non-physician practitioner services (including primary care), dental services, prescription drugs, and imaging and laboratory testing. These acute care services accounted for 74 percent of Medicaid spending for this population in fiscal year 2008 (MACPAC 2012).

Persons with disabilities may also need other services not examined here in order to maintain function and independence. These services—referred to as long-term services and supports (LTSS)—usually include home health, durable medical equipment, personal attendant care, residential habilitation, minor home modifications, and other services. Average Medicaid spending on LTSS for Medicaid-only enrollees is relatively low compared to spending on acute care services (MACPAC 2012), and only a small share (16 percent) of the Medicaid-only population with disabilities uses Medicaid-covered LTSS (MACPAC 2013).

Sources. We reviewed published studies and critical reviews on access to care for adults with disabilities under age 65, drawing from quantitative and qualitative research. These sources included peer-reviewed journals, federal and state government sources, independent federal agencies or advisory bodies, and web-based published literature from universities and non-partisan independent research organizations and foundations.

A Framework for Examining Access to Health Care

The access framework previously developed by MACPAC informs this assessment of the literature on access. The framework recognizes three main elements of a health care coverage program as essential to examining access to care: (1) the unique characteristics of enrollees, (2) provider availability and other health care system arrangements, and (3) utilization or realized access, including enrollees' experiences with the health care system (MACPAC 2011). For the purposes of this review, we first briefly summarize the unique characteristics of the population of interest, and then look more systematically at the current knowledge and supporting evidence of the factors influencing provider availability and service use as they relate to enrollees with disabilities.

Characteristics of the Population

The health characteristics and health needs of persons with disabilities in Medicaid vary widely. Importantly, having a disability is not equivalent to ill-health or incapacity. Persons with disabilities can be both healthy and well (CDC 2005). Some persons with disabilities have a disability that is stable and unrelated to any chronic disease process (e.g., deafness present at birth) (CDC 2005). Other individuals are medically fragile or have a medically complex disease or disorder underlying the disability. In these cases, inattention to routine or minor medical problems can result in further functional decline or life-threatening infections and other complications (CDC 2005, Neri and Kroll 2003, Rimmer 1999).

Health needs and risk factors

Persons with disabilities often have health and medical needs stemming from the disability itself, an underlying condition, or common risk factors and co-occurring conditions. Among Medicaid-only enrollees with disabilities, there is a high prevalence of cardiovascular and central nervous system diseases, in addition to mental and behavioral diagnoses (Kronick et al. 2009).

To address these health needs and risk factors appropriately, some patients may require special equipment or additional time with practitioners. For other patients, time and equipment may not be a factor. Instead, practitioners may need specialized training or need to tailor the clinical process or communication strategy to meet the patient's clinical needs.

Selected examples of the health needs and risk factors common to persons with specific disabilities include the following:

- Persons with intellectual disabilities have difficulty recognizing and communicating symptoms (DFCM 2011), are at increased risk of osteoporosis (Fisher and Kettl 2005, Center et al. 1998), and are highly susceptible to dental disease (Fisher 2012).
- Persons with neurodevelopmental disabilities such as cerebral palsy may be medically complex and require ongoing care from specialists, they may take medications that increase fall risk, and physicians may encounter challenges attributing symptoms to the disabling condition or another emerging condition (DFCM 2011).
- Individuals with spinal cord injury and those dependent on wheelchairs are at risk of osteoporosis, bowel dysfunction, and loss of muscle tone. An inability to feel pain (due to paralysis) places these individuals at risk of unknowingly injuring themselves and developing major infections (McColl et al. 2008, CDC 2005).

Prevention and wellness

Persons with disabilities have the same general need for health prevention and wellness services as persons without disabilities (McColl et al. 2008, CDC 2005). In addition, prevention of secondary conditions and the maintenance of functional independence are vitally important to the well-being of persons with disabilities. Health prevention services for adults and youth with disabilities may include prescribing exercise in a health care setting, and counseling and guidance to change eating habits or take measures to avoid injury (CDC 2005).[4]

Women with disabilities require the full spectrum of reproductive and family planning health care services, just as women without disabilities do. For older women, this would include information related to menopause, including osteoporosis and insomnia (NCD 2009, Wilkinson and Cerreto 2008).

Socioeconomic characteristics

Individuals with disabilities are more likely than non-disabled individuals to face socioeconomic disadvantages that create additional challenges to obtaining medical care, and this is true within the Medicaid population as well.

Income and education. Medicaid enrollees with disabilities are more likely than enrollees without disabilities to face economic and educational disadvantages. Adults receiving Supplemental Security Income (SSI) and enrolled in Medicaid are among the poorest Medicaid enrollees, and just over 40 percent have no high school degree.[5]

In addition, low health literacy and lack of English language proficiency are also challenges.

Health literacy. Health literacy—the ability to read and understand health care information—is reported to be a common challenge within disabled populations (NCD 2009). Low literacy may stem from difficulties with communication over a lifetime related to auditory processing disabilities, cognitive limitations, and neuromuscular limitations (NCD 2012).

People with specific disabilities that limit the ability to read (e.g., blindness, traumatic brain injury, stroke, Down syndrome, cerebral palsy) may have difficulty understanding written materials (NCD 2012). People who are deaf or hard-of-hearing may lack exposure to the popular media due to the auditory format, which limits the opportunity to learn about health promotion activities or health services (Steinberg et al. 1998).

Individuals with low health literacy are less likely to be responsive to health education, to use disease prevention services, and to successfully manage their chronic illnesses (Dewalt et al. 2004).

English proficiency. Lack of English proficiency can be an additional barrier for persons whose primary language is American Sign Language (ASL) or Braille. ASL and Braille are recognized as "succinct and separate from English under federal regulation and guidance."[6] ASL does not have a written form and does not have syntax equivalent to English syntax (NCD 2012). ASL does not have signs for many common medical terms like "cholesterol." Deaf individuals who use ASL as their primary language may lack English proficiency and have low health literacy as a result. A survey among deaf individuals in Chicago found that one-third could not define the word "cancer" (Margellos et al. 2004).

A Review of Research Findings on Access to Care

Information about access to care among persons with disabilities enrolled in Medicaid is based primarily on four kinds of data sources: (1) large-scale population surveys, (2) provider and stakeholder data, (3) consumer interviews and other qualitative data, and (4) state Medicaid program data. The summary of the research presented in this section is organized into four subsections based on each of these four types of data sources. Given that research studies from common types of sources often share the same limitations in the scope and generalizability of their findings, each subsection of this chapter concludes with a discussion about the strengths and limitations of the literature with respect to this chapter's objective.

Findings from large-scale population surveys

Several large-scale population surveys have supported general research on access to care for non-institutionalized individuals with disabilities. Two federal surveys permit comparisons between individuals covered by Medicaid and individuals with other forms of health coverage. The National Health Interview Survey (NHIS) can produce national and state-level estimates (NCHS 2010), while the Medical Expenditure Panel Survey (MEPS) is designed to be nationally representative (AHRQ 2009). The survey items on disability in the NHIS and in the household component of the MEPS allow a variety of definitions of disability with respect to degree of dependency, domains of disability, and source of disability (NCHS 2010).[7] The surveys collect data on respondents' limitations in activities of daily living (e.g., dressing) and functional activities (e.g., climbing a flight of stairs); impairments in mobility, cognition, vision, and hearing; as well as conditions that cause these limitations.

Although the NHIS and the MEPS differ somewhat in wording and scope of questions, both surveys ask about the respondent's experiences with regular providers and about barriers to care. Specifically, surveys collect self-reported data about characteristics of the respondent's usual place of care; reasons for not having one; problems experienced obtaining needed medical, mental health, dental, and prescription care; and reasons for not getting needed care, as examples. Both the NHIS and the MEPS also collect self-reported data on utilization of preventive visits and preventive care, doctor visits, emergency department visits, inpatient hospital stays, and contact with other providers (AHRQ 2011, NCHS 2010).

The Behavioral Risk Factors Surveillance System (BRFSS) was established by the Centers for Disease Control and Prevention and is fielded on an ongoing basis by all 50 states, the District of Columbia, and the U.S. Territories. The BRFSS provides state estimates of basic access measures for individuals with activity limitations. It does not capture Medicaid coverage but allows comparison between individuals with public, private, and no coverage (CDC 2012). Three other national surveys are no longer fielded, but have supported analysis cited in this review (Box 3-1).

There are few studies that focus specifically on Medicaid enrollees with disabilities under age 65 that draw data from large-scale surveys. However, when complemented by additional studies of the broader population of adults with disabilities, survey analyses consistently draw the same conclusions about persons with disabilities enrolled in Medicaid. These conclusions are summarized below.

BOX 3-1. Other Large-Scale Surveys Supporting Analyses of Medicaid Enrollees with Disabilities Cited in This Chapter

National Survey of SSI Children and Families (NSCF). This nationally representative survey of current and former recipients of Supplemental Security Income (SSI) was last fielded from 2001 to 2002 (SSA 2012). The NSCF provided a rich source of information on health services use and access to care among children and young adults in the SSI program (and enrolled in Medicaid) and a comparison group of young adults who had recently exited the program (former Medicaid enrollees).

Henry J. Kaiser Family Foundation (KFF)/ICR 2003 Survey. This one-time national telephone survey of adults ages 18 through 64 with permanent physical and mental disabilities was fielded from 2002 to 2003 for the purpose of comparing access to care and unmet needs for persons with severe disabilities based on source of insurance coverage (KFF 2003).

National Survey of American Families (NSAF). This national survey was fielded in 1997, 1999, and 2003 by the Urban Institute as part of its Assessing the New Federalism project. The NSAF provided national and state-level estimates (for 13 states) of adults and children with different forms of health insurance coverage, including Medicaid. The NSAF captured disability through a question on work limitations and included a rich set of questions about access to care and service use, as well as other topics (Coughlin et al. 2005).

Access to health care among persons with disabilities enrolled in Medicaid is comparable to that of persons with other sources of coverage. The percentage of individuals reporting that they have a usual place to go when they need care or have a regular doctor are commonly cited measures of potential access to care. In a national survey of persons with severe and permanent disabilities, the percentage of persons who reported having no regular doctor was the same— 15 percent—for persons with Medicaid-only coverage, persons with Medicare-only or private-only insurance, and those dually enrolled in Medicare and Medicaid (Hanson et al. 2003). Persons with Medicare and supplemental private insurance had the lowest percentage (7 percent) with no regular doctor. In contrast, 69 percent of uninsured persons with disabilities had no regular doctor.

Medicaid enrollees appear to face similar challenges as persons with Medicare and private coverage in finding a regular doctor whom they perceive as competent to treat them. In the same study, the percentage of Medicaid-only respondents who reported trouble finding a doctor who understood their disability (25 percent) was not significantly different from respondents with other forms of coverage (Hanson et al. 2003).

Studies also show that a greater or equal percentage of persons with disabilities report having a usual source of care relative to persons without disabilities but with similar incomes, education, and health conditions (NCHS 2008, Iezzoni and O'Day 2006). However, few studies have controlled adequately for age and insurance type (Coughlin et al. 2008, Parish and Ellison-Martin 2007).

For some persons with disabilities, the lack of a usual source of care may have serious health consequences. Young adults with developmental disabilities are an especially vulnerable population because they rely on an array of public programs and services, frequently face challenges being actively engaged as patients, and upon adulthood must leave specialized pediatric clinics familiar with their condition and find adult care physicians who can meet their unique care needs (DFCM 2009). For such vulnerable groups, having no established source of care might signal disruptions in care that could present particular risks.

Unmet need among persons with disabilities enrolled in Medicaid is lower compared to those with other sources of coverage. Studies comparing persons with disabilities covered by Medicaid to those covered by private insurance or Medicare, or who are uninsured show Medicaid reduces unmet need and unmet need due to cost. A national study of youth with disabilities transitioning into adulthood estimated that continuing Medicaid coverage after age 18 had a major impact on access to care (Hemmeter 2011). The study analyzed the experiences of SSI recipients after turning age 18 and found that, relative to youth who continued Medicaid insurance after age 18, the uninsured were 42 percentage points more likely to report an unmet medical need, 33 percentage points more likely to report an unmet dental need, and 27 percentage points more likely to report an unmet prescription drug need.

In another study of working-age persons with severe and permanent disabilities, those with Medicaid-only coverage were significantly less likely than those with either Medicare-only or private insurance to report postponing care or skimping on medications due to cost (Hanson et al. 2003). Medicare-only enrollees were more than 12 times as likely as Medicaid-only enrollees to postpone care due to cost, despite the fact that Medicaid-only enrollees in this sample were much poorer. Having unmet need has been linked to higher use of hospital care and emergency departments in the following year among disabled Medicaid enrollees (Long et al. 2005).

Unmet need among persons with disabilities enrolled in Medicaid is higher than among Medicaid enrollees without disabilities. In a national sample of working-age women from the 1999 National Survey of American Families, women with work limitations who were covered by Medicaid reported lower rates of receiving medical care and medications when needed, were less likely to have cervical cancer screenings, and were less satisfied with their care than were other women covered by Medicaid, controlling for the usual type of care reported (Parish and Ellison-Martin 2007).

In a 2003 national telephone survey of working-age adults with severe and permanent disabilities, one-fourth of adults covered by Medicaid reported having postponed care, 40 percent had gone without needed equipment, and 28 percent had skipped doses of their medications (Hanson et al. 2003). Studies have also identified disparities in access between Medicare enrollees with and without disabilities (Iezzoni et al. 2003) and among the uninsured with and without disabilities (Sommers 2006). Among persons with disabilities, those with greater impairment report more unmet need and difficulty accessing care than do those with less impairment (Sommers 2006, Long et al. 2002).

Use of many health services among persons with disabilities enrolled in Medicaid is high compared to service use among those without disabilities. A recent national study of working-age adults with disabilities found that having a disability is associated with more difficulty accessing needed care, higher emergency department use, and higher hospitalization rates than having multiple conditions but no disability (Gully et al. 2011). According to these data, persons with disabilities also reported more chronic and acute conditions, obesity, physical inactivity, and smoking when compared to persons without disabilities. The same study found substantially higher ambulatory health care visits to a wider array of physicians and other providers among persons with disabilities than among those with no disability but similar health conditions. This pattern of high physician contact and high unmet need among persons with disabilities is documented in other surveys as well (Gully and Altman 2008).

Studies have also reported higher hospital readmission rates among Medicaid and other insured beneficiaries with disabilities relative to their counterparts without disabilities (Sommers and Cunningham 2011, Gilmer and Hamblin 2010). Lack of engagement among patients and their community providers may contribute to high hospitalization rates. Both readmission studies found that a significant share of Medicaid patients did not have a physician visit within 30 days after discharge.

Other research has estimated that the independent effect of disability doubles the risk of high use of services, after accounting for chronic conditions and disease severity (McColl and Shortt 2006). The authors attribute the higher consumption of services to needs directly related to the disability, as well as conditions exacerbated by social factors.

Preventive services are potentially underused among Medicaid enrollees with disabilities, though findings vary by service. The possible exception to the pattern of high use documented above is preventive services. In the few surveys that support comparisons in preventive screenings, women with disabilities have consistently reported lower rates of routine screening for breast cancer and cervical cancer than have women without disabilities (Armour et al. 2009, Parish and Ellison-Martin 2007, Smeltzer 2006, Wei et al. 2006, Ramirez et al. 2005). A similar pattern is apparent with respect to PSA tests for prostate cancer among men with and without disabilities (Ramirez et al. 2005). Only one of these studies tested and found statistically significant disparities among Medicaid enrollees (Parish and Ellison-Martin 2007). In one national study, women with disabilities were more likely than those without disabilities to receive influenza immunizations, cholesterol screenings, and colorectal screenings after controlling for insurance status (Wei et al. 2006). None of these studies directly compared the experiences of persons with disabilities enrolled in Medicaid to similarly disabled individuals with private insurance.

Findings are inconclusive regarding the effect of Medicaid managed care on access to care among persons with disabilities. Most states have only recently begun to transition a large share of adults with disabilities into partial or full-risk managed care (MACPAC 2011, Gifford and Paradise 2011). The only two national studies that have examined the experiences of persons with disabilities in managed care report conflicting results. Using survey data from 1996 to 2004, Burns (2009) found that adults with disabilities in counties with mandatory Medicaid managed care were more likely to wait over 30 minutes to see a provider or report a problem accessing a specialist, and less likely to receive a flu shot, relative to adults with disabilities living in counties with voluntary managed care or fee for service (FFS).

Using other survey data from the same time period, Coughlin and colleagues (2008) found that adult Medicaid enrollees with disabilities living in urban counties with Medicaid managed care reported better access to care than their FFS counterparts on three measures: (1) having a usual source of preventive care, (2) contact with a general medical doctor or specialist, and (3) receipt of flu shots. The study found no improvement in the use of other preventive services, and no gains in access in rural managed care counties.

Neither study could capture enrollment in managed care at the individual level and instead used county-level managed care status as a proxy for individual experience. In one study of California's voluntary Medicaid managed care program in which individual enrollment was observed, there were no differences in any measures of access to care or quality of care for Medicaid enrollees who enrolled voluntarily into managed care compared to those who remained in FFS (Graham et al. 2011).

Limitations of large-scale population surveys

Population surveys typically used in national studies of access to health care are limited in their ability to explain why individuals experience barriers to care because these sources do not measure such details as the percentage of individuals who delayed care or reported unmet need due to lack of accommodation for a disability.

With respect to the performance of managed care plans, research based on population surveys can provide only the broadest picture of the access experience and does not identify plan-level factors that could drive results (e.g., member services such as case management or transportation, and enrollee use of these services). In summary, national studies to date on access to care among persons with disabilities have consistently identified overall patterns that would benefit from further investigation into the factors driving them. These patterns include: (1) high unmet need, (2) high utilization rates, and (3) low preventive care use.

Findings from provider and stakeholder data

A small number of statewide provider surveys have captured providers' perceptions of access to medical facilities and clinical practices for persons with disabilities. Other studies have drawn on in-depth interviews with primary care physicians (McColl et al. 2008) and other key informants—such as subject matter experts, non-physician providers, health plans, program managers, and agency directors—to identify critical barriers to access and quality of care for persons with disabilities (Engquist et al. 2012, NCD 2009, Harder and Company 2008). These stakeholders share three areas of concern summarized below.

Disability competency training in medical schools for non-pediatric specialties. Disability competency in the medical setting refers to several aspects of care, including how to perform basic procedures; disability-specific clinical training, such as awareness of atypical risk factors; cultural competency in the treatment of persons with disabilities; and gaining experience in the diagnosis and treatment of persons with a variety of disabilities.

In its 2009 report, the National Council on Disability concluded: "The absence of professional training on disability competency issues for health care practitioners is one of the most significant barriers that prevent persons with disabilities from receiving appropriate and effective health care" (NCD 2009). This conclusion was based on a literature review and interviews with subject matter experts, including federal agency officials and health care practitioners. A workgroup of California stakeholders, including representatives from county health departments, health plans, clinicians, and community-based organizations drew similar conclusions (Harder and Company 2008).

Surveys of practicing physicians provide additional support for closer attention to disability competency in medical school curriculum; however, none of the data gathered pertains specifically to Medicaid providers. A 2003 survey of primary care physicians in California found that, among those interacting with persons with physical disabilities, 68 percent had not received education or training on physical disability issues (McNeal et al. 2002). A 2004 survey of primary care physicians in Connecticut found that 91 percent of physicians treating adults with intellectual disabilities had no formal training in the care of this population (Kerins et al. 2004).

A 2001 survey of diverse health care delivery sites across Massachusetts provides a somewhat different picture (Bachman et al. 2006). The large majority of responding sites served persons with disabilities on a daily or weekly basis. Three-quarters of the responding providers reported they had received training in disability-related issues over the previous year, including cognitive impairments, severe psychiatric impairments, and communication impairments.

Accessibility of medical equipment and service delivery processes. Provider surveys that have collected information on providers' perceptions of the accessibility of facilities indicate that medical equipment and delivery processes that are not disability-compliant continue to persist as barriers to care (NCD 2009, Harder and Company 2008, McNeal et al. 2002). Three 2006 case studies of tertiary care hospitals found a range of deficiencies related to accessibility, including lack of accessible call systems, diagnostic equipment, and examination tables (Kirschner et al. 2007). This finding is consistent with qualitative interviews with consumers reporting a lack of accommodation in medical settings (Wilkinson et al. 2011, Scheer et al. 2003).

In a recently published "secret shopper" survey of 256 subspecialty practices in four U.S. cities, only 9 percent of practices reported the ability to use a height-adjustable table or mechanical lift to accommodate a patient in a wheelchair unable to self-transfer (Lagu et al. 2013). Another 40 percent could schedule appointments with such patients, but reported the patient would be transferred manually to a standard table, and 29 percent offered to examine the patient without transfer.[8, 9] The remaining 22 percent of the practices reported they would not schedule appointments with such patients, explaining that they could not accommodate patients in wheelchairs unable to self-transfer or that the building was inaccessible.[10]

Access to dental services. The oral health needs among persons with disabilities is high. Research documents a combination of high incidence of oral disease, poor oral hygiene, and greater treatment needs in this population (HRSA 2001).

Quantitative data documenting access to dental services nationwide for adults with disabilities enrolled in Medicaid is scant (Stiefel 2002) due in part to the limited scope of adult dental benefits in most state Medicaid programs (Wall 2012, McGinn-Shapiro 2008). Specialty care dentists and other provider advocates have raised concern that access to dental services is poor for adults with disabilities (Waldman and Perlman 2012), and unmet need for dental care is high (Fisher 2012).

Studies of broader populations inclusive of the study population are consistent with this assertion but do not directly answer this question. In one qualitative study, persons with disabilities generally reported difficulty finding a dentist willing to treat them (Drainoni et al. 2006). In a national analysis of outpatient visit data, a significant number of individuals in the United States, including those covered by private insurance and Medicaid, were found to have sought care for avoidable dental problems in hospital emergency rooms (Elangovan et al. 2011, Nalliah et al. 2010). In another nationwide study comparing Medicaid-covered adults to low-income privately insured adults, Medicaid-covered adults reported poorer access to dental services (Coughlin et al. 2005). Neither study was specific to persons with disabilities covered by Medicaid.

Poor access is generally attributed to: documented evidence of the small number of dentists who are trained to provide specialty care dentistry to persons with developmental disabilities (Waldman and Perlman 2012); inadequate training in general dentistry education on treating persons with special health care needs (Davis 2009); and the small share of dentists who participate in Medicaid (GAO 2010).

Limitations of provider and stakeholder data

Data from physicians, other providers, and stakeholders complement data collected from consumers on access issues and help form a clearer picture of delivery- and program-level barriers to receiving appropriate, quality care, as well as interventions that have facilitated access to care. Provider studies specific to the Medicaid program, however, are sparse and other studies are dated, leaving an unclear picture of the current state of access to care for persons with disabilities enrolled in Medicaid. Another limitation of provider surveys is that person-level estimates cannot be derived. Thus, the proportion of Medicaid enrollees who are served by physicians with disability competency (or other characteristics) cannot be estimated from them.

Findings from consumer interviews

Qualitative studies using in-depth interviews and focus groups of consumers with disabilities provide insights into the barriers that individuals confront, and the mechanisms by which individuals' disability characteristics and related factors (e.g., poverty) compound the daily challenges they face in meeting their health and medical needs (Drainoni et al. 2006, Iezzoni and O'Day 2006, Iezzoni et al. 2006, Iezzoni et al. 2003, Neri and Kroll 2003, Scheer et al. 2003). Participants were usually recruited on a voluntary basis from multiple sites in a selected community to seek a diversity of perspectives. Study participants were also recruited based on characteristics such as their disability attributes, income, insurance status, age, race, managed care enrollment, or geography to represent individuals with different experiences with the health system. Almost all of these studies include individuals with a mix of sources of insurance coverage and little ability to stratify by source, and thus do not allow detailed analysis of the experiences of those with Medicaid coverage.

Several access barriers figure prominently in qualitative studies of adults with disabilities and are summarized below. However, most findings on this topic do not establish the barriers most common to Medicaid enrollees with disabilities. Moreover, qualitative studies are not designed to assess the relative importance of these barriers. As a result, these studies simply identify barriers that need to be investigated further to establish their importance for Medicaid program management.

Scheduling appointments and receiving timely primary care. In several qualitative studies, some persons with disabilities describe multiple barriers when scheduling appointments, including problems finding a doctor who accepts Medicaid and difficulties getting an appointment in a timely manner (Drainoni et al. 2006, Scheer et al. 2003). Difficulty getting an appointment can be related to the challenge of finding a facility that can provide physical access for a procedure or test, with one study pointing to the accessibility of dental services as a significant challenge (Drainoni et al. 2006).

Factors reportedly contributing to delays in getting timely care have been fear or distrust of one's physician based on prior negative encounters, or known problems with an inaccessible provider office, leading patients to avoid seeking needed medical care in the first place (Drainoni et al. 2006, Neri and Kroll 2003). Other factors relate to process or practice at the provider's office, including staff untrained in the use of text telephone (TTY), telephone menu options that do not accommodate a relay service, and lack of same-day appointments (Drainoni et al. 2006, Neri and Kroll 2003).[11]

The same studies have also documented serious health consequences that some persons with disabilities have suffered when small issues were not addressed in a timely manner, leading to unnecessary hospitalizations, avoidable surgeries, and permanent losses of function in some cases (Drainoni et al. 2006, Neri and Kroll 2003), with the frequency of these consequences unknown.

Communication with providers and support staff. Communication difficulties may complicate the scheduling of appointments, completing a visit with a provider, and obtaining appropriate care during a visit or procedure. Persons with disabilities have described communication barriers with staff and practitioners due to the lack of auxiliary aids, lack of interpreters, and staff untrained in the use of TTY phone systems for the deaf or hearing-impaired (Drainoni et al. 2006, Iezzoni et al. 2004). Rushed physicians or short appointment slots can also be barriers to obtaining appropriate care for persons with other disabilities, simply due to the complexity of their health care needs and the additional time needed to address all of their concerns (McColl et al. 2008, Drainoni et al. 2006).[12]

Communication difficulties can pose challenges for individuals whose primary language is ASL or Braille; persons who are hard-of-hearing; and persons with cognitive impairment, neuromuscular disorders, or voice and speech disorders (e.g., traumatic brain injury, stroke, cerebral palsy) who depend on alternative methods and devices to communicate.[13] To effectively communicate with these patients, providers may need to modify their own speech, written materials may need to be adapted to accessible formats, and alternative modalities such as video, photos, or demonstration may need to be used to relay important health information (NCD 2012).

For persons who are deaf or hard-of-hearing, repeated communication difficulties can lead to fear and mistrust of practitioners in general (Steinberg et al. 2006). Lack of adequate communication assistance has been documented by consumers in specific cases to have led to allergic reactions, fear for safety and confusion during and after procedures, and medication errors (Drainoni et al. 2006).

Physical accessibility of health care facilities and services. Persons with disabilities, without respect to insurance status and source of coverage, describe physical barriers to accessing medical facilities (Iezzoni et al. 2006). Persons with mobility impairments report additional barriers once inside provider offices due to the physical layout of the facility, inaccessible equipment, and lack of adaptive devices. Examples include exam rooms that are too small to accommodate a wheelchair, exam tables and diagnostic equipment that are not height-adjustable (Iezzoni and O'Day 2006), weight scales that do not accommodate a wheelchair (Iezzoni et al. 2010), and lack of nurse call bells or bed adjustment controls (Drainoni et al. 2006). Patients report fears of being injured when being lifted from a wheelchair if they cannot transfer themselves (Iezzoni et al. 2010).

Inaccessible equipment in office-based practices is one reason cited by physicians for refusing to schedule appointments for persons with disabilities, and thus may contribute to patients' difficulties in finding a doctor (Lagu et al. 2013). Mammography and other x-ray machines that do not accommodate persons with a range of mobility impairments and the absence of height-adjustable exam tables are described by women with disabilities as a barrier to obtaining screenings for breast and cervical cancer (Wilkinson et al. 2011, Mele et al. 2005), and as a barrier to obtaining treatment for breast cancer (Iezzoni et al. 2010).

Finding a doctor who understands their disability. Physicians' understanding of patients' disabilities encompasses several aspects of care, including how to perform basic procedures, knowledge of each patient's unique medical history, and disability-specific clinical training, such as cultural competence and experience distinguishing symptoms directly related to the underlying disability from those related to an emerging medical problem.

Persons with disabilities interviewed in depth describe difficulties finding physicians who understand their disabilities (Iezzoni et al. 2006). They also describe physicians' misconceptions about persons with disabilities and their health needs (Wilkinson and Cerreto 2008, Drainoni et al. 2006), and in specific cases, health problems that have gone undetected due to lack of training or clinical experience (Scheer et al. 2003).

Transportation to provider settings. Some persons with disabilities identify transportation as an issue in accessing primary and specialty care practices (Scheer et al. 2003). Transportation is reported to be a challenge for individuals with different kinds of disabilities across regions, especially for persons with mobility impairments (Iezzoni and O'Day 2006) and persons with intellectual disabilities (Havercamp et al. 2004).

As rural communities often lack extensive public transportation, persons with disabilities living in these areas may be more dependent on family or friends to drive them. Individuals living in rural areas have also reported difficulty gaining access to medical facilities in older buildings (Iezzoni et al. 2006).

Limitations of consumer interview data

In general, qualitative studies using voluntary methods of recruitment are subject to participant bias, in which those choosing to participate may place higher value on the subject matter of the study or offer perspectives different in scope or intensity from those of people who could have been chosen randomly from the wider population. Studies advertised as an opportunity to discuss problems with access to care may attract individuals with a poor history of access.

In many cases, qualitative studies provide the only information about certain barriers to care. Surveys do not collect the same details about barriers (e.g., the percentage of persons who missed an appointment due to unreliable transportation services). Without such representative data, it is not possible to draw conclusions as to how common these barriers are for persons with disabilities (e.g., what percentage of individuals confront inaccessible facilities or equipment when seeking appointments, what percentage of individuals delay care due to provider difficulty scheduling a certified interpreter). Finally, little is known about the extent to which individuals successfully overcome these barriers and obtain needed care.

State Medicaid program data

Studies using Medicaid program data usually examine the experience of program enrollees in one state or locale (Blecker et al. 2010, Allen et al. 2009, Banta et al. 2009, Long et al. 2005, Mitchell et al. 2004, Long et al. 2002), a subpopulation eligible for certain services or waiver programs (Chalmers et al. 2011, Bershadsky and Kane 2010, Hall et al. 2007, Krahn et al. 2007, Krahn et al. 2006), or enrollees eligible for managed care (Graham et al. 2011, Burns 2009, Coughlin et al. 2008). These studies draw from medical claims and encounters or other program data to describe participation, service levels, or referral rates, and some include interviews with participating enrollees or providers about access experiences with the program.

Studies of state Medicaid programs provide little information on access to care for Medicaid enrollees with disabilities. Study populations and access measures have varied widely, and rarely include comparison groups. Selected examples include the following:

- In a Florida home and community-based services (HCBS) waiver program for adults with intellectual and developmental disabilities (I/DD), 40 percent of the adults enrolled did not see a primary care provider between 1999 and 2003 (Hall et al. 2007). The study did not report on use of specialists.

- In Iowa, among adults under age 65 with I/DD either enrolled in a Medicaid HCBS waiver or receiving case management services, over 80 percent received a preventive dental visit in 2005 (Chalmers et al. 2011).

- In New York City during 1999 and 2000, among SSI beneficiaries under age 65 in FFS Medicaid, 25 percent of adults with mental illness had no outpatient mental health visits (Long et al. 2002). The study did not report comparable estimates for adults with other forms of coverage.

- In rural counties of Kentucky with only FFS Medicaid, more than 95 percent of SSI recipients had a usual source of primary care in 1999. Among persons with mental illness, 60 percent had a usual source of mental health care (Mitchell et al. 2004).

- Two studies that include multistate comparisons among persons with disabilities documented wide variations in Medicaid-covered maternity care across states in terms of access and service use (Gavin et al. 2006) and in diabetes care among persons taking antipsychotic medications (Morrato et al. 2008).

Well-designed evaluations in the published literature are rare. In one comprehensive evaluation of substance abuse treatment services for Medicaid-eligible adults in Oregon, adults eligible on the basis of disability accessed treatment services at about half the rates of two other Medicaid comparison groups (Krahn et al. 2007). Interviews with participants, providers, and agency staff identified multiple patient-, provider-, and program-level barriers to participation for persons with disabilities, including family support for treatment, staff training about disability, and route of referrals (Krahn et al. 2006).

One nationwide effort to collect access measures for a portion of our study population is the National Core Indicators Project (NCI). To our knowledge, NCI supports the only ongoing, large-scale, multi-state comparison on acute care access for Medicaid enrollees with disabilities at the subpopulation level. NCI reports underscore the variability in access experiences reported in other state program data (HSRI 2013). Because the sample represents the most severely disabled persons with developmental disabilities who receive long-term care services and case management, a small portion of all persons enrolled in Medicaid on the basis of disability, we do not report on those findings here.[14]

Limitations of program studies

The overall quality, depth, and scope of studies using state program data are generally poor and the most recent data on some topics are over 10 years old. Virtually no studies assess the relationship between state program elements and access to care. Typically, studies provide descriptive information about service use without investigating the factors contributing to utilization or describing the characteristics of persons who did not receive services. Studies do not have comparison groups of similarly situated persons with other forms of coverage and include no data on service use among Medicaid enrollees prior to enrollment. Thus, they do not allow conclusions as to whether access levels are due to community factors that would affect all individuals with disabilities or to program factors that affect only Medicaid enrollees. Moreover, without comparison groups, it is unclear whether to interpret access levels as "low," "improved," or "high." Finally, these studies are not representative of Medicaid programs or enrollee experiences nationally.

Further Research Needed

This review serves to inform the Commission's future activities in its examination of access to appropriate care. Major gaps are evident in the research and evidence base about access to care for persons with disabilities, in part because there are too few studies posing access questions about Medicaid enrollees with disabilities to assess which barriers are significant problems for this population. Additionally, access issues especially important to this population have not been explored.

Enabling services. Various studies identify lack of non-emergency transportation and difficulty obtaining sign and oral interpretation services as barriers for persons with disabilities generally. State Medicaid programs offer these enabling services to specifically address these barriers. While the utilization of some enabling services financed by Medicaid and consumer satisfaction with these services has been documented in state reports, the focus of these evaluations is on cost and service process, not the effect of the service on medical care.[15]

Federal Medicaid rules require that states "ensure necessary transportation for recipients to and from providers."[16] States have several options through which to provide transportation services, and this choice determines the federal matching rate for these services and the amount of flexibility a state has in the provision of services. In addition, states may choose to carve-in or carve-out transportation from managed care contracts (Hilltop Institute 2008).

With respect to translation and interpretation services, states face similar choices in service provision and payment. State Medicaid agencies and their subcontractors are required to "take reasonable steps to provide meaningful access to Limited English Proficient (LEP) persons," including individuals with impaired hearing, vision, or speech.[17, 18, 19] The Children's Health Insurance Program Reauthorization Act allowed the costs incurred by state Medicaid programs for translation and interpretation services for LEP persons—including persons whose primary or spoken language is ASL or Braille—to be matched at the enhanced State Children's Health Insurance Program (CHIP) federal medical assistance percentage (FMAP) (CMS 2010).[20] CMS guidance further clarified that the enhanced match was available to assist CHIP and adult Medicaid enrollees to "access covered services" (CMS 2010).

These major design elements—payment, carve-out contracts, capitation, and waiver design—would affect plan and provider incentives for delivering enabling services and are expected to affect access. The impact of enabling services on improved access to medical care has not been independently evaluated to our knowledge.

Medicaid provider networks. A small number of physicians participating in Medicaid serve a disproportionately large share of Medicaid enrollees, relative to physicians participating in Medicare or commercial markets (Cunningham and May 2006). Further research is needed on the disability competency of the clinicians serving the largest share of Medicaid enrollees with disabilities, on the accessibility of diagnostic equipment, and on clinical and staff practices in these settings.

A study using a nationally representative sample of practicing physicians confirmed that the small percentage of primary care physicians serving Medicaid patients differs in many respects from physicians disproportionately serving privately insured patients or accepting few or no Medicaid patients (Sommers et al. 2011).[21] Physicians serving Medicaid patients more frequently reported having an interpreter available at their main practice, and that the settings in which they work are community health clinics and hospital-based practices, or practices owned in part by a hospital.[22] These entities generally have other incentives to comply with federal laws requiring physical accommodation for persons with disabilities.

Medicaid managed care. With a few exceptions, states have only recently begun to enroll a larger number of persons with disabilities into full- and partial-risk Medicaid managed care (MACPAC 2011, Gifford and Paradise 2011). Therefore, states' experiences with setting capitation rates and managed care plans' corresponding experiences serving high-cost, high-need populations vary considerably. Best practices and evaluations of risk-based managed care could help states improve managed care contracting practices and potentially improve oversight of risk-based managed care programs as they expand to serve these populations.

Additional areas of research that would be especially critical for building an evidence base to support Medicaid policy include:

- the role of non-physician practitioners in access to appropriate care for subpopulations with disabilities, and capacity to draw state comparisons using standard measures;

- studies evaluating the effects of program changes on access to care and service use;
- studies exploring the links between barriers to care, service use, and the appropriateness of care, cost, and efficiency of care delivery; and
- evidence from best practices in service delivery for persons with disabilities to produce access, quality, and health outcomes.

Access to care for children with special health care needs falls outside the scope of this chapter. Nonetheless, the program's performance in meeting the needs of these children also deserves attention.

Endnotes

[1] MACPAC analysis of Medicaid Statistical Information System annual person summary data and CMS-64 Financial Management Report net expenditure data, as shown in Figure 1b-2 on p. 45 of MACPAC's March 2012 report to the Congress.

[2] Box 1a-1 of MACPAC's March 2012 report to the Congress (p. 19) provides examples of Medicaid enrollees with disabilities.

[3] The five most common physical conditions are asthma/chronic obstructive pulmonary disease, congestive heart failure, coronary heart disease, diabetes, and hypertension.

[4] Exercise prescription refers to an individualized plan for fitness-related activities designed for a specific purpose, often developed by a fitness or rehabilitation specialist for a patient with chronic illness or disability. This prescription looks much like a drug prescription, indicating the type of activity, duration, frequency, intensity, and precautions (Suleman et al. 2012, HHS 2008, Moore 2004).

[5] MACPAC calculations based on the 2009–2011 NHIS.

[6] Subregulatory guidance defines a "limited English proficient individual" (LEP individual) (HHS 2003). Individuals whose primary language is ASL or Braille are identified as LEP individuals by CMS guidance (CMS 2010).

[7] For a description of questionnaire items in the MEPS, see the Medical Expenditure Panel Survey, Questionnaire Section: Health Status (AHRQ 2011).

[8] Manual transfer of a person with a disability by medical staff places the patient at risk of being dropped or hurt in the process (DOJ 2010). Lifting and transferring patients is a major risk factor for back injury among nurses and health aides (Hedge 2009).

[9] Guidance from the U.S. Department of Justice states that "examining a patient in their wheelchair usually is less thorough than on the exam table, and does not provide the patient equal medical services" (DOJ 2010).

[10] In accordance with federal laws, physicians cannot deny service to a patient who they would otherwise serve because the patient has a disability (DOJ 2010).

[11] A TTY, also known as a telecommunication device for the deaf, is a device that could be used by people who are deaf, hard-of-hearing, or speech-impaired. The telephone handset allows people to communicate over a telephone line by typing messages instead of speaking. A TTY is required at both ends in order to communicate. An alternative to TTY is the Telephone Relay Service, which requires a special operator. See http://www.abouttty.com for more information.

[12] For a more detailed discussion, see pp. 57–66 (Iezzoni and O'Day 2006).

[13] For a description of many of the devices used for augmentative and alternative communication, see the Assistech article on deaf communication (Assistech 2013).

[14] The NCI is a collaborative effort between the National Association of State Directors of Developmental Disabilities Services (NASDDDS) and the Human Services Research Institute (HSRI) and supports the quality management systems for 36 participating states and 22 sub-state regions or counties. More information about NCI can be found at http://www.nationalcoreindicators.org/about. The NCI Adult Consumer Survey interviews persons with developmental disabilities receiving publicly funded and case management services. In 2011-2012, a total of 19 states and one sub-state region participated in this survey. These data are limited for our purposes because states do not report the insurance status of respondents, although about 70 percent of respondents participate in an HCBS waiver program. The generalizability of report findings to non-participating states and to other persons with disabilities has not been established.

[15] See, as an example, a review of state reports on Medicaid non-emergency transportation by The Hilltop Institute (Hilltop Institute 2008).

[16] 45 CFR 1902(a)(70).

[17] State Medicaid agencies and their subcontractors are required to take these steps as recipients of federal financial assistance from the U.S. Department of Health and Human Services (HHS) under Title VI and HHS regulations, 45 CFR 80.3(b)(2).

[18] According to the Office of Civil Rights, recipients of federal financial assistance may include hospitals, nursing homes, home health agencies, managed care organizations, state Medicaid agencies, physicians, and other entities (OCR 2013).

[19] The accessibility of health care facilities is further mandated for people with disabilities under Section 504 of the Rehabilitation Act, which prohibits programs that receive federal financial assistance, as well as federally conducted programs and activities, from discriminating against individuals with disabilities; and Titles II and III of the Americans with Disabilities Act of 1990, which prohibits disability discrimination and requires health care providers to be physically and programmatically accessible to people with disabilities.

[20] Section 201(b) of the Children's Health Insurance Program Reauthorization Act of 2009, Pub. L. No. 111-3, enacted February 4, 2009.

[21] The study analyzed data from the 2008 Center for Studying Health System Change Health Tracking Physician Survey, which includes 1,460 primary care physicians (internists, family practice physicians, and general practitioners) who treat adults in outpatient settings.

[22] Authors found similar results for non-pediatric specialists in unpublished analysis.

References

Agency for Healthcare Research and Quality (AHRQ), U.S. Department of Health and Human Services. 2011. Medical Expenditure Panel Survey (MEPS), MEPS survey questionnaires. http://meps.ahrq.gov/survey_comp/survey.jsp.

Agency for Healthcare Research and Quality (AHRQ), U.S. Department of Health and Human Services. 2009. Medical Expenditure Panel Survey (MEPS), Survey background. http://meps.ahrq.gov/mepsweb/about_meps/survey_back.jsp.

Allen, S.M., A.L. Croke, et al. 2000. *The faces of Medicaid: The complexities of caring for people with chronic illnesses and disabilities*. Princeton, NJ: Center for Health Care Strategies, Inc. http://www.chcs.org/usr_doc/Chartbook.pdf.

Allen, S.M., S. Wieland, et al. 2009. Continuity in provider and site of care and preventive services receipt in an adult Medicaid population with physical disabilities. *Disability and Health Journal* 2, no. 4: 180e–187e.

American Therapeutic Recreation Association (ATRA). 2009. What is TR? Hattiesburg, MS: ATRA. http://www.atra-online.com/displaycommon.cfm?an=12.

Anderson, W.L., B.S. Armour, et al. 2010. Estimates of state-level health-care expenditures associated with disability. *Public Health Reports* 125, no. 1: 44–51. http://www.publichealthreports.org/issueopen.cfm?articleID=2328.

Armour, B.S., J.M. Thierry, and L.A. Wolf. 2009. State-level differences in breast and cervical cancer screening by disability status: United States, 2008. *Women's Health Issues* 19, no. 6: 406–414.

Assistech Special Needs. 2013. Deaf communication. http://www.assistech.com/deaf-communication.htm.

Bachman, S.S., M. Vedrani, M. Drainoni, et al. 2006. Provider perceptions of their capacity to offer accessible health care for people with disabilities. *Journal of Disability Policy Studies* 17, no. 3: 130–136.

Banta, J., E.H. Morrato, et al. 2009. Retrospective analysis of diabetes care in California Medicaid patients with mental illness. *Journal of General Internal Medicine* 24, no. 7: 802–808.

Bershadsky, J., and R.L. Kane. 2010. Place of residence affects routine dental care in the intellectually and developmentally disabled adult population on Medicaid. *Health Services Research* 45, no. 5 – Part 1: 1376–1389.

Blecker, S., Y. Zhang, et al. 2010. Quality of care for heart failure among disabled Medicaid recipients with and without severe mental illness. *General Hospital Psychiatry* 32, no. 3: 255–261.

Boyd, C., B. Leff, C. Weiss, et al. 2010. *The faces of Medicaid: Clarifying multimorbidity patterns to improve targeting and delivery of clinical services for Medicaid populations*. Hamilton, NJ: Center for Health Care Strategies, Inc. http://www.chcs.org/publications3960/publications_show.htm?doc_id=1261201.

Burns, M.E. 2009. Medicaid managed care and health care access for adult beneficiaries with disabilities. *Health Services Research* 44, no. 5 – Part 1: 1521–1541.

Center, J., H. Beange, and A. McElduff. 1998. People with mental retardation have an increased prevalence of osteoporosis: A population study. *American Journal of Mental Retardation* 103, no. 1: 19–28.

Center for Medicare & Medicaid Services (CMS), U.S. Department of Health and Human Services. 2010. Letter from Cindy Mann to State Medicaid Directors and State Health Officials regarding "Increased Federal Matching Funds for Translation and Interpretation Services under Medicaid and CHIP." July 1, 2010. http://www.hhs.gov/ocr/civilrights/resources/specialtopics/hospitalcommunication/cmsletteronincreasefunds.pdf.

Centers for Disease Control and Prevention (CDC), U.S. Department of Health and Human Services. 2012. *Behavioral Risk Factors Surveillance System (BRFSS) 2011 codebook report*. Atlanta, GA: CDC. http://www.cdc.gov/brfss/annual_data/annual_2011.htm.

Centers for Disease Control and Prevention (CDC), U.S. Department of Health and Human Services. 2005. *The Surgeon General's call to action to improve the health and wellness of persons with disabilities*. Atlanta, GA: CDC. http://www.surgeongeneral.gov/library/calls/disabilities/healthwellness.html.

Chalmers, J.M., R.A. Kuthy, E.T. Momany, et al. 2011. Dental utilization by adult Medicaid enrollees who have indicators of intellectual and developmental disabilities. *Specialty Care Dentistry* 31, no. 1: 18–26.

Coughlin, T.A., S.K. Long, and J.A. Graves. 2008. Does managed care improve access to care for Medicaid beneficiaries with disabilities? A national study. *Inquiry* 45 no. 4: 395–407.

Coughlin, T.A., S.K. Long, and Y.C. Shen. 2005. Assessing access to care under Medicaid: Evidence for the nation and thirteen states. *Health Affairs* 24, no. 4: 1073–1083. http://content.healthaffairs.org/content/24/4/1073.full.pdf+html.

Cunningham, P.J., and J.H. May. 2006. *Medicaid patients increasingly concentrated among physicians*. Tracking report no. 16. Washington, DC: Center for Studying Health System Change. http://www.hschange.com/CONTENT/866/.

Davis, M.J. 2009. Issues in access to oral health care for special care patients. *Dental Clinics of North America* 53, no. 2: 169–181.

Department of Family and Community Medicine (DFCM). 2011. *Health care maintenance guidelines for adults with developmental disabilities*. San Francisco, CA: University of California-San Francisco. http://developmentalmedicine.ucsf.edu/odpc/docs/pdf/practice_pearls/health-care-maintenance-guidelines-adults-with-dd.pdf.

Department of Family and Community Medicine (DFCM). 2009. *A hole in the safety net: Health care for transition age youth and adults with developmental disabilities*. San Francisco, CA: University of California-San Francisco. http://developmentalmedicine.ucsf.edu/odpc/docs/pdf/policy/Hole_in_Safety_Net.pdf.

Dewalt, D.A., N.D. Berkman, S. Sheridan, et al. 2004. Literacy and health outcomes: A systematic review of the literature. *Journal of General Internal Medicine* 19, no. 12: 128–139.

Drainoni, M., E. Lee-Hood, C. Tobias, et al. 2006. Cross-disability experiences of barriers to health-care access: Consumer perspectives. *Journal of Disability Policy Studies* 17, no. 2: 101–115.

Elangovan, S., R. Nalliah, V. Allareddy, et al. 2011. Outcomes in patients visiting hospital emergency departments in the United States because of periodontal conditions. *Journal of Periodontology* 82, no. 6: 809–819.

Engquist, G., C. Johnson, and W.C. Johnson. 2012. *Systems of care for individuals with intellectual and developmental disabilities: A survey of states*. Hamilton, NJ: Center for Health Care Strategies, Inc. http://www.chcs.org/usr_doc/IDD_State_Priorities_and_Barriers_Snapshot2_082812.pdf.

Fisher, K. 2012. Is there anything to smile about? A review of oral care for individuals with intellectual and developmental disabilities. *Nursing Research and Practice* 2012. http://www.hindawi.com/journals/nrp/2012/860692/.

Fisher, K., and P. Kettl. 2005. Aging with mental retardation: Increasing population of older adults with MR require health interventions and prevention strategies. *Geriatrics* 60, no. 4: 26–29.

Gavin, N.I., M.B. Benedict, and E.K. Adams. 2006. Health service use and outcomes among disabled Medicaid pregnant women. *Women's Health Issues* 16, no. 6: 313–322.

Gifford, K., and J. Paradise. 2011. *A profile of Medicaid managed care programs in 2010: Findings from a 50-state survey.* Washington, D.C.: Kaiser Commission on Medicaid and the Uninsured. http://kaiserfamilyfoundation.files.wordpress.com/2013/01/8220.pdf.

Gilmer, T., and A. Hamblin. 2010. *Hospital readmissions among Medicaid beneficiaries with disabilities: Identifying targets of opportunity.* Hamilton, NJ: Center for Health Care Strategies, Inc. http://www.chcs.org/usr_doc/CHCS_readmission_101215b.pdf.

Goldstein, M.F., E.A. Eckhardt, et al. 2006. An HIV knowledge and attitude survey of deaf U.S. adults. *Deaf Worlds* 22, no. 1: 163–183.

Grabois, E.W., M.A. Nosek, and C.D. Ross. 1999. Accessibility of primary care physicians' offices for people with disabilities: An analysis of compliance with the Americans with Disabilities Act. *Archives of Family Medicine* 8, no. 1: 44–51.

Graham C.L., E. Kurtovich, S.L. Ivey, et al. 2011. Fee-for-service and managed care for seniors and people with disabilities on Medicaid: Implications for the managed care mandate in California. *Journal of Health Care for the Poor and Underserved* 22, no. 4: 1413–1423.

Gully, S.P., and B.M. Altman. 2008. Disability in two health care systems: Access, quality, satisfaction, and physician contacts among working-age Canadians and Americans with disabilities. *Disability and Health Journal* 1, no. 4: 196–208.

Gully, S.P., E.K. Rasch, and L. Chan. 2011. The complex web of health: Relationships among chronic conditions, disability, and health services. *Public Health Reports* 126, no. 4: 495–507.

Hall, A., D. Wood, et al. 2007. Patterns in primary health care utilization among individuals with intellectual and developmental disabilities in Florida. *Intellectual Developmental Disability* 45, no. 5: 310–322.

Hanson, K.W., P. Neuman, et al. 2003. Uncovering the health challenges facing people with disabilities: The role of health insurance. *Health Affairs* (November 19): 552e–565e. http://content.healthaffairs.org/content/early/2003/11/19/hlthaff.w3.552/suppl/DC1.

Harder and Company Community Research. 2008. *A blind spot in the system: Health care for people with developmental disabilities. Findings from stakeholder interviews.* San Francisco, CA: Harder and Company Community Research. http://familymedicine.medschool.ucsf.edu/odpc/docs/pdf/A%20Blind%20Spot%20in%20the%20System.pdf.

Harmer, L. 1999. Health care delivery and deaf people: practice, problems, and recommendations for change. *Journal of Deaf Studies and Deaf Education* 4, no. 2: 73–110.

Havercamp, S.M., D. Scandlin, and M. Roth. 2004. Health disparities among adults with developmental disabilities, adults with other disabilities, and adults not reporting disability in North Carolina. *Public Health Reports* 119, no. 4: 418–426.

Health Resources and Services Administration (HRSA). 2001. *Dental care considerations of disadvantaged and special care populations: Proceedings of the conference held April 18–19, 2011 in Baltimore, MD,* eds. A.J. Bonito and L.Y. Cooper. Rockville, MD: HRSA. http://ask.hrsa.gov/detail_materials.cfm?ProdID=417.

Hedge, A. 2009. Back care for nurses. http://www.spineuniverse.com/wellness/ergonomics/back-care-nurses.

Hemmeter, J. 2011. Health-related unmet needs of Supplemental Security Income youth after the age-18 redetermination. *Health Services Research* 46, no. 4: 1224–1239.

Hilltop Institute. 2008. *Non-emergency medical transportation (NEMT) study report.* Baltimore, MD: University of Maryland, Baltimore County. http://www.hilltopinstitute.org/publications/Non-EmergencyMedicalTransportationStudyReport-September2008.pdf.

Human Services Research Institute (HSRI) and National Association of State Directors of Developmental Disabilities Services (NASDDDS). 2013. *National Core Indicators (NCI): Adult consumer survey 2011-12.* Final report. Cambridge, MA: HSRI. http://www.nationalcoreindicators.org/resources/reports/.

Huffman, L.C., B.A. Brat, et al. 2010. Impact of managed care on publicly insured children with special health care needs. *Academic Pediatrics* 10, no. 1: 48–55.

Iezzoni, L.I., R.B. Davis, et al. 2003. Quality dimensions that most concern people with physical and sensory disabilities. *Archives of Internal Medicine* 163, no. 17: 2086–2092.

Iezzoni, L.I., K. Kilbridge, and E.R. Park. 2010. Physical access barriers to care for diagnosis and treatment of breast cancer among women with mobility impairments. *Oncology Nursing Forum* 37, no. 6: 711–717.

Iezzoni, L.I., M.J. Killeen, and B.L. O'Day. 2006. Rural residents confront substantial barriers to obtain primary care. *Health Services Research* 41, no. 4 – Part 1: 1258–1275.

Iezzoni, L.I., and B.L. O'Day. 2006. *More than ramps: A guide to improving health care quality and access for people with disabilities.* New York, NY: Oxford University Press.

Iezzoni, L.I., B.L. O'Day, et al. 2004. Communicating about health care: Observations from persons who are deaf or hard of hearing. *Annals of Internal Medicine* 140, no. 5: 356–362.

Institute of Medicine (IOM). 2007. *The future of disability in America*. Washington, DC: National Academies Press.

Institute of Medicine (IOM). 1991. *Disability in America: Toward a national agenda for prevention*. Washington, DC: National Academies Press.

Kaiser Commission on Medicaid and the Uninsured (KCMU). 2011. *Faces of Medicaid*. Washington, DC: Kaiser Family Foundation. http://kff.org/interactive/faces-of-medicaid/.

Kaiser Family Foundation (KFF). 2003. *Understanding the health-care needs and experiences of people with disabilities: Findings from a 2003 survey*. Washington, DC: KFF. http://kff.org/medicaid/report/understanding-the-health-care-needs-and-experiences/.

Kerins, G., K. Petrovic, J. Gianesini, et al. 2004. Physician attitudes and practices on providing care to individuals with intellectual disabilities: An exploratory study. *Connecticut Medicine* 68, no. 8: 485–490.

Kinne S., D.L. Patrick, and D.L. Doyle. 2004. Prevalence of secondary conditions among people with disabilities. *American Journal of Public Health* 94, no. 3: 443–445.

Kirschner, K.L., M.L. Breslin, and L.I. Iezzoni. 2007. Structural impairments that limit access to health care for patients with disabilities. *Journal of the American Medical Association* 297, no. 10: 1121–1125.

Krahn, G., R. Deck, et al. 2007. A population-based study on substance abuse treatment for adults with disabilities: Access, utilization, and treatment outcomes. *American Journal of Drug and Alcohol Abuse* 33, no. 6: 791–798.

Krahn, G., N. Farrell, et al. 2006. Access barriers to substance abuse treatment for persons with disabilities: An exploratory study. *Journal of Substance Abuse Treatment* 31, no. 4: 375–384.

Kronick, R.G., M. Bella, and T.P. Gilmer. 2009. *The faces of Medicaid III: Refining the portrait of people with multiple chronic conditions*. Hamilton, NJ: Center for Health Care Strategies, Inc. http://www.chcs.org/usr_doc/Faces_of_Medicaid_III.pdf.

Kronick, R.G., M. Bella, et al. 2007. *The faces of Medicaid II: Recognizing the care needs of people with multiple chronic conditions*. Hamilton, NJ: Center for Health Care Strategies, Inc. http://www.chcs.org/usr_doc/Full_Report_Faces_II.pdf.

Lagu, T., N.S. Hannon, M.B. Rothberg, et al. 2013. Access to subspecialty care for patients with mobility impairment: A survey. *Annals of Internal Medicine* 158, no. 6: 441–446.

Li, C., E.S. Ford, et al. 2008. Prevalence of depression among U.S. adults with diabetes: Findings from the 2006 Behavioral Risk Factor Surveillance System. *Diabetes Care* 31, no. 1: 105–107.

Long, S.K., T.A. Coughlin, and S.J. Kendall. 2002. Access to care among disabled adults on Medicaid. *Health Care Financing Review* 23, no. 4: 159–173.

Long S.K., J. King, and T.A. Coughlin. 2005. The implications of unmet need for future health care use: Findings for a sample of disabled Medicaid beneficiaries in New York. *Inquiry* 42, no. 4: 413–420.

MacMahon, P., and A. Jahoda. 2008. Social comparison and depression: People with mild and moderate intellectual disabilities. *American Journal of Mental Retardation* 113, no. 4: 307–318.

Margellos H., T. Hedding, et al. 2004. *Improving access to health and mental health for Chicago's deaf community: A survey of deaf adults*. Chicago, IL: Sinai Health System and Advocate Health Care. http://www.suhichicago.org/files/publications/C.pdf.

Margellos-Anast, H., M. Estarziau, and G. Kaufman. 2006. Cardiovascular disease knowledge among culturally deaf patients in Chicago. *Preventive Medicine* 42, no. 3: 235–239.

McColl, M., and S. Shortt. 2006. Another way to look at high service utilization: The contribution of disability. *Journal of Health Services Research and Policy* 11, no. 2: 74–80.

McColl, M.A., D. Forster, et al. 2008. Physician experiences providing primary care to people with disabilities. *Healthcare Policy* 4, no. 1: e129–e147.

McGinn-Shapiro, M. 2008. *Medicaid coverage of adult dental services*. Washington, DC: National Academy for State Health Policy. http://www.nashp.org/publication/medicaid-coverage-adult-dental-services.

McNeal, M.A., L. Carrothers, and B. Premo. 2002. *Providing primary health care for people with physical disabilities: A survey of California physicians*. Pomona, CA: Center for Disability Issues and the Health Professions, Western University of Health Services. www.cdihp.org/pdf/ProvPrimeCare.pdf.

Medicaid and CHIP Payment and Access Commission (MACPAC). 2013. *Report to the Congress on Medicaid and CHIP*. March 2013. Washington, DC: MACPAC. http://www.macpac.gov/reports.

Medicaid and CHIP Payment and Access Commission (MACPAC). 2012. *Report to the Congress on Medicaid and CHIP.* March 2012. Washington, DC: MACPAC. http://www.macpac.gov/reports.

Medicaid and CHIP Payment and Access Commission (MACPAC). 2011. *Report to the Congress on Medicaid and CHIP.* March 2011. Washington, DC: MACPAC. http://www.macpac.gov/reports.

Mele, N., J. Archer, and B.D. Pusch. 2005. Access to breast cancer screening services for women with disabilities. *Journal of Obstetric and Gynecological Neonatal Nursing* 34, no. 4: 453–464.

Mitchell, J.B., S. Hoover, and A. Bir. 2004. *Access to care for Medicaid beneficiaries with disabilities in rural Kentucky.* Report to CMS, contract no. 500-95-0040. Waltham, MA: RTI International. http://www.cms.gov/Research-Statistics-Data-and-Systems/Statistics-Trends-and-Reports/Reports/downloads/mitchell2.pdf.

Moore, G.E. 2004. The role of exercise prescription in chronic disease. *British Journal of Sports Medicine* 38, no. 1: 6-7.

Morrato, E.H., J.W. Newcomer, R.R. Allen, et al. 2008. Prevalence of baseline serum glucose and lipid testing in users of second-generation antipsychotic drugs: A retrospective, population-based study of Medicaid claims data. *Journal of Clinical Psychiatry* 69, no. 2: 316–322.

Nalliah, R., V. Allareddy, S. Elangovan, et al. 2010. Hospital based emergency department visits attributed to dental caries in the United States in 2006. *Journal of Evidence Based Dental Practice* 10, no. 4: 212–222.

National Center for Health Statistics (NCHS), Centers for Disease Control and Prevention, U.S. Department of Health and Human Services. 2010. *Data file documentation, National Health Interview Survey, 2009* (machine readable data file and documentation). Hyattsville, MD: NCHS. http://www.cdc.gov/nchs/nhis.htm.

National Center for Health Statistics (NCHS), Centers for Disease Control and Prevention, U.S. Department of Health and Human Services. 2008. *Disability and health in the United States, 2001–2005.* Hyattsville, MD: NCHS. http://www.cdc.gov/nchs/data/misc/disability2001-2005.pdf.

National Center on Health, Physical Activity, and Disability (NCHPAD). Physical activity, leisure and recreation for youth with disabilities: A primer for parents. http://www.ncpad.org/90/686/Physical~Activity~~Leisure~and~Recreation~for~Youth~with~Disabilities~~A~Primer~for~Parents.

National Council on Disability (NCD). 2012. *Rocking the cradle: Ensuring the rights of parents with disabilities and their children.* Chapter 9. Washington, DC: NCD. http://www.ncd.gov/publications/2012/Sep272012/.

National Council on Disability (NCD). 2009. *The current state of health care for people with disabilities.* Washington, DC: NCD. http://www.ncd.gov/publications/2009/Sept302009.

Neri, M.T., and T. Kroll. 2003. Understanding the consequences of access barriers to health care: Experiences of adults with disabilities. *Disability and Rehabilitation* 25, no. 2: 85–96.

Office for Civil Rights (OCR), U.S. Department of Health and Human Services. 2013. *Guidance to federal financial assistance recipients regarding Title VI prohibition against national origin discrimination affecting Limited English Proficient (LEP) persons.* Washington, DC: OCR. http://www.hhs.gov/ocr/civilrights/resources/specialtopics/lep/policyguidancedocument.html.

O'Hearn, A. 2006. Deaf women's experiences and satisfaction with prenatal care: A comparative study. *Family Medicine* 38, no. 10: 712–716.

Okoro, C.A., L.R. McKnight-Eily, et al. 2011. State and local area estimates of depression and anxiety among adults with disabilities in 2006. *Disability and Health Journal* 4, no. 2: 78–90.

Parish, S.L., and M.J. Ellison-Martin. 2007. Health-care access of women Medicaid recipients. *Journal of Disability Policy Studies* 18, no. 2: 109–116.

Patchias, E., and M. Birnbaum. 2011. *Providing care to Medicaid beneficiaries with behavioral health conditions: Challenges for New York.* New York, NY: Medicaid Institute at United Hospital Fund. http://www.uhfnyc.org/assets/879.

Ramirez, A., G.C. Farmer, D. Grant, et al. 2005. Disability and preventive cancer screening: Results from the 2001 California Health Interview Survey. *American Journal of Public Health* 95, no. 11: 2057–2064.

Rimmer, J.H. 1999. Health promotion for people with disabilities: The emerging paradigm shift from disability prevention to prevention of secondary conditions. *Physical Therapy* 79, no. 5: 495–502.

Scheer, J.M, T. Kroll, et al. 2003. Access barriers for persons with disabilities. *Journal of Disability Policy Studies* 13, no. 4: 221–230.

Scott, K.M., M. Von Korff, et al. 2009. Mental-physical co-morbidity and its relationship with disability: Results from the World Mental Health Surveys. *Psychological Medicine* 39, no. 1: 33–43.

Shier, G., M. Ginsburg, et al. 2013. Strong social support services, such as transportation and help for caregivers, can lead to lower health care use and costs. *Health Affairs* 32, no. 3: 544–551.

Smeltzer, S.C. 2006. Preventive health screening for breast and cervical cancer and osteoporosis in women with physical disabilities. *Family Community Health* 29, no. 1: 35s–43s.

Social Security Administration (SSA). 2012. *National survey of SSI children and families (NSCF): User's manual for the public use file.* Baltimore, MD: SSA. http://www.ssa.gov/disabilityresearch/documents/nscf/Documentation/NSCF_PUF_Users_Manual.pdf.

Sommers, A.S. 2006. Access to health insurance, barriers to care, and service use among adults with disabilities. *Inquiry* 43, no. 4: 393–405.

Sommers, A.S., and P.J. Cunningham. 2011. *Physician visits after hospital discharge: Implications for reducing readmissions.* Research brief no. 6. Washington, DC: Center for Studying Health System Change. http://www.nihcr.org/Reducing_Readmissions.html.

Sommers, A.S., J. Paradise, and C. Miller. 2011. *Physician willingness and resources to serve more Medicaid patients: Perspectives from primary care physicians.* Washington, DC: Kaiser Commission on the Uninsured. http://kff.org/disparities-policy/issue-brief/physician-willingness-and-resources-to-serve-more/.

Steinberg, A.G., S. Barnett, et al. 2006. Health care system accessibility: Experiences and perceptions of deaf people. *Journal of General Internal Medicine* 21, no. 3: 260–266.

Steinberg, A.G., V.J. Sullivan, and R.C. Loew. 1998. Cultural and linguistic barriers to mental health services: The deaf consumer's perspective. *American Journal of Psychiatry* 155, no. 7: 982–984.

Stiefel, D.J. 2002. Dental care considerations for disabled adults. *Special Care Dentistry* 22, no. 3: 26S–39S.

Suleman, A., K.D. Heffner, and S.W. Sherwin. 2012. Medscape reference: Exercise prescription. http://emedicine.medscape.com/article/88648-overview.

Sullivan, W.F., J.M. Berg, et al. 2011. Primary care of adults with developmental disabilities: Canadian consensus guidelines. *Canadian Family Physician* 57, no. 5: 541–553.

Taylor, D.H., and H. Hoenig. 2006. Access to health care services for the disabled elderly. *Health Services Research* 41, no. 3, Part 1: 743–758.

U.S. Department of Health and Human Services (HHS). 2008. Additional considerations for some adults. In *2008 physical activity guidelines for Americans.* Washington, DC: HHS. http://www.health.gov/paguidelines/guidelines/chapter7.aspx.

U.S. Department of Health and Human Services. 2003. Guidance to federal financial assistance recipients regarding Title VI prohibition against national origin discrimination affecting limited English proficient persons. Policy guidance document. *Federal Register* 68, no. 153 (August 8): 47311–47323.

U.S. Department of Justice (DOJ). 2010. *Access to medical care for individuals with mobility disabilities.* Washington, DC: DOJ. http://www.ada.gov/medcare_mobility_ta/medcare_ta.pdf.

U.S. Government Accountability Office (GAO). 2010. *Efforts under way to improve children's access to dental services, but sustained attention needed to address ongoing concerns.* Washington, DC: GAO. http://www.gao.gov/new.items/d1196.pdf.

Van Winkel, R., M. De Hert, et al. 2008. Prevalence of diabetes and the metabolic syndrome in a sample of patients with bipolar disorder. *Bipolar Disorder* 10, no. 2: 342–348.

Waldman, H.B., and S.P. Perlman. 2012. Individuals with disabilities: What about dental services? *The Exceptional Parent* 42, no. 4: 17–18.

Wall, T.P. 2012. *Dental Medicaid 2012. Dental analysis health policy series.* Chicago, IL: American Dental Association. http://www.ada.org/sections/professionalResources/pdfs/12_med.pdf.

Wei, W., P.A. Findley, and U. Sambamoorthi. 2006. Disability and receipt of clinical preventive services among women. *Womens Health Issues* 16, no. 6: 286–296.

Wilkinson, J.E., and M.C. Cerreto. 2008. Primary care for women with intellectual disabilities. *Journal of the American Board of Family Medicine* 21, no. 3: 215–222.

Wilkinson, J.E., C.E. Deis, D.J. Bowen, et al. 2011. "It's easier said than done": Perspectives on mammography from women with intellectual disabilities. *Annals of Family Medicine* 9, no. 2: 142–147.

CHAPTER 4

Update on Medicaid and CHIP Data for Policy Analysis and Program Accountability

Key Points

Update on Medicaid and CHIP Data for Policy Analysis and Program Accountability

- Data on Medicaid and the State Children's Health Insurance Program (CHIP) play a key role in answering policy questions that affect program enrollees, states, the federal government, health care providers, and others—and in ensuring accountability for taxpayer dollars. This chapter provides an update on efforts to improve the timeliness, quality, and availability of federal administrative data on the programs, which MACPAC first addressed in its March 2011 report to the Congress.

- Federal administrative data on Medicaid and CHIP are meant to provide comparable information across states, which maintain their own disparate data systems. These federal data are necessary to fully understand the programs and to make evidence-based policy decisions.

- Since the Commission last reported on the topic in March 2011, the Centers for Medicare & Medicaid Services (CMS) has taken steps to improve federal Medicaid and CHIP data through initiatives that include:

    - MACPro, a web-based system designed to collect state plan, waiver, and other programmatic documents in a structured and consistent format;

    - the Transformed Medicaid Statistical Information System (T-MSIS), a data source building on existing person-level and claims-level MSIS data submitted by states; and

    - Medicaid Information Technology Architecture (MITA), which establishes national guidelines and standards for state-operated Medicaid and CHIP data systems that are funded with federal dollars.

- Improvements to Medicaid and CHIP data will not occur overnight, and they will require significant federal and state resource investments. MACPro and T-MSIS are scheduled for roll-out in 2013, with full implementation expected to take at least two years. MITA is an ongoing effort with states, whose data systems are at varying levels of modernization.

CHAPTER 4

Update on Medicaid and CHIP Data for Policy Analysis and Program Accountability

In its inaugural report to the Congress, MACPAC described the key role that Medicaid and State Children's Health Insurance Program (CHIP) data play in answering policy questions that affect program enrollees, states, the federal government, health care providers, and others—and in ensuring accountability for taxpayer dollars. In that report, the Commission:

- highlighted ways in which existing federal administrative data on Medicaid and CHIP can help to answer key policy and accountability questions;

- identified major federal administrative data sources that are used for most national and cross-state analyses of Medicaid and CHIP; and

- noted areas where better data on the programs are needed (MACPAC 2011).

Consistent with MACPAC's statutory charge to review national and state-specific Medicaid and CHIP data and to submit reports and recommendations based on such reviews (§1900(b)(3) of the Social Security Act), this chapter describes recent efforts by the Centers for Medicare & Medicaid Services (CMS) to improve the timeliness, quality, and availability of federal administrative data on the programs.

The Commission strongly supports continued improvements to federal Medicaid and CHIP data, and encourages CMS to continue seeking input from states and other stakeholders as it implements its new initiatives. As the timeliness, quality, and availability of data improve, so will the ability of the Commission and others to address questions that are currently difficult to answer. For example, do enrollees receive appropriate care in both fee-for-service and managed care settings? To what extent does provider participation in Medicaid vary? Can the impact of policy changes, such as the current increase in payment rates for certain primary care providers, be assessed in a timely manner?

Brief Overview of Federal Administrative Data on Medicaid and CHIP

In the course of administering the Medicaid and CHIP programs, states and the federal government receive and generate large amounts of data. Sources include:

- **State plan and waiver documents.** States describe a wide range of program policies—such as eligibility levels and covered benefits—in state plan and waiver documents that must be approved by CMS.
- **Eligibility information.** Individuals report information such as income, age, and other personal and family characteristics in the process of applying for coverage.
- **Claims.** Health care providers submit claims that document the services provided to enrollees, and, in turn, states (as well as managed care plans under contract with states) process payments for those claims.
- **Accounting statements.** States complete detailed quarterly accounting statements to obtain federal funds for a share of their Medicaid and CHIP costs.

State data systems

All states maintain comprehensive and detailed data on their individual Medicaid and CHIP programs, and are statutorily required to maintain a Medicaid Management Information System (MMIS) to process claims from providers and to perform a variety of information retrieval and reporting functions (§1900(r) of the Social Security Act). However, each state's MMIS reflects its own administrative structures and processes, even when multiple states contract with the same private vendor for MMIS support. In addition, MMIS and other data are often housed in multiple systems that are fragmented within states and in formats that limit their comparability across states. Some of the issues include:

- **Unique billing codes.** Some states create state-specific billing codes for certain services. This is particularly an issue for services that are unique to Medicaid, such as long-term services and supports provided in home and community-based settings.
- **Payments not based on claims.** Not all payments to providers are processed through a state's MMIS. Examples may include: retrospective settlement amounts for providers who are paid on the basis of costs, rather than a fee schedule; supplemental payments to providers made under various statutory authorities; and payments to certain public providers who receive funding through state or local budget processes, sometimes in lieu of direct payments by the state Medicaid agency.
- **Eligibility data coming from different systems.** Although federal law requires states to operate their Medicaid programs under the authority of a single state agency, multiple state and local government entities may have responsibility for different program functions. State MMISs typically receive and store data extracts containing eligibility-related information to ensure that payments are made only for services provided to current Medicaid and CHIP enrollees. However, state eligibility systems generally operate separately and distinctly from MMISs, in part because they may be used to enroll individuals in public programs other than Medicaid and CHIP.

As acknowledged in MACPAC's March 2011 report to the Congress, states have their own data that paint a rich picture of their individual Medicaid and CHIP programs but that may not always be reflected in federal sources. Encounter data, which provide a record of the services furnished to Medicaid and CHIP enrollees in managed care plans, are one such example. Historically, these data were underreported by states (OIG 2009), and their quality and completeness at the federal level went largely unexamined (Byrd and Verdier 2011). However, all states with managed care programs obtain encounter data in some form, and many have had years of experience in using the data for a variety of purposes that include setting capitation rates for plans, calculating performance measures, and generating ad hoc reports for state agencies, legislatures, and external constituencies. The ongoing use of encounter data by states provides a continuing check on its quality at the state level, but the federal government is only now beginning to examine these data—an important change, since data that are not used tend not to improve (Byrd and Verdier 2011).

Federal administrative data systems

At the federal level, most administrative data on Medicaid and CHIP consist of information reported by states to CMS on their program policies, the characteristics and service use of their enrollees, and their program spending (Table 4-1).

These federal administrative data are critical because they are the only source that can provide a comprehensive picture of the Medicaid and CHIP programs, which cost nearly $450 billion in fiscal year (FY) 2012 and were estimated to serve about 80 million people for at least part of the year (MACPAC 2013). Unlike the data held by states, federal sources are meant to provide comparable information in a standard format, allowing for national and cross-state examinations of program issues. In addition, researchers may link administrative and survey data sources to provide more detailed information—for example, on the health and other characteristics of program enrollees (Dodd and Gleason 2013)—than can be obtained from a single source in isolation.

In addition to serving as an important resource for program oversight by CMS and others, some general uses of the data for analytic purposes include:

- **Projections.** Historical data are a key source of information used in projections of future enrollment and spending, under both current law and alternative proposals, by CMS and other agencies such as the Congressional Budget Office (Truffer 2013).

- **Spending growth.** Data can be used to identify enrollee subgroups and services that account for a disproportionate share of program spending, and also to examine the extent to which spending is driven by increases in enrollment versus increases in spending per enrollee. This information provides a focus for cost-control policies.

- **Continuity of coverage.** Data can show the extent to which individuals experience churn in their Medicaid and CHIP enrollment—a consideration in analyses of access to and use of services (Czajka 2012a, 2012b).

- **Quality and appropriateness of care.** Claims and encounter data that provide information on service use can be used to examine receipt of recommended care, such as well-child and preventive dental visits for children (Bouchery 2012a, 2012b).

- **Provider participation.** Data on providers can inform efforts to examine their participation in Medicaid, as well as enrollees' access to and use of services (Baugh and Verghese 2012).

TABLE 4-1. Key Sources of Federal Administrative Data on Medicaid and CHIP

Source	Brief Description
Medicaid and CHIP Budget and Expenditure System (MBES/CBES)	Reports (Forms CMS-64, CMS-21, and CMS-37) detailing aggregate spending that are submitted by states to receive federal reimbursement for a share of their Medicaid and CHIP spending
Medicaid Statistical Information System (MSIS)	Demographic and enrollment-related information on each person enrolled in Medicaid and, at state option, separate CHIP programs, as well as a record of each claim paid for most services an enrollee receives
Statistical Enrollment Data System (SEDS)	Aggregate statistics on CHIP and child Medicaid enrollment
Form CMS-416	Aggregate statistics on children receiving Early and Periodic Screening, Diagnostic, and Treatment (EPSDT) services
Form CMS-372	Aggregate statistics on enrollment and spending under home and community-based services waivers
Medicaid Drug Rebate (MDR) System	Aggregate statistics on drug utilization and payments, used for calculating rebates to states from drug manufacturers
State Medicare Modernization Act (MMA) files	Monthly eligibility-related information on individuals dually enrolled in Medicaid and Medicare, used for Medicare Part D purposes
State plan documents	Documents that describe a state's Medicaid and CHIP policies under regular state plan (i.e., non-waiver) rules
Waiver documents	Documents that describe a state's Medicaid and CHIP waiver programs, including those operating under Section 1115, 1915(b), and 1915(c) authorities
Medicaid Managed Care Data Collection System (MMCDCS)	Aggregate statistics on managed care enrollment, along with basic descriptive information on each managed care plan and program within a state
CHIP Annual Report Template System (CARTS)	Information on CHIP programs, such as policies on eligibility and cost sharing, as well as performance measures regarding receipt of care

Note: For more information on each of these data sources, see MACPAC's March 2011 report to the Congress.

▶ **Program characteristics.** Qualitative information on service delivery and payment mechanisms, such as capitated managed care, provide important context when examining spending and utilization across states.

▶ **Program integrity.** CMS is exploring how to make better use of federal data sources for purposes of identifying billing and utilization patterns that indicate potential fraud and abuse in Medicaid and CHIP. (See Chapter 5 on program integrity.)

Recent Federal Efforts to Improve Data Timeliness, Quality, and Availability

As outlined in MACPAC's March 2011 report to the Congress, Medicaid and CHIP data are collected from states at different times, in different formats, for different purposes. States report some information on their programs more than once, while gaps remain that limit the usefulness of various data sources. In its report, the Commission noted a number of areas where better federal administrative data on Medicaid and CHIP were needed and provided examples of how improvements in these data could allow for better analysis of policy and program accountability issues. These areas included:

- the ability to understand service use among managed care enrollees, children eligible for Early and Periodic Screening, Diagnostic, and Treatment (EPSDT) benefits, and children in separate CHIP programs;
- the timeliness and consistency of various data sources; and
- the availability of information on state program policies.

At the time of MACPAC's March 2011 report to the Congress, CMS had established a Medicaid and CHIP Business Information Solutions (MACBIS) Council to oversee a transformation of the agency's data strategy and environment (Plewes 2010, Thompson 2010). As part of this effort, the Council commissioned a review of existing Medicaid and CHIP data sources and their uses (Borden et al. 2010). CMS had also released a plan for modernizing its computer and data systems (CMS 2010a). The Commission noted that CMS activities to inventory its existing data sources provided a valuable starting point for addressing both redundancies and gaps in the information reported by states, and encouraged the agency to continue its development of a strategic plan for Medicaid and CHIP data.

In a February 2013 presentation to the Commission, CMS highlighted two major initiatives aimed at improving Medicaid and CHIP data that are scheduled for roll-out in 2013, with full implementation to follow in coming years (Boughn 2013). The first is MACPro, a web-based system designed to collect state plan, waiver, and other programmatic documents in a structured and consistent format. The second is the Transformed Medicaid Statistical Information System (T-MSIS), which builds on existing person-level and claims-level MSIS data submitted by states. CMS is also using its ongoing Medicaid Information Technology Architecture (MITA) initiative to establish national guidelines and standards for state-operated Medicaid and CHIP data systems that are funded with federal dollars (CMS 2013a). The following sections describe these initiatives, provide information on their anticipated improvements to Medicaid and CHIP data, and highlight areas where additional attention may be warranted. Although not discussed here in detail, CMS has also been providing technical assistance to states and their contractors on a variety of issues such as managed care encounter data, separate CHIP program data, and individuals dually eligible for Medicare and Medicaid (CMS 2013c, Camillo 2012, Byrd and Verdier 2011).

MACPro

MACPro is a web-based system under development at CMS to collect state plan, waiver, and other programmatic documents in a structured and consistent format (Boughn 2013). Capturing information in this manner has been cited as a critical need for CMS (Borden et al. 2010). With the exception of certain waivers related to home and community-based services and managed care, current Medicaid and CHIP program data are largely submitted, reviewed, and approved in paper or electronic formats that cannot be easily summarized or linked with other data sources.

In 2013, CMS expects that MACPro will be used for the submission of state plan amendments (SPAs) related to the eligibility and benefit package provisions of the Patient Protection and Affordable Care Act (ACA, P.L. 111-148, as amended). CMS expects to roll out additional components of the system on a two-year schedule. During this time, the agency will maintain its existing processes for state plan and waiver approvals alongside MACPro.

As previously noted by the Commission, modernizing the data systems that collect programmatic information on Medicaid and CHIP would be beneficial for several reasons. The federal government could strengthen its program oversight by providing consistent and comprehensive information on state activities for use by CMS and other agency staff. Second, states could more easily learn about the policy choices made by others as they consider their own program changes. In addition, analysts could better identify the range of policies in place across states as they relate to the number of people who are covered by Medicaid and CHIP, the services they use, and the amount spent on those services—and use this information to identify possible best practices or program improvements.

As pieces of the system are implemented over the next two years, the Commission encourages CMS to make the information collected in MACPro publicly available in a timely and transparent manner. The Commission also encourages CMS to ensure that existing information be made more readily available during the transition to MACPro. For example, prior to making the entirety of state plans available on the CMS website using MACPro, the agency could compile links to the location of this information on state websites or post scanned electronic versions of the hard-copy documents that it now maintains at its regional offices. Historically, CMS has been inconsistent in its efforts to keep the SPAs and waiver documents on its website complete and up to date.

In a 2010 letter to state Medicaid directors describing its process for reviewing SPAs, CMS acknowledged that the submission of a SPA may sometimes lead to the identification of existing state plan provisions that appear to be contrary to federal statute, regulations, or established guidance (CMS 2010b). In such cases, the potentially non-compliant state plan provisions must also be reviewed and resolved. For states, one area of concern about MACPro may be that the process of converting existing state plan documents could lead to an increase in the number of state plan provisions that are questioned by CMS and potentially reopened for consideration, some of which may have been approved under a previous administration's statutory or regulatory interpretation.

T-MSIS

MSIS is a data source compiled by CMS from detailed demographic, enrollment, and claims information reported by all states since FY 1999. Currently, states must submit five MSIS files every quarter: one containing eligibility-related information on each person enrolled in Medicaid—and optionally CHIP—and four containing information on paid claims for inpatient hospital services, institutional long-term care, drugs, and all other services. T-MSIS will expand the data to include three additional files with information on providers, third-party payers, and managed care plans.

The expanded system will also include changes to address several concerns about current MSIS data (Boughn 2013):

- **Timeliness.** T-MSIS will move states from quarterly to monthly data submissions and will replace manual reviews of the data with automated quality checks that provide states with real-time feedback.

- **Reliability.** Data reliability will be addressed in a number of ways, but a key component will be an up-front mapping effort that requires states to document their source data and processes for populating each of the nearly 800 data elements in T-MSIS (CMS 2013a). Assuring consistency of this mapping across states will be a significant challenge.

- **Completeness.** CMS will be working with states to ensure that existing requirements for managed care encounter data are met, along with new requirements for the reporting of provider and other data. However, the extent to which states currently collect and use these data for their own purposes will affect their T-MSIS submissions.

In its March 2011 report to the Congress, the Commission identified how data improvements of the sort currently contemplated for T-MSIS would be beneficial. For example:

- CMS could reduce reporting burdens by directly calculating certain measures reported elsewhere by states. These might include EPSDT statistics reported for children on the CMS-416, as well as certain child and adult quality measures that would otherwise be voluntarily reported by states (HHS 2012a, 2012b).

- Encounter data could be used to make national and cross-state comparisons of the care received by Medicaid and CHIP enrollees whose benefits are delivered through fee-for-service versus managed care systems, which some states already do on an individual basis (Ku et al. 2009, Thomson Medstat 2006). Although these data are currently reported by many states, their quality and completeness vary (Borck et al. 2013, Byrd and Dodd 2012, Byrd et al. 2012, Dodd et al. 2012, Nysenbaum et al. 2012).

- Complete enrollment and claims data for separate CHIP enrollees could be used to help CMS and states understand the effectiveness of enrollment strategies like express lane eligibility, program transitions, and payment variation by state (Camillo 2012).

- Results from the measurement and monitoring of enrollees' service use could be used to better target outreach efforts for individuals most in need of services.

- More timely data would give administrators and legislators a clearer picture of the programs as they operate now—rather than as they did two or three years ago. The availability of current data may be particularly important for program integrity efforts such as the identification of potential fraud and abuse by providers and enrollees. (See Chapter 5 on program integrity.)

An initial version of T-MSIS was tested as a pilot in 12 states beginning in 2011 (Gorman 2012). CMS made changes to the data dictionary as part of the pilot process and anticipates that full implementation of T-MSIS may take up to two years, with some states beginning to submit the data in 2013.

CMS has recently added the submission of T-MSIS data as a condition on approvals for states that receive enhanced federal match for significant upgrades to their data systems (see discussion of MITA below), as well as for certain eligibility-related activities (CMS 2013b). However, as with the current MSIS, T-MSIS will not serve as the basis for calculating federal reimbursement to states—a use that could provide the most powerful incentive for states to submit high-quality data in a timely manner. To the extent that T-MSIS data are used for statistical reporting rather than federal funding purposes, states may continue to view T-MSIS data as a low priority relative to the many competing pressures they face. As noted in the MITA discussion below, the spending amounts reported in today's MSIS data are not always consistent with those reported in the CMS-64 data that are used to calculate federal matching funds.

T-MSIS will require a significant investment of resources at the state level, both in the initial stages of mapping data from multiple systems into the federally required format and in the ongoing maintenance and submission of the data. States may have a number of concerns about T-MSIS implementation:

- **Staff resources.** Given the many activities related to ACA implementation currently under way, a small number of state staff may be responsible for implementing a wide range of systems changes other than those related to T-MSIS. In addition, many states' current MSIS submissions are extracted from legacy systems using coding that is not well understood. In some cases, T-MSIS will not be a modification of an existing process, but a completely new development effort.

- **Data mapping.** Data mapping may be particularly challenging for states contracting with several managed care plans or in cases where Medicaid services are coordinated and paid through a different state agency, such as the department of mental health. It may be difficult for a state to coordinate the collection and validate the quality and consistency of data coming from the other agencies or managed care plans. States may also have to update the data maps periodically, if they make changes to their MMIS systems or contract with new managed care plans.

- **Unavailable data.** States have some concerns about the level of completeness that may be required in T-MSIS. States may be missing certain data elements, or, even if they are collecting information for a particular data element, it may be that not all records have a valid value within that field. None of the T-MSIS pilot states were able to provide all of the data elements required for T-MSIS, leading CMS to indicate that it will need to identify items with a low submission or population rate and assess how this will impact the ability to analyze the data (Gorman 2012).

- **Continued duplication.** While T-MSIS will provide more robust analytic capabilities for CMS, states have some concerns that it may not provide all of the necessary information to eliminate additional data requests for other CMS activities, such as the Payment Error Rate Measurement (PERM) program for Medicaid and CHIP.

Some activities related to the collection and submission of T-MSIS data may be eligible for enhanced federal matching funds. Among other purposes, states may be able to use the enhanced federal funds to improve and standardize Medicaid and CHIP data for T-MSIS. This includes improving encounter data, which would also help states with their managed care oversight and monitoring capabilities. However, even with the availability of enhanced federal matching funds, states may still struggle to finance their share of these and other Medicaid and CHIP costs.

MITA

MITA is a CMS initiative to establish national guidelines and standards for state-operated Medicaid and CHIP data systems that are funded with federal dollars. As noted earlier, each state is required to have an MMIS that processes claims from providers and performs a variety of other functions. Historically, MMISs were primarily designed to serve as financial and accounting systems for provider payments. As additional

Medicaid functions (such as managed care oversight, clinical support, data analysis, fraud management, non-emergency transportation coordination, and prior authorization) became automated, some were added as separate systems while others were added into the MMIS. Some of these fragmented systems had difficulty communicating, lost information in the process of exchanging data, and could not provide a consolidated overview of all provider and beneficiary activity.

MITA efforts are intended to ensure the use of standard data definitions and processes so that disparate state systems can operate together as a virtual MMIS, and so that federal data reported by states is comparable. Toward that goal, CMS has developed a framework for the standardization and interoperability of state data systems (CMS 2012).

Enhanced federal funding is available for MMIS upgrades (at a 90 percent match) or the operation of a federally certified MMIS (at a 75 percent match). To receive this enhanced funding, states are required to submit advance planning documents (APDs) that describe how their systems will meet MITA goals and objectives. These goals currently include the submission of T-MSIS data, which has been added as a condition for obtaining APD approval from CMS (CMS 2013a).

MACPAC's March 2011 report to the Congress cited a lack of consistency in state-reported information on Medicaid and CHIP as an ongoing issue that limits the usefulness of federal data for analytic and oversight purposes. A prominent example arises in comparisons of the spending amounts reported in CMS-64 data (which are used by states to obtain federal matching funds) and MSIS data (which are used for statistical and research purposes). Even after adjusting for differences in scope and design (such as the treatment of drug rebates and administrative costs), the MSIS generally produce lower spending figures than the CMS-64 (GAO 2012). Structural differences will always exist between these data sources. However, as part of its MITA efforts, CMS could include an examination of inconsistencies that remain unexplained.

As noted by states, the challenges associated with MITA include organizational resistance when collaborating across state agencies, a need to modernize both their technology and business processes, and the long time-frame required to implement programs—often through changing political administrations (NASCIO 2008). However, there is recognition that improving the use of information technology is a way for states to cut costs, increase productivity, and concentrate efforts where they are most needed (NGA 2012).

Looking Forward

Consistent with previous reporting by the Commission, CMS is taking a number of steps to improve the timeliness, quality, and availability of federal administrative data on the Medicaid and CHIP programs. The Commission supports these efforts and encourages the agency to continue seeking input from states and other stakeholders. Adequate staffing, funding, and support at both the federal and state levels will be critical to ensuring that the best possible information is collected on Medicaid and CHIP and that it is disseminated in an efficient manner—for example, by making use of technology that allows users to generate key indicators and summary reports with minimal need to sift through large volumes of raw data. Given that plans to modernize the agency's Medicaid and CHIP data systems currently rely on a patchwork of program integrity, quality measurement, health information technology, and CHIP reauthorization funds (CMS 2013a), the Commission urges CMS to assess whether its available resources will be sufficient for this purpose.

References

Baugh, D., and S. Verghese. 2012. *Physician service use and participation in Medicaid, 2009.* Issue brief no. 11. Princeton, NJ: Mathematica Policy Research, Inc. http://www.cms.gov/Research-Statistics-Data-and-Systems/Computer-Data-and-Systems/MedicaidDataSourcesGenInfo/Downloads/MAX_IB11_PhysicianParticipation.pdf.

Borck, R., A. Zlatinov, and S. Williams. 2013. *Medicaid analytic eXtract 2008 encounter data Chartbook.* Report to CMS, contract no. HHSM-500-2005-00025I. Princeton, NJ: Mathematica Policy Research, Inc. http://www.cms.gov/Research-Statistics-Data-and-Systems/Computer-Dataand-Systems/MedicaidDataSourcesGenInfo/Downloads/MAX_2008_Encounter_Data_Chartbook_Appendix_Tables.zip.

Borden, W.S., C.A. Camillo, M. Potts, et al. 2010. *Improving the completeness, accuracy and timeliness of Medicaid data.* Princeton, NJ: Mathematica Policy Research, Inc.

Bouchery, E. 2012a. *Utilization of dental services among Medicaid enrolled children.* Issue brief no. 9. Princeton, NJ: Mathematica Policy Research, Inc. http://www.cms.gov/Research-Statistics-Data-and-Systems/Computer-Data-and-Systems/MedicaidDataSourcesGenInfo/Downloads/MAX_IB9_DentalCare.pdf.

Bouchery, E. 2012b. *Utilization of well-child care among Medicaid enrolled children.* Issue brief no. 10. Princeton, NJ: Mathematica Policy Research, Inc. http://www.cms.gov/Research-Statistics-Data-and-Systems/Computer-Data-and-Systems/MedicaidDataSourcesGenInfo/Downloads/MAX_IB10_WellChild.pdf.

Boughn, J. 2013. Presentation before the Medicaid and CHIP Payment and Access Commission, February 12, 2013, Washington, DC. http://www.macpac.gov/home/meetings.

Byrd, V.L.H., and J. Verdier. 2011. *Collecting, using, and reporting Medicaid encounter data: A primer for states.* Final report. Report to CMS, contract no. HHSM-500-2005-00025I. Washington, DC: Mathematica Policy Research, Inc. http://www.cms.gov/Research-Statistics-Data-and-Systems/Computer-Data-and-Systems/MedicaidDataSourcesGenInfo/Downloads/MAX_PDQ_Task_X_EncounterDataPrimerforStates.pdf.

Byrd, V.L.H., and A.H. Dodd. 2012. *Assessing the usability of encounter data for enrollees in comprehensive managed care across MAX 2007–2009.* Issue brief no. 15. Princeton, NJ: Mathematica Policy Research, Inc. http://www.cms.gov/Research-Statistics-Data-and-Systems/Computer-Data-and-Systems/MedicaidDataSourcesGenInfo/Downloads/MAX_IB_15_AssessingUsability.pdf.

Byrd, V.L.H., A.H. Dodd, et al. 2012. *Assessing the usability of MAX 2008 encounter data for enrollees in comprehensive managed care.* Issue brief no. 7. Princeton, NJ: Mathematica Policy Research, Inc. http://www.cms.gov/Research-Statistics-Data-and-Systems/Computer-Data-and-Systems/MedicaidDataSourcesGenInfo/Downloads/MAX_IB7_EncounterData_071312.pdf.

Camillo, C.A. 2012. *CHIP Data in the Medicaid Statistical Information System (MSIS): Availability and uses.* Issue brief no. 12. Princeton, NJ: Mathematica Policy Research, Inc. http://www.cms.gov/Research-Statistics-Data-and-Systems/Computer-Data-and-Systems/MedicaidDataSourcesGenInfo/Downloads/MAX_IB12_CHIPData.pdf.

Centers for Medicare & Medicaid Services (CMS), U.S. Department of Health and Human Services. 2013a. Communication with MACPAC staff.

Centers for Medicare & Medicaid Services (CMS), U.S. Department of Health and Human Services. 2013b. *Affordable Care Act: State resources FAQ.* Baltimore, MD: CMS. http://www.medicaid.gov/State-Resource-Center/FAQ-Medicaid-and-CHIP-Affordable-Care-Act-ACA-Implementation/Downloads/Affordable-Care-Act_-Newest-Version.pdf.

Centers for Medicare & Medicaid Services (CMS), U.S. Department of Health and Human Services. 2013c. Medicare data for dual eligibles for states. Baltimore, MD: CMS. http://www.cms.gov/Medicare-Medicaid-Coordination/Medicare-and-Medicaid-Coordination/Medicare-Medicaid-Coordination-Office/MedicareDataforStates.html.

Centers for Medicare & Medicaid Services (CMS), U.S. Department of Health and Human Services. 2012. MITA information series: What is MITA? An overview. http://www.medicaid.gov/Medicaid-CHIP-Program-Information/By-Topics/Data-and-Systems/Downloads/mitaoverview.pdf.

Centers for Medicare & Medicaid Services (CMS), U.S. Department of Health and Human Services. 2010a. *Modernizing CMS computer and data systems to support improvements in care delivery.* Baltimore, MD: CMS. http://www.cms.gov/Research-Statistics-Dataand-Systems/CMS-Information-Technology/CIO-Directivesand-Policies/Downloads/CMSSection10330Plan.pdf.

Centers for Medicare & Medicaid Services (CMS), U.S. Department of Health and Human Services. 2010b. Letter from Cindy Mann to State Medicaid Directors and State Health Officials regarding "Revised State Plan Amendment Review Process." October 1, 2010. http://downloads.cms.gov/cmsgov/archived-downloads/SMDL/downloads/SMD10020.pdf.

Czajka, J.L. 2012a. *Medicaid enrollment gaps, 2005–2007*. Issue brief no. 6. Princeton, NJ: Mathematica Policy Research, Inc. http://www.cms.gov/Research-Statistics-Data-and-Systems/Computer-Data-and-Systems/MedicaidDataSourcesGenInfo/Downloads/MAX_IB6_EnrollGaps.pdf.

Czajka, J.L.. 2012b. *Movement of children between Medicaid and CHIP, 2005–2007*. Issue brief no. 4. Princeton, NJ: Mathematica Policy Research, Inc. http://www.cms.gov/Research-Statistics-Data-and-Systems/Computer-Data-and-Systems/MedicaidDataSourcesGenInfo/Downloads/Medicaid_and_CHIP_Transitions.pdf.

Dodd, A.H., and P.M. Gleason. 2013. *Using the MAX-NHANES merged data to evaluate the association of obesity and Medicaid costs*. Issue brief no. 16. Princeton, NJ: Mathematica Policy Research, Inc. http://www.cms.gov/Research-Statistics-Data-and-Systems/Computer-Data-and-Systems/MedicaidDataSourcesGenInfo/Downloads/MAX_IB16_MAX_NHANES.PDF.

Dodd, A.H., J. Nysenbaum, and A.Zlatinov. 2012. *Assessing the usability of the MAX 2007 inpatient and prescription encounter data for enrollees in comprehensive managed care*. Issue brief no. 5. Princeton, NJ: Mathematica Policy Research, Inc. http://www.cms.gov/Research-Statistics-Data-and-Systems/Computer-Data-and-Systems/MedicaidDataSourcesGenInfo/Downloads/MAXTA_Usability_MAX_2007_IP_and_RX_EncounterData.pdf.

Gorman, J. 2012. T-MSIS pilot overview. Presentation at Medicaid Enterprise Systems Conference, August 2012, Boston, MA. http://www.mesconference.org/wp-content/uploads/2012/08/Monday_TMSIS_Gorman.pdf.

Ku, L., P. MacTaggart, et al. 2009. *Improving Medicaid's continuity of coverage and quality of care*. Washington, DC: Association for Community Affiliated Plans (ACAP). http://www.ahcahp.org/Portals/0/ACAP%20Docs/Improving%20Medicaid%20Final%20070209.pdf.

Medicaid and CHIP Payment and Access Commission (MACPAC). 2013. *Report to the Congress on Medicaid and CHIP*. March 2013. Washington, DC: MACPAC. http://www.macpac.gov/reports/2013-03-15_MACPAC_Report.pdf?attredirects=0&d=1.

Medicaid and CHIP Payment and Access Commission (MACPAC). 2011. *Report to the Congress on Medicaid and CHIP*. March 2011. Washington, DC: MACPAC. http://www.macpac.gov/reports/MACPAC_March2011_web.pdf?attredirects=0&d=1.

National Association of State Chief Information Officers (NASCIO). 2008. *The MITA touch: State CIOs and Medicaid IT transformation*. Lexington, KY: NASCIO. http://www.nascio.org/publications/documents/NASCIO-MITA.pdf.

National Governors Association (NGA). 2012. *Top IT actions to save states money and boost efficiency*. Washington, DC: NGA. http://www.nga.org/cms/home/nga-center-for-best-practices/center-publications/page-ehsw-publications/col2-content/main-content-list/top-it-actions-to-save-states-mo.html.

Nysenbaum, J., E. Bouchery, and R. Malsberger. 2012. *The availability and usability of behavioral health organization encounter data in MAX 2009*. Issue brief no. 14. Princeton, NJ: Mathematica Policy Research, Inc. http://www.cms.gov/Research-Statistics-Data-and-Systems/Computer-Data-and-Systems/MedicaidDataSourcesGenInfo/Downloads/MAX_IB14_BHO.pdf.

Office of Inspector General (OIG), U.S. Department of Health and Human Services. 2009. *Medicaid managed care encounter data: Collection and use*. Washington, DC: OIG. http://oig.hhs.gov/oei/reports/oei-07-06-00540.pdf.

Plewes, T.J. 2010. *Databases for estimating health insurance coverage for children: A workshop summary*. Washington, DC: The National Academies Press. http://www.nap.edu/catalog/13024.html.

Thomson Medstat. 2006. *Thirteen state Medicaid core performance measure reporting summary: Highlighting model practices*. Baltimore, MD: Centers for Medicare & Medicaid Services. https://www.cms.gov/MedicaidCHIPQualPrac/Downloads/13.pdf.

Thompson, P. 2010. Presentation before the Medicaid and CHIP Payment and Access Commission, October 28, 2010, Washington, DC. http://www.macpac.gov/home/meetings/2010_10.

Truffer, C. 2013. Medicaid expenditures outlook. Presentation before the Medicaid and CHIP Payment and Access Commission, January 2013, Washington, DC. http://www.macpac.gov/home/meetings.

U.S. Department of Health and Human Services (HHS). 2012a. Medicaid program: Initial core set of health quality measures for Medicaid-eligible adults. Final notice. *Federal Register* 77, no. 2 (January 4): 286–291.

U.S. Department of Health and Human Services (HHS). 2012b. *2012 Annual report on the quality of care for children in Medicaid and CHIP*. Washington, DC: HHS. http://www.medicaid.gov/Medicaid-CHIP-Program-Information/By-Topics/Quality-of-Care/Downloads/2012-Ann-Sec-Rept.pdf.

U.S. Government Accountability Office (GAO). 2012. *Medicaid: Data sets provide inconsistent picture of expenditures*. Washington, DC: GAO. http://www.gao.gov/assets/650/649733.pdf.

CHAPTER 5

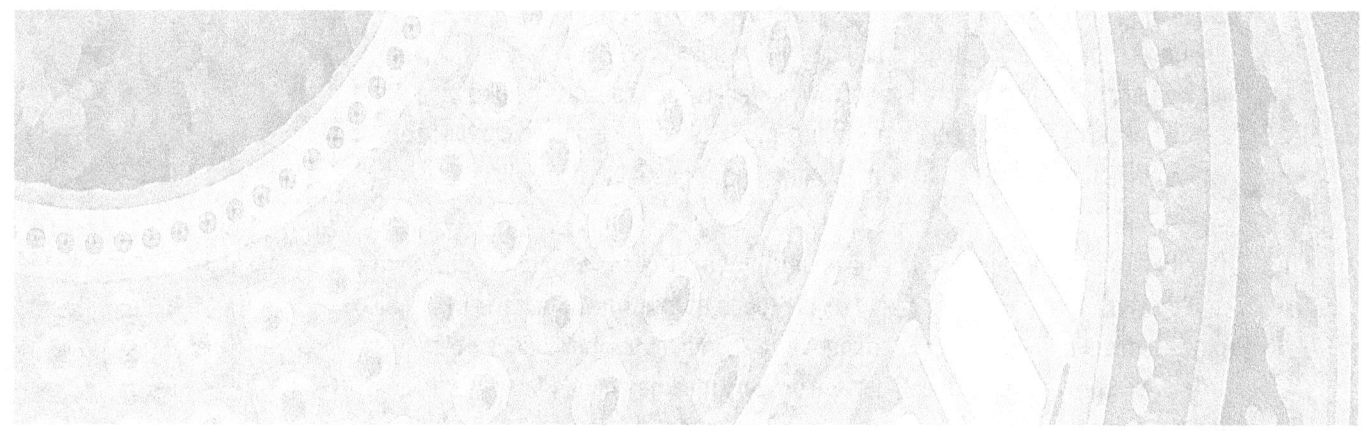

Update on Program Integrity in Medicaid

Key Points

Update on Program Integrity in Medicaid

- Program integrity activities are intended to ensure that public dollars are spent appropriately on delivering high-quality, medically necessary care. An effective program integrity approach should prevent improper payments, reduce waste and abuse particularly when it leads to patient harm, and help achieve value.

- An effective program integrity strategy in Medicaid requires coordination among state and federal agencies, a task complicated by the fact that current activities are governed by multiple federal statutes and regulations. Each state develops its own approach to program integrity, while federal activities are guided by a comprehensive plan that was last updated in 2009. A new plan, which will take into account lessons learned from prior initiatives, is expected to be released in the fall of 2013.

- Program integrity includes both a discrete set of activities related to the detection and prevention of fraud, waste, and abuse (such as post-payment review) but also other aspects of Medicaid program administration such as individual enrollment (eligibility), provider enrollment, service delivery, and payment. States and the federal government conduct mandatory and optional activities in all of these areas.

- In some programmatic areas such as eligibility determination, there are multiple program integrity initiatives, while other areas, such as managed care, receive comparatively little attention. Attention should be paid to identifying opportunities to better distribute and coordinate resources and shift focus to higher-value activities.

- The Medicaid Eligibility Quality Control (MEQC) and Payment Error Rate Measurement (PERM) eligibility reviews are an example of duplicative program integrity initiatives. While both programs review the accuracy of individual Medicaid and CHIP eligibility determinations, the rules for the two programs overlap and do not align well with each other.

- Future Commission work will focus on identifying specific opportunities to streamline regulatory requirements, and point the way to eliminating redundant functions, promoting greater integration of state and federal activities, or investing additional resources.

CHAPTER 5

Update on Program Integrity in Medicaid

This chapter continues MACPAC's work on program integrity in Medicaid and the State Children's Health Insurance Program (CHIP). As described in the Commission's March 2012 report to the Congress, program integrity consists of initiatives to detect and deter fraud, waste, and abuse (Box 5-1). These problems exist throughout the health care system, not just in Medicaid and CHIP. Even so, maintaining the ability to ensure that federal and state dollars are spent appropriately on delivering quality, necessary care to eligible individuals in Medicaid and CHIP is a priority for policymakers.[1]

Although estimates vary, the size and reach of the Medicaid program is expected to increase substantially due to changes made by the Patient Protection and Affordable Care Act (ACA, P.L. 111-148, as amended): in 2014, the Centers for Medicare & Medicaid Services (CMS) estimates that the program will cover an additional 11.5 million people on average over the course of the calendar year, while the Congressional Budget Office (CBO) estimates that Medicaid and CHIP together will cover an additional 9 million people on average (CMS 2013a and CBO 2013). In addition to preparing for enrollment growth, states are implementing a variety of policy and operational changes to manage interactions with exchange coverage and shift to value-based payment methods (KFF 2013). An effective program integrity approach will be essential to preventing improper payments, protecting enrollees, and achieving value as Medicaid and CHIP evolve.

Successful program integrity efforts depend on coordination among various state and federal agencies. The size and diversity of the 56 state and territorial Medicaid programs makes these efforts complex (GAO 2012a). Furthermore, within and among individual states and within the federal government, program integrity activities require coordination among a variety of discrete monitoring and detection activities and administrative processes (e.g., eligibility determinations, provider enrollment, service delivery, and claims payment).

The success of these efforts will also depend on investment in activities known to work. Many program integrity strategies have been conceived as independent efforts and may require rethinking or revisions to stay current as the evidence base grows or newer strategies emerge. A broad view of Medicaid program integrity activities across a range of programmatic areas at the state and federal levels can help identify opportunities to better distribute and coordinate resources and shift focus to higher-value activities. For example, many program integrity efforts remain focused on fee-for-service (FFS) payments, while states are increasingly shifting to capitated and other payment approaches. The Commission plans to look more carefully at program integrity issues related to managed care in future reports.

Previous Commission Review and Recommendations

Over the past two decades, but particularly since the passage of the Deficit Reduction Act of 2005 (P.L. 109-107) and creation of the federal Medicaid Integrity Program, there has been growing interest in Medicaid program integrity at the federal level and greater investment by states in a range of activities. In our March 2012 report, we described the status of those activities, provided an overview of federal and state oversight responsibilities, summarized how various federal agencies and states coordinate program integrity activities, described the challenges associated with quantifying program integrity outcomes, and discussed how managed care plans address program integrity. We identified a number of challenges associated with implementation of an effective and efficient Medicaid program integrity strategy, including:

- overlap between federal and state responsibilities;
- insufficient collaboration and information sharing among federal agencies and states;
- diffusion of authority among multiple federal and state agencies;

BOX 5-1. Regulatory Definitions of Fraud and Abuse

Medicaid regulations define fraud and abuse as follows:

- **Fraud:** "An intentional deception or misrepresentation made by a person with the knowledge that the deception could result in some unauthorized benefit to himself or some other person. It includes any act that constitutes fraud under applicable federal or state law."

- **Abuse:** "Provider practices that are inconsistent with sound fiscal, business, or medical practices, and result in an unnecessary cost to the Medicaid program, or in reimbursement for services that are not medically necessary or that fail to meet professionally recognized standards for health care."

- **Waste,** which is not defined in federal Medicaid regulations, is not a criminal or intentional act but results in unnecessary expenditures to the Medicaid program. Examples include avoidable hospitalizations, duplication of services, and the use of emergency departments for non-emergent care.

Both providers and enrollees can contribute to waste, fraud, and abuse.

Source: 42 CFR 433.304 and 42 CFR 455.2.

- lack of information on the effectiveness of program integrity initiatives and appropriate performance measures;
- lower federal matching rates for state activities not directly related to fraud control;
- incomplete and outdated data; and
- few program integrity resources for delivery system models other than FFS (e.g., managed care).

To address these issues, the Commission made two recommendations related to program integrity.

First, in order to ensure that current program integrity requirements make efficient use of federal resources and do not place undue burden on states or providers, the Commission recommended that the Secretary of the U.S. Department of Health and Human Services (HHS) (the Secretary) should collaborate with states to "create feedback loops to simplify and streamline program integrity requirements, determine which current federal program integrity initiatives are most effective, and take steps to eliminate programs that are redundant, outdated, or not cost-effective" (MACPAC 2012).

Second, in order to enhance states' abilities to detect and deter fraud and abuse, the Commission recommended that the Secretary should "develop methods for better quantifying the effectiveness of program integrity activities, assess analytic tools for detecting and deterring fraud and abuse and promote the use of those tools that are most effective, improve dissemination of best practices in program integrity, and enhance program integrity training programs" (MACPAC 2012).

Current Status of Federal Medicaid Program Integrity Activities

Federal Medicaid program integrity activities are guided by a Comprehensive Medicaid Integrity Plan, which is developed by the Medicaid Integrity Group (MIG) within CMS (CMS 2009a). The plan was last updated in 2009; CMS is in the process of updating its strategy, and a new comprehensive plan is expected to be released in the fall of 2013 (CMS 2013c).

In addition to the Commission, others have also questioned the effectiveness and efficiency of the current federal approach as outlined in the 2009 plan. In a series of reviews published in 2012, the Government Accountability Office (GAO) found that the hiring of separate contractors for the National Medicaid Audit Program was inefficient and led to duplication. Other MIG oversight and support activities, such as the Medicaid Integrity Institute and State Program Integrity Assessments, showed mixed results (GAO 2012a, GAO 2012b).

CMS concurred with many of the suggestions GAO provided to improve the efficiency of federal Medicaid program integrity activities, and as part of a broader effort to increase program efficiency, has begun revising its approach to program integrity and expanding efforts to support states (CMS 2013c). This new federal approach aligns with the recommendations made by the Commission in 2012 (Table 5-1).

The new comprehensive plan will include additional changes based on the lessons learned from various initiatives implemented over the last eight years, including:

- ensuring that new Medicaid initiatives, particularly those based on Medicare approaches, are appropriately tailored and take into account the diversity of state programs;

- aligning and coordinating federal resources around program integrity functions and goals instead of individual statutes and initiatives;
- promoting collaboration between federal staff (including contractors) and states and among states; and
- using risk assessment to identify areas of focus, rather than taking a "one size fits all" approach.

This updated approach to federal Medicaid program integrity efforts will also leverage improvements in Medicaid and CHIP data described by CMS in a February 2013 presentation

TABLE 5-1. Updates to CMS Medicaid Program Integrity Activities

MACPAC Recommendation	Recent CMS Actions Related to Recommendations
Determine which federal program integrity activities are most effective and eliminate programs that are redundant, outdated, or not cost-effective	Shifting the focus of the National Medicaid Audit Program from independent audits based on federal data to collaborative audits that leverage state expertise and state data
	Suspending collection of the annual State Program Integrity Assessment dataset while CMS streamlines questionnaires to eliminate duplication
Assess analytic tools and promote use of those that are most effective	Working with states to develop new provider screening tools
	Using state-supplied Medicaid Management Information System (MMIS) data to support federal Medicaid Integrity Contractor audits while CMS separately works to improve the quality and timeliness of federal Medicaid Statistical Information System (MSIS) data
Improve dissemination of best practices	Launched a Medicaid program integrity workgroup to identify best practices for financial management and provide input for a CMS framework to strengthen the federal-state Medicaid program oversight partnership
	Providing a secure online platform for states to exchange best practices and documents on program integrity
	Published prescriber guidelines to promote best practices for therapeutic drug classes identified as high risk
Enhance program integrity training programs	Created a new managed care program integrity curriculum for states and the first Certified Program Integrity Professional program of study through the Medicaid Integrity Institute
	Offering distance learning webinars to increase access to training opportunities for state Medicaid staff

Sources: GAO 2012b; Thompson 2012

to the Commission (Boughn 2013). The Transformed Medicaid Statistical Information System (T-MSIS), which will begin incorporating state data later in 2013, builds on existing person-level and claims-level MSIS data submitted by states and will provide more robust analytic capabilities for CMS. See Chapter 4: *Update on Medicaid and CHIP Data for Policy Analysis and Program Accountability* for more details on T-MSIS and other CMS data improvement initiatives.

Key Programmatic Areas in Program Integrity

In our March 2012 report, we highlighted federal-state coordination as a particular concern for program integrity efforts. In this section, we present an overview of program integrity activities from a state program administration point of view, while highlighting strategies that are embedded in larger program functions (e.g., individual and provider enrollment, service delivery, and payment) and dedicated program integrity activities that cross multiple functions (e.g., post-payment review, reporting, and follow-up).

As CMS continues to refine and implement a national Medicaid program integrity strategy, it must balance the need to comply with existing statutory and regulatory requirements with the goals of making efficient use of federal resources and avoiding undue burden on states and providers. This is a delicate balancing act for two reasons.

First, program integrity relates to all aspects of the program, including eligibility, provider enrollment, claims payment, managed care oversight, and federal claiming. However, states must continually strike a balance between tight front-end controls in each programmatic area and other program goals, particularly access to a sufficient network of providers and efficient program administration.

Second, a Medicaid program integrity strategy must be executed within a state-federal program structure, where the federal government and states have shared responsibility for financing and administering the program. Because federal and state dollars are used to pay for Medicaid services, both levels of government have a strong interest in program integrity. However, state and federal government roles and responsibilities sometimes diverge and sometimes overlap, complicating their ability to jointly implement a program integrity strategy.

Seven programmatic areas are integral to a comprehensive program integrity approach: program integrity operations, individual enrollment, provider enrollment, service delivery, payment, post-payment review, and reporting and follow-up. States and the federal government conduct mandatory and optional activities in each area (Table 5-2); this section briefly reviews activities in each area. There are duplicative initiatives as well as areas that receive relatively little attention. There are also areas where state and federal responsibilities align and others where they overlap.

This section is followed by a more detailed discussion of one specific area of overlap and duplication—eligibility review—as an example of challenges states face in trying to comply with federal program integrity requirements that may be outdated and redundant. Future Commission work will investigate potential concerns surfaced by this analysis and help policymakers identify specific opportunities to streamline regulatory requirements, eliminate redundant functions, promote greater integration of state and federal activities, or invest additional resources.

Program integrity operations

Program integrity is identified in Title XIX of the Social Security Act (the Act) as an essential

TABLE 5-2. Overview of State and CMS Program Integrity Activities

	State	CMS
Program integrity operations	Establish overall strategy Develop operational plans Obtain necessary authorities Hire and train staff Obtain necessary data Develop appropriate linkages among state and federal agencies	Establish overall strategy Develop and implement curricula for the Medicaid Integrity Institute, provide no-cost training to state staff Review and approve state information system plans Develop and publish performance standards and best practices Provide individual and provider education regarding program integrity issues Develop appropriate linkages among state and federal agencies
Individual enrollment	Determine eligibility Collect third-party liability (TPL) information and coordinate benefits Verify reported information	Provide access to federal databases to verify individuals' reported application or redetermination information Support cross-state information sharing of individual application verification information through the Public Assistance Reporting Information System
Provider enrollment	Enroll providers Check exclusion lists Conduct onsite inspections and verifications Report any adverse provider application actions to the Office of Inspector General Contract with managed care plans	Provide access to Medicare provider databases and risk screen findings Support cross-state information sharing of provider application verification information Review managed care contracts
Service delivery	Develop and document coverage, billing, and payment policies Restrict (lock in) to certain providers those individuals prone to abusing services Verify eligibility at point of service Review prior authorization requests Review prospective drug utilization review requests	Review proposed Medicaid state plan amendments that relate to services

TABLE 5-2, Continued

	State	CMS
Payment	Apply prepayment edits Process service and payment edits Apply TPL information Use predictive modeling to flag potential errors Suspend potential fraudulent claims Adjudicate final payments Issue Explanation of Benefits statements Submit claims for federal matching funds	Develop, publish, and update National Correct Coding Initiative edits based on typical billing issues Develop, publish, and update predictive modeling algorithms to be applied pre-payment Review state claims for federal matching funds
Post-payment review	Conduct Medicaid Eligibility Quality Control (MEQC) and Payment Error Rate Measurement (PERM) eligibility reviews Participate in federal PERM fee-for-service (FFS) and managed care measurement Pursue third-party payments when available Perform retrospective reviews of care Conduct surveillance and utilization review Audit payments Support federal Medicaid Integrity Contractor (MIC) audits Contract with Recovery Audit Contractors (RACs) Supply data for Medicare-Medicaid (Medi-Medi) matches Identify potential fraud	Review MEQC and PERM sampling plans Conduct federal PERM FFS and managed care measurement Conduct federal MIC audits Conduct federal Medi-Medi data matches Review claims data for potential fraud and abuse Provide staff and other resources to support state field investigations
Reporting and follow-up	Refer suspected fraud to law enforcement Provide support for fraud investigations Terminate fraudulent providers and contracts Recoup overpayments from providers Return federal share of overpayments Calculate return on investment Compile program integrity statistics Complete federal State Program Integrity Assessment surveys Participate in comprehensive State Program Integrity Reviews Identify and implement corrective actions Report the identification and collection of overpayments due to waste, fraud, and abuse Report administrative expenses associated with program integrity activities	Conduct comprehensive State Program Integrity Reviews Conduct annual State Program Integrity Assessments Develop and implement national PERM corrective action plan Develop Medicaid integrity review "lessons learned" reports Facilitate access to federal databases and web portals for reporting payment suspensions, provider terminations, and state Recovery Audit Contractor activity

program function, and all Medicaid programs must have "methods and procedures relating to the utilization of and payment for care and services....as may be necessary to safeguard against unnecessary utilization of such care and services and to assure that payments are consistent with efficiency, economy, and quality of care" (§1902(a)(30)).

Over time, many additional statutory and regulatory requirements for how states must monitor, detect, and measure fraud, waste, and abuse have been added to statute and regulation. States have developed a variety of strategies to implement these rules, ranging from largely decentralized to highly coordinated program integrity functions. States' resource constraints are a fundamental issue: with limited budgets, states must often shift limited resources to mandated activities in lieu of other preferred activities.

With the creation of the MIG in 2005 and the allocation of substantially greater resources to support Medicaid program integrity, the federal government has increased its support for state program integrity activities. In September 2007, CMS established the Medicaid Integrity Institute, a national Medicaid program integrity training center for states that has provided no-cost training to over 3,000 state employees and is highly regarded by states (GAO 2012a). The federal government has also created new initiatives that require state resources, such as the comprehensive State Program Integrity Reviews (MACPAC 2012).

Other federal efforts to support states in building internal program integrity infrastructure and capacity have had more limited impact. The federally contracted Education Medicaid Integrity Contractor (Education MIC) provides support for the MIG in developing materials and conducting training on Medicaid fraud, waste, and abuse. As of April 2013, the Education MIC had developed and broadly disseminated guidance on a small number of topics (CMS 2013d). CMS has also used information collected during periodic reviews of state Medicaid program integrity activities to identify three sets of best practices and provide technical guidance for other states (CMS 2013e). States, through the National Association of Medicaid Directors, have asked that CMS devote a greater share of contractor resources to support training, education, and implementation of state-level tools (NAMD 2012).

Individual and provider enrollment

One of the strongest tools that state Medicaid agencies have to prevent fraud, waste, and abuse is the ability to conduct initial and periodic assessments of individuals and providers and exclude ineligible, unqualified, or inappropriate individuals from participation. Long-standing federal policies require states to verify and validate individual eligibility at the time of application and periodically thereafter and to promptly disenroll persons who are not eligible. In recent years, greater focus has been placed on screening providers who seek to participate in the program, routinely verifying their continuing eligibility to bill Medicaid, and promptly suspending or removing providers who are suspected or convicted of defrauding the program.

States must balance their interest in excluding ineligible persons with the responsibility to ensure that eligible persons are not inappropriately denied participation or dissuaded from completing the application process due to rules designed to protect program integrity. This applies to providers as well: states must verify that only providers who meet program criteria are allowed to bill the program, but must also take care that the process does not deter qualified providers from participation and negatively affect enrollee access to care.

Medicaid enrollee eligibility. In order to support state efforts to ensure that only persons who meet eligibility criteria are enrolled in the program, the federal government provides access to national data sources to facilitate state validation of individual application enrollment information. For example, the HHS maintains a database of income and program participation information from multiple states and federal programs. States can access the data to determine duplicate program enrollment or the accuracy of application information. CMS is in the process of developing a comprehensive federal eligibility data hub to support real-time, electronic verification of enrollee eligibility information beginning in late 2013 (CMS 2013f). The availability of systems to automate the validation of data that are available electronically, once fully implemented, could reduce burden on state staff and eventually support the reallocation of resources that would have been spent collecting and reviewing paper-based information to other activities.

State Medicaid programs are federally required to conduct two different types of retrospective reviews of eligibility determinations.

- **Medicaid Eligibility Quality Control (MEQC).** All states are required to conduct monthly MEQC reviews of active Medicaid cases to determine whether eligibility decisions were made correctly: whether enrollees were eligible for services, and whether denied or terminated Medicaid applications were correctly processed. States calculate and report state-specific error rates.

- **Payment Error Rate Measurement (PERM).** States must also participate in the federal PERM eligibility measurement every three years. One requirement of the program is to sample and review a small number of eligibility cases each month. PERM error findings are reported to CMS for inclusion (along with the FFS and managed care findings) in the state and national error rates and are used at the state level to inform corrective action.

PERM and MEQC are discussed in greater detail later in this chapter.

Provider enrollment. States must ensure that providers comply with state rules regarding qualification to participate in the Medicaid program. States must also ensure that they do not enroll or make payments to providers excluded by the Medicare program or other state Medicaid programs and terminate providers whose billing privileges have been revoked by other programs for cause (42 CFR 455(e)). In 2011, CMS expanded the provider screening rules for Medicare and required states to implement them in the Medicaid program; specifically, states must obtain certain disclosures from providers upon enrollment (and periodically thereafter), search exclusion and debarment lists and databases, and take action to exclude providers who appear on such lists. Medicaid managed care organizations (MCOs) must also conduct routine screens to ensure that excluded providers are not permitted to participate. States are now required not only to check federal databases but also to share information on provider enrollment decisions proactively with federal program administrators (42 CFR 1002.3(b)(3)).

States report that current processes to conduct the required checks are difficult to implement and time consuming to operate (NAMD 2013). Systems that streamline application data collection, automate exclusion checks, and target enhanced checks at riskier providers could help to reduce state and provider burden and improve efficiency. Because all states must comply with the same provider screening rules and conduct the same database checks, and because most of these databases are federally maintained, a comprehensive system to support states in the Medicaid provider enrollment process could greatly improve efficiency.

CMS has implemented a system that provides some information to states, but it is incomplete. The web-based application allows states to share information regarding Medicaid providers who have been terminated for cause and to view information on Medicare providers and suppliers who have had their billing privileges revoked for cause. However, the system does not provide information on other types of exclusions (Budetti 2013). The available systems are also not updated in real time (some only monthly). Thus, states must conduct additional checks to exclude ineligible providers.

Service delivery

Program integrity activities at the time of service delivery (often referred to as the point of service) focus on confirming enrollee eligibility to receive a particular service and ensuring that services provided are medically necessary, appropriate, and provided in accordance with program rules. In FFS Medicaid, states determine which services are covered and what restrictions or limitations apply to each service. Medicaid covers a broader range of rehabilitative, habilitative, and support services than most private insurers and has many unique coverage and payment rules, so states provide written guidance (in the form of manuals and bulletins) to providers and conduct periodic training to help promote understanding of and compliance with program rules.

States can also require providers to receive prior approval for some services, but the approval process can be costly to the state, create burdens for providers, and delay the initiation of treatment. States must weigh all of these factors when determining which front-end controls to implement.

CMS reviews state policy change requests to ensure that covered services and payment mechanisms comply with federal laws and regulations and that proposed payment strategies align with Medicaid financing rules (HHS and DOJ 2012). However, CMS does not typically review—or even collect—the detailed guidance that states develop to instruct providers on what can be covered, nor does it assess the extent to which states impose pre-payment controls apart from those explicitly required by federal statute. CMS has provided detailed policy guidance for states to support accurate coverage and payment determinations and to decrease fraud, waste, and abuse associated with prescription drugs, but has not broadly disseminated guidance for most Medicaid-covered services, including those known to be vulnerable to fraud and abuse such as certain home and community-based services (CMS 2013d). CMS, like states, generally relies on post-payment audits (discussed in greater detail below) to assess the degree to which paid claims comply with state and federal coverage and billing requirements.

Payment

In most cases, Medicaid provider payments are triggered by the submission of a claim by a provider indicating that a service has been provided, and the systems that adjudicate most payment requests have numerous controls built in to support program integrity. States use the information presented on a claim and other data contained in their systems to adjudicate the claim and determine the appropriate payment.

Federal statute and rules mandate many of the checks that states must conduct, including requirements to verify provider authorization, check for logical consistency (e.g., whether the patient on an obstetrical claim is a woman), prevent duplicate payments, and verify payment amounts (42 CFR 447.45(f)). States must also develop and apply edits to ensure that appropriate limitations are put on claims submitted on behalf of enrollees who are eligible for a restricted or alternate benefit package, who have third-party coverage (including Medicare), or who are enrolled in a Medicaid managed care plan (42 CFR 433.137). Most of these checks and reviews are automatically conducted by the claims processing system and the majority of claims are processed without any manual intervention. Because Medicaid claims are subject to complex adjudication rules, consistent and accurate application of these rules is a critical aspect of program integrity.

Every state claims payment system must meet certain requirements in order to be approved by CMS and receive enhanced federal funding. These requirements generally pertain to specific functionality that the system must support, including having a surveillance and utilization review component to support program integrity (42 CFR 456). Beginning in 2010, the Congress created two new requirements that extend Medicare program integrity strategies to state Medicaid payment systems. These are:

- **National Correct Coding Initiative (NCCI).** NCCI promotes national correct coding methodologies and reduces improper coding, which may result in inappropriate payments. The ACA required state Medicaid programs to incorporate compatible NCCI methodologies in their systems for processing Medicaid claims by October 1, 2010.

- **Predictive modeling.** As part of the Small Business Jobs Act of 2010 (P.L. 111-240), the Congress mandated that CMS implement predictive modeling technologies (i.e., analyze large datasets for suspicious patterns, anomalies, or other factors that may be linked to fraud, waste, and abuse) to help identify potential fraud prior to making Medicare payments. By April 1, 2015, CMS must begin expanding the program to Medicaid and CHIP and apply lessons learned from the use of predictive modeling in Medicare (Budetti 2012).

Post-payment review

A variety of post-payment reviews are conducted to correct over- and underpayments and identify potential fraud and abuse.

Federal rules require states to conduct post-payment reviews of provider payments to assure appropriate utilization and to identify potential fraud and abuse.

Routine reviews of accuracy and quality. States conduct a variety of limited-scope analyses of provider records, claims, and supporting documentation after they have issued payments. States use both automated computer analysis and manual review to assure proper utilization and payment. These analyses may not be as extensive as an audit, but seek to determine quality of care, compliance with accepted standards of care, program compliance, and validity of services.

States can also provide state claims data and payment policies to the federal Medicare-Medicaid Data Matching Project (Medi-Medi), which combines Medicaid and Medicare claims and identifies data patterns indicating improper payments that previously went undetected in either program.

Audits. States conduct a variety of post-payment reviews to verify the accuracy of payments made for certain services or to certain types of providers. Many of these audits are federally required, each authorized through separate legislation and many being implemented in different centers within CMS.[2] Key requirements include the following:

- States must audit any provider that is paid on a cost-related basis and audit payments made to disproportionate share hospitals.
- States are required to participate in the periodic PERM error rate measurement, where federal contractors conduct audits of a random sample of claims to assess whether payments were made in accordance with federal and state requirements.
- States are required to cooperate with federal Medicaid Integrity Contractors (MICs), which are under contract to CMS to review provider claims, audit providers, identify overpayments, and educate providers, payers, and enrollees about program integrity.
- States are required to contract with a Recovery Audit Contractor (RAC) to identify underpayments and overpayments and to recoup overpayments on a contingency basis.

Fraud detection. State Medicaid agencies use many of the post-payment data analysis activities described above to identify potential fraud. States must also verify with enrollees whether services billed by providers were received (42 CFR 455.20). States that use managed care delivery systems must require MCOs to have a fraud and abuse or compliance plan, or both, and to report promptly any instances of provider fraud and abuse to the state.

When any of these activities uncover potential fraud, states must make referrals to appropriate external entities for investigation and prosecution. States also provide support to fraud investigators (e.g., provide access to claims data) and recoup improper payments.

As the number of federal Medicaid-related post-payment review activities has grown over time, states and others (including the Commission) have raised concerns about duplication of effort. For example, PERM, MICs, and RACs all audit FFS providers, but CMS has not created a mechanism for the various contractors to coordinate with each other or with state program integrity reviews to ensure that the same providers are not reviewed multiple times (NAMD 2012).

Reporting and follow-up

Federal rules require states to take certain actions when they identify improper payments, whether due to fraud, abuse, or inadvertent errors. States are also required to return the federal share of any identified overpayments within one year of identification—whether or not the state is able to recoup the erroneously paid amount from the provider. To prevent future improper payments, states use findings from program integrity activities to strengthen program controls, such as implementing new claims payment edits or conducting additional provider screenings. They may also analyze the outcomes of program integrity efforts to assess the return on staff and technology investments.

Every state must have a Medicaid Fraud Control Unit (MFCU), an entity of state government that investigates program administration and health care providers, prosecutes (or refers to prosecutors) those defrauding the programs, and collects overpayments. Federal regulation requires states to refer all cases of suspected provider fraud to the MFCU, comply with document requests from the MFCU, and initiate administrative or judicial action for cases referred to the state by the MFCU. When providers are convicted of fraud, the state must terminate the providers' participation in Medicaid, place them on exclusion lists, and notify the federal HHS Office of Inspector General (OIG). States also cooperate with a variety of other federal fraud task forces such as the Health Care Fraud Prevention and Enforcement Action Team (HEAT), a partnership between the federal HHS and the U.S. Department of Justice designed to gather resources across the federal government to prevent fraud, waste, and abuse in Medicare and Medicaid.

At the federal level, CMS collects a variety of Medicaid program integrity information. The MIG conducts a comprehensive review of each state integrity program every third year to assess the effectiveness of state program integrity activities and compliance with federal program integrity laws. Findings from these reviews are published on the MIG website. Until recently, the MIG conducted an annual State Program Integrity Assessment for all states, which collected statistics about program integrity staffing, expenditures, audits, and recoveries. This process has been temporarily suspended while CMS streamlines the questionnaire to eliminate duplication (GAO 2012a). Information from these reviews and from other MIG activities is used to develop descriptive reports for each state, identify areas for technical assistance, and assess state performance over time. CMS also reviews state claims for program integrity expenditures and periodic reports on recoveries, which states report separately for certain defined program integrity activities (e.g., National Medicaid Audit Program, state-initiated activities, and OIG-initiated audits).

PERM and MEQC: An Opportunity to Streamline

As noted earlier, states must strike a balance between front-end controls to support program integrity and other program goals, such as access. These competing priorities can be seen in the area of individual eligibility determinations: while states are required to verify eligibility, they also have the responsibility to ensure that enrollment of eligible persons is not inappropriately denied or delayed due to rules designed to protect program integrity. Retrospective eligibility reviews, conducted after an eligibility determination is made, can help states maintain program integrity without complicating or delaying the eligibility determination process. However, current federal rules regarding retrospective eligibility reviews are perceived by states to be costly and difficult to implement (CMS 2009b).

States must conduct two different types of retrospective reviews of eligibility determinations, MEQC and PERM. The rules for these two programs are overlapping and do not align well with each other (Table 5-3). They also have not been aligned with changes that have been made in eligibility policies and processes, particularly the significant changes required by the ACA. The result is illustrative of the challenges states face in trying to comply with federal program integrity requirements that may be outdated and redundant.

Medicaid Eligibility Quality Control

The MEQC program was created in 1978 to monitor the accuracy and timeliness of Medicaid eligibility determinations in order to avoid inappropriate payments and eligibility decision delays (§1903(u) of the Act). MEQC was also intended to identify methods to reduce and prevent errors related to incorrect eligibility determinations. The program is implemented by the states and overseen by CMS, per federal regulations at 42 CFR 431.800ff.

In the traditional MEQC program, states select a sample of eligibility cases over each six-month period. The sample includes both active cases (cases in which the individual or family was found to be eligible) and negative cases (cases in which Medicaid eligibility was denied). Only Medicaid cases are selected for review. Stand-alone CHIP programs are not subject to MEQC. Reviewers independently verify eligibility information as of the review month (the month in which the case is sampled), including interviewing enrollees and applicants and conducting home visits.

States are required to report their findings to CMS at the end of each six-month period, and then CMS calculates an error rate. Per the statute, states with error rates over 3 percent are subject to disallowances of federal matching funds, but states are permitted to request good faith waivers of disallowances. By the end of 1994 most states reduced and maintained their error rates to less than 2 percent, and only one state has been liable for disallowances since 1996 (CMS 2000).

Due to the consistently low error rates, in 1994 CMS developed criteria that allowed states to freeze their error rates as of the most recent completed MEQC period and develop pilot programs to find alternate ways to identify and reduce erroneous payments (CMS 2000). Over time, most states elected to conduct pilots under MEQC or an 1115 waiver; as of 2013, only eight states still conducted traditional MEQC reviews. (This number can fluctuate from year to year.) In the pilots, which must be approved by CMS, states can use a different sample size, focus on specific eligibility subgroups, and implement alternate review methodologies.

Payment Error Rate Measurement

PERM eligibility measurement was implemented in 2006 to comply with the Improper Payments Information Act of 2002 (P.L. 107-300) and related guidance, which identified Medicaid and CHIP as susceptible to significant erroneous payments. Among other requirements, CMS must produce an annual estimate of the amount of improper payments in Medicaid and CHIP and report on actions to reduce them.[3] The eligibility portion of the measurement is conducted by the states and overseen by CMS, per federal regulations at 42 CFR 431.950ff.

One third of states are included in the PERM measurement each year. Every three years, the state must measure error rates for a full 12-month period. States select a sample of eligibility cases, drawing separate samples for Medicaid and CHIP. Children enrolled in Medicaid-expansion CHIP programs are included in the CHIP sample. Like MEQC, the sample includes both active and negative cases.

Unlike MEQC, reviewers rely on information in the case record to determine whether the last action on a case was determined accurately. Reviewers only independently verify eligibility criteria where evidence is missing or outdated and likely to change, or if the last action was more than 12 months prior.

States are required to report their findings to CMS on a monthly basis and CMS calculates an error rate at the end of each measurement cycle. Overpayments identified based on PERM eligibility review are subject to disallowances (§1903(u) of the Act).

Initial PERM eligibility review guidance did not allow states to accept an applicant's self-declaration or self-certification of various eligibility criteria, although many states relied extensively on self-declaration to expedite the enrollment process, particularly for CHIP programs (HHS 2009). Many PERM eligibility reviews were consequently "undetermined" and counted as errors, leading to high error rates in many states. The Children's Health Insurance Program Reauthorization Act of 2009 (CHIPRA, P.L. 111-3) required that the payment error rate not take into account payment errors resulting from failure to validate self-declared eligibility information, if the self-declaration was provided in accordance with federal rules. CHIP programs were excluded from the PERM measurement until after CMS promulgated regulations implementing the CHIPRA provisions in 2010.

TABLE 5-3. Comparison of Payment Error Rate Measurement (PERM) and Medicaid Eligibility Quality Control (MEQC)

	Traditional MEQC	PERM
Time period	Six months, continuous	Twelve months, every third year
Sampling	Fixed sample size for each state, varies by state size (for most states, 550 active and 210 negative cases each year) Medicaid samples only	State-specific sample sizes recalculated each cycle based on statistical precision in prior cycle (base sample size is 504 active and 204 negative cases each year) Separate Medicaid and CHIP samples
Populations excluded	Children in foster care Supplemental Security Income (SSI) beneficiaries in states with an agreement with the Social Security Administration under §1634 of the Social Security Act Enrollees in separate CHIP programs Programs that are 100 percent federally funded	Children in foster care or adoption assistance SSI beneficiaries in §1634 agreement states Cases under active fraud investigation Cases approved using Express Lane eligibility Cases for which the state received no federal match
Verifications	Independently verify actual circumstances Applicant interviews and home visits required	Review case record and independently verify eligibility criteria only where evidence is missing, outdated and likely to change, or otherwise needed
Review period	Review eligibility in month sampled	Review eligibility as of date of last action on a case, up to 12 months prior to the sample month
Incomplete reviews	Cases can be dropped from review if beneficiary does not cooperate, cannot be located, or has moved out of state	Cases cannot be dropped Cases that cannot be completed are considered "undetermined" and counted as errors
Payment reviews	Collect payments for services received by sampled enrollees in the sample month (if paid in that month or the following four months)	Collect payments for services received by sampled enrollees in the sample month (if paid in that month or the following four months)
Error tolerance	Errors less than $5 are not counted	No tolerance for errors
Error rate calculation	Lower limit of statistical confidence interval used to calculate rate	Midpoint of statistical confidence interval used to calculate rate
Corrective action	Must take action to correct issues Correction plan must be submitted to CMS within 60 days of identification of error	Must take action to correct issues Correction plan must be submitted to CMS within 90 days of official notification of error rate

Note: As of 2013, only eight states still conducted traditional MEQC reviews. This number can fluctuate from year to year. Other states conduct pilots that may use a different sample size, focus on specific eligibility subgroups, or implement alternate review methodologies.

Source: CMS 2012a.

Due to substantial overlap in the MEQC and PERM eligibility review requirements and resulting burden on states, CHIPRA also directed CMS to take steps to harmonize the two programs and allow states the option of using PERM eligibility review findings to meet MEQC requirements and vice versa. While CMS has been able to implement the substitution requirement of CHIPRA, it has been unable to substantially harmonize the two programs due in part to other statutes and rules that were not changed by CHIPRA. States remain burdened by duplicative requirements.[4]

The process that CMS developed to allow states to use MEQC results to meet PERM requirements and vice versa requires states to draw a sample that meets the requirements of both traditional MEQC and PERM (CMS 2012a). For example, PERM measures Medicaid and CHIP separately, so enrollees in a Medicaid-expansion CHIP program must be excluded from an MEQC sample before it can be used to meet the PERM requirement. However, because all but a small number of states conduct MEQC pilots that cannot be substituted for PERM findings, most states must still conduct both MEQC and PERM reviews in the PERM measurement years.

Recent changes in eligibility policy may further complicate efforts to harmonize the programs or facilitate substitution. For example, MEQC excludes from the review persons whose Medicaid costs are borne completely by the federal government. Historically, this has included only a small proportion of enrollees eligible through special federal programs (e.g., American Indians receiving treatment in an Indian Health Service facility). However, under the ACA, the federal government will initially pay 100 percent of the cost of coverage for most persons in the adult expansion group. Although estimates of the number of individuals gaining Medicaid coverage under the ACA vary, CMS expects that the majority will be newly eligible adults for whom increased federal match is available (CMS 2013a). If these enrollees are excluded from MEQC but not PERM, it could be difficult for states to develop a sampling plan that would satisfy both programs.

It is also unclear how PERM and MEQC will be impacted by ACA-driven changes to the eligibility determination process. Beginning in 2014, Medicaid decisions can be made by state or federal exchanges in addition to state Medicaid agencies. CMS is evaluating the impact of the ACA on the PERM and MEQC eligibility measurements. However, at this time CMS has not issued rules or published guidance to indicate whether persons determined eligible by an exchange will be excluded from MEQC and PERM reviews, whether exchanges must share case information with states for purposes of eligibility review, or whether states will be accountable for verification or calculation errors made by exchanges. States must submit sampling plans for reviews that will take place in 2014 no later than August 1, 2013, but may have to amend these plans or obtain additional review resources depending on how CMS decides exchange-determined cases should be treated for purposes of MEQC and PERM reviews.

The Commission's Program Integrity Focus for the Coming Year

During the coming year, the Commission will continue to review Medicaid program integrity activities and highlight potential areas for program improvement. Specific areas of focus will include:

▶ **State and federal division of responsibilities.** Starting with the administrative perspective outlined in this chapter, we will look for opportunities to improve efficiency by clarifying federal and state roles relating to Medicaid program integrity. We will isolate specific areas of overlap and redundancy that can be eliminated and identify areas in statute or regulation where a more rational allocation of state and federal responsibilities may result in greater efficiency and effectiveness.

- **Effectiveness of current efforts.** We will evaluate information on the effectiveness of various program integrity initiatives and identify successful initiatives that should be expanded and programs that are not cost-effective and should be eliminated. We also will identify where better performance measures or improved data are necessary to evaluate the effectiveness of certain activities.

- **Openings for additional guidance and support.** We will examine Medicaid program integrity activities associated with various program areas to determine if there are areas where additional guidance or greater cross-state consistency would support overall program integrity, or where improved technology could better support both integrity and efficiency. We will specifically consider Medicaid program integrity approaches for managed care delivery systems, which now enroll a majority of Medicaid enrollees (CMS 2012b). We will also consider emerging payment and delivery models and the extent to which new program integrity approaches may be required.

Endnotes

[1] State Children's Health Insurance Programs (CHIP) that are part of a Medicaid expansion are included in that state's Medicaid program integrity efforts. A separate CHIP program likely enrolls its enrollees in managed care, so some program integrity activities are carried out by the health plan.

[2] See Chapter 4, Annex 1 to MACPAC's March 2012 report to the Congress for a list of the corresponding statutes.

[3] PERM also measures the accuracy of FFS claims payments and managed care capitation payments through reviews conducted by federal contractors. Findings from the federal contractor review of FFS and managed care payments are combined with findings from state review of eligibility determinations to produce national Medicaid and CHIP program error rates.

[4] CMS estimated that the burden for a single state to conduct 504 active case reviews and 204 negative case reviews for both Medicaid and CHIP under the PERM methodology would be 9,980 labor hours (CMS 2010).

References

Boughn, J. 2013. Presentation before the Medicaid and CHIP Payment and Access Commission, February 12, 2013, Washington, DC. http://www.macpac.gov/home/meetings/2013-02/2013-02_Session3.pdf.

Budetti, P. 2013. Statement on Fostering Innovation to Fight Waste, Fraud, and Abuse in Health Care before the Committee on Energy and Commerce, Subcommittee on Health, U.S. House of Representatives, February 27, 2013, Washington, DC. http://docs.house.gov/meetings/IF/IF14/20130227/100329/HMTG-113-IF14-Wstate-BudettiP-20130227.pdf.

Budetti, P. 2012. Statement on Assessing Medicare and Medicaid Program Integrity before the Committee on Oversight and Government Reform, Subcommittee on Government Organization, Efficiency, and Financial Management, U.S. House of Representatives, June 7, 2012, Washington, DC. http://www.hhs.gov/asl/testify/2012/06/t20120607a.html.

Centers for Medicare & Medicaid Services (CMS), U.S. Department of Health and Human Services. 2013a. 2012 *Actuarial report on the financial outlook for Medicaid*. Baltimore, MD: CMS. http://medicaid.gov/Medicaid-CHIP-Program-Information/By-Topics/Financing-and-Reimbursement/Downloads/medicaid-actuarial-report-2012.pdf.

Centers for Medicare & Medicaid Services (CMS), U.S. Department of Health and Human Services. 2013b. *Medicaid moving forward: Opportunities for achieving improvements in care and program efficiency*. Baltimore, MD: CMS. http://www.medicaid.gov/State-Resource-Center/Events-and-Announcements/Downloads/MMF_Jan-Dec-2012_FINAL.pdf.

Centers for Medicare & Medicaid Services (CMS), U.S. Department of Health and Human Services. 2013c. Communication with MACPAC staff, March 22, 2013.

Centers for Medicare & Medicaid Services (CMS), U.S. Department of Health and Human Services. 2013d. Medicaid integrity provider education program. Baltimore, MD: CMS. http://www.cms.gov/Medicare-Medicaid-Coordination/Fraud-Prevention/MedicaidIntegrityProgram/Medicaid-Integrity-Provider-Education-Program.html.

Centers for Medicare & Medicaid Services (CMS), U.S. Department of Health and Human Services. 2013e. Medicaid guidance fraud prevention. Baltimore, MD: CMS. http://www.cms.gov/Medicare-Medicaid-Coordination/Fraud-Prevention/FraudAbuseforProfs/MedicaidGuidance.html.

Centers for Medicare & Medicaid Services (CMS), U.S. Department of Health and Human Services. 2013f. *MAGI-based eligibility verification plans*. Baltimore, MD: CMS. http://www.medicaid.gov/Federal-Policy-Guidance/Downloads/CIB-02-21-13.pdf.

Centers for Medicare & Medicaid Services (CMS), U.S. Department of Health and Human Services. 2012a. *Payment Error Rate Measurement (PERM)—Eligibility review guidance for Medicaid and CHIP benefits*. Baltimore, MD: CMS. http://www.cms.gov/Research-Statistics-Data-and-Systems/Monitoring-Programs/PERM/Downloads/PERM-elig-rev-guide-13.pdf.

Centers for Medicare & Medicaid Services (CMS), U.S. Department of Health and Human Services. 2012b. Medicaid managed care enrollment report summary statistics as of July 1, 2011. Baltimore, MD: CMS. http://www.medicaid.gov/medicaid-CHIP-Program-Information/By-Topics/Data-and-Systems/Downloads/2011-Medicaid-MC-Enrollment-Report.pdf.

Centers for Medicare & Medicaid Services (CMS), U.S. Department of Health and Human Services. 2010. Medicaid program and Children's Health Insurance Program (CHIP); Revisions to the Medicaid Eligibility Quality Control and Payment Error Rate Measurement programs. Final rule. *Federal Register* 75, no. 154 (August 11): 48815–48852.

Centers for Medicare & Medicaid Services (CMS), U.S. Department of Health and Human Services. 2009a. *Comprehensive Medicaid integrity plan of the Medicaid Integrity Program, FYs 2009–2013*. Baltimore, MD: CMS. http://www.cms.gov/Regulations-and-Guidance/Legislation/DeficitReductionAct/Downloads/CMIP2009-2013.pdf.

Centers for Medicare & Medicaid Services (CMS), U.S. Department of Health and Human Services. 2009b. Medicaid program and Children's Health Insurance Program (CHIP); Revisions to the Medicaid Eligibility Quality Control and Payment Error Rate Measurement programs. Proposed rule. *Federal Register* 74, no. 134 (July 15): 34482–34487.

Centers for Medicare & Medicaid Services (CMS), U.S. Department of Health and Human Services. 2000. *Medicaid Eligibility Quality Control (MEQC) and simplification of application and enrollment processes*. Baltimore, MD: CMS. http://www.cms.gov/smdl/downloads/smd091200.pdf.

Congressional Budget Office (CBO). 2013. *CBO's May 2013 estimate of the effects of the Affordable Care Act on health insurance coverage*. Washington, DC: CBO. http://cbo.gov/sites/default/files/cbofiles/attachments/44190_EffectsAffordableCareActHealthInsuranceCoverage_2.pdf.

Kaiser Family Foundation (KFF). 2013. *The public's health care agenda for the 113th Congress*. Washington, DC: KFF. http://kff.org/health-reform/poll-finding/the-publics-policy-agenda-for-the-113th-congress.

Medicaid and CHIP Payment and Access Commission (MACPAC). 2012. *Report to the Congress on Medicaid and CHIP*. March 2012. Washington DC: MACPAC. http://www.macpac.gov/reports.

National Association of Medicaid Directors (NAMD). 2013. *Rethinking Medicaid program integrity: States identify opportunities to improve federal-state program integrity collaboration*. Washington, DC: NAMD. http://medicaiddirectors.org/sites/medicaiddirectors.org/files/public/pi_survey_summary_130314.pdf.

National Association of Medicaid Directors (NAMD). 2012. *Rethinking Medicaid program integrity: Eliminating duplication and investing in effective, high-value tools*. Washington, DC: NAMD. http://medicaiddirectors.org/sites/medicaiddirectors.org/files/public/namd_medicaid_pi_position_paper_final_120319.pdf.

Thompson, P. 2012. Statement on Medicaid Financial Management in New York State Developmental Centers before the Committee on Oversight and Government Reform, U.S. House of Representatives, September 20, 2012, Washington, DC. http://oversight.house.gov/wp-content/uploads/2012/09/9-20-12-HC-Thompson.pdf.

U.S. Department of Health and Human Services (HHS) and the U.S. Department of Justice (DOJ). 2012. *Health care fraud and abuse control program annual report for fiscal year 2011*. Washington, DC: HHS and DOJ. https://oig.hhs.gov/publications/docs/hcfac/hcfacreport2011.pdf.

U.S. Government Accountability Office (GAO). 2012a. *Medicaid Integrity Program (MIP): CMS should take steps to eliminate duplication and improve efficiency*. Report no. GAO-13-50. Washington, DC: GAO. http://www.gao.gov/assets/650/649964.pdf.

U.S. Government Accountability Office (GAO). 2012b. *National Medicaid Audit Program (NMAP): CMS should improve reporting and focus on audit collaboration with states*. Report no. GAO-12-627. Washington, DC: GAO. http://www.gao.gov/assets/600/591601.pdf.

Appendix

Acronym List

ADD	Attention Deficit Disorder
ADHD	Attention Deficit Hyperactivity Disorder
ADL	Activities of Daily Living
AAP	American Academy of Pediatrics
ABMS	American Board of Medical Specialties
ABPS	American Board of Physician Specialties
ACA	Patient Protection and Affordable Care Act
ACNM	American College of Nurse-Midwives
ACOG	American Congress of Obstetricians and Gynecologists
AFDC	Aid to Families with Dependent Children
AHRQ	Agency for Healthcare Research and Quality
AOA	American Osteopathic Association
APD	Advance Planning Document
ASL	American Sign Language
BRFSS	Behavioral Risk Factor Surveillance System
CAHMI	Child and Adolescent Health Measurement Initiative
CARTS	CHIP Annual Report Template System
CBO	Congressional Budget Office
CCCESUN	Children with Chronic Conditions and Elevated Service Use or Need
CDC	U.S. Centers for Disease Control and Prevention
CHIP	State Children's Health Insurance Program
CHIPRA	Children's Health Insurance Program Reauthorization Act
CMS	Centers for Medicare & Medicaid Services
COBRA	Consolidated Omnibus Budget Reconciliation Act
CPT	Current Procedural Terminology
CSHCN	Children with Special Health Care Needs
CY	Calendar Year
DRA	Deficit Reduction Act
DRG	Diagnosis Related Group
DSH	Disproportionate Share Hospital
ED	Emergency Department
EPSDT	Early and Periodic Screening, Diagnostic, and Treatment
FFS	Fee for Service
FMAP	Federal Medical Assistance Percentage

FPL	Federal Poverty Level
FY	Fiscal Year
GAO	U.S. Government Accountability Office
GEMS	Moms Getting Early Maternity Services
GME	Graduate Medical Education
HCBS	Home and Community-based Services
HCUP	Healthcare Cost and Utilization Project
HEAT	Health Care Fraud Prevention and Enforcement Action Team
HHS	U.S. Department of Health and Human Services
HMO	Health Maintenance Organization
HPV	Human Papillomavirus
HRSA	Health Resources and Services Administration
I/DD	Intellectual and Developmental Disabilities
ICD-9-CM	International Classification of Diseases, Ninth Revision, Clinical Modification
ICF/ID	Intermediate Care Facility for Persons with Intellectual Disabilities
IHS	Indian Health Service
IOM	Institute of Medicine
KFF	Kaiser Family Foundation
LBW	Low Birth Weight
LEP	Limited English Proficient
LTSS	Long-term Services and Supports
MACBIS	Medicaid and CHIP Business Information and Solutions
MACPAC	Medicaid and CHIP Payment and Access Commission
MAGI	Modified Adjusted Gross Income
MAX	Medicaid Analytic eXtract
MBES/CBES	Medicaid and CHIP Budget and Expenditure System
MCCA	Medicare Catastrophic Coverage Act
MCHB	Maternal and Child Health Bureau
MCO	Managed Care Organization
MDR	Medicaid Drug Rebate
Medi-Medi	Medicare-Medicaid Data Match Program
MEPS	Medical Expenditure Panel Survey
MEQC	Medicaid Eligibility Quality Control
MFCU	Medicaid Fraud Control Unit
MIC	Medicaid Integrity Contractor
MIG	Medicaid Integrity Group
MITA	Medicaid Information Technology Architecture
MMA	Medicare Modernization Act
MMCDCS	Medicaid Managed Care Data Collection System
MMIS	Medicaid Management Information System

MQCC	California Maternal Quality Care Collaborative
MSIS	Medicaid Statistical Information System
NASCIO	National Association of State Chief Information Officers
NASDDDS	National Association of State Directors of Developmental Disabilities Services
NCCI	National Correct Coding Initiative
NCD	National Council on Disability
NCI	National Core Indicators
NGA	National Governors Association
NHIS	National Health Interview Survey
NICU	Neonatal Intensive Care Unit
NINT	Neonatal Intermediate Care Unit
NIS	Nationwide Inpatient Sample
NQF	National Quality Forum
NSAF	National Survey of American Families
NSCF	National Survey of SSI Children and Families
NTSV	Nulliparous Term Singleton Vertex
OB/GYN	Obstetrician and Gynecologist
OBRA	Omnibus Budget Reconciliation Act
OIG	Office of Inspector General
OPQC	Ohio Perinatal Quality Collaborative
PAHP	Prepaid Ambulatory Health Plan
PCCM	Primary Care Case Management
PERM	Payment Error Rate Measurement
PHP	Prepaid Health Plan
PIHP	Prepaid Inpatient Health Plan
PMH	Pregnancy Medical Home
PRWORA	Personal Responsibility and Work Opportunity Reconciliation Act
QMB	Qualified Medicare Beneficiary
RAC	Recovery Audit Contractor
SEDS	Statistical Enrollment Data System
SID	State Inpatient Databases
SPA	State Plan Amendment
SSDI	Social Security Disability Insurance
SSI	Supplemental Security Income
STD	Sexually Transmitted Disease
T-MSIS	Transformed Medicaid Statistical Information System
TPL	Third Party Liability
TDD	Telecommunication Device for the Deaf
TTY	Text Telephone
VFC	Vaccines for Children

Authorizing Language from the Social Security Act (42 U.S.C. 1396)

MEDICAID AND CHIP PAYMENT AND ACCESS COMMISSION

(a) ESTABLISHMENT.—There is hereby established the Medicaid and CHIP Payment and Access Commission (in this section referred to as 'MACPAC').

(b) DUTIES.—

(1) REVIEW OF ACCESS POLICIES FOR ALL STATES AND ANNUAL REPORTS.—MACPAC shall—

(A) review policies of the Medicaid program established under this title (in this section referred to as 'Medicaid') and the State Children's Health Insurance Program established under title XXI (in this section referred to as 'CHIP') affecting access to covered items and services, including topics described in paragraph (2);

(B) make recommendations to Congress, the Secretary, and States concerning such access policies;

(C) by not later than March 15 of each year (beginning with 2010), submit a report to Congress containing the results of such reviews and MACPAC's recommendations concerning such policies; and

(D) by not later than June 15 of each year (beginning with 2010), submit a report to Congress containing an examination of issues affecting Medicaid and CHIP, including the implications of changes in health care delivery in the United States and in the market for health care services on such programs.

(2) SPECIFIC TOPICS TO BE REVIEWED.—Specifically, MACPAC shall review and assess the following:

(A) MEDICAID AND CHIP PAYMENT POLICIES.—Payment policies under Medicaid and CHIP, including—

(i) the factors affecting expenditures for the efficient provision of items and services in different sectors, including the process for updating payments to medical, dental, and health professionals, hospitals, residential and long-term care providers, providers of home and community based services, Federally-qualified health centers and rural health clinics, managed care entities, and providers of other covered items and services;

(ii) payment methodologies; and

(iii) the relationship of such factors and methodologies to access and quality of care for Medicaid and CHIP beneficiaries (including how such factors and methodologies enable such beneficiaries to obtain the services for which they are eligible, affect provider supply, and affect providers that serve a disproportionate share of low-income and other vulnerable populations).

(B) ELIGIBILITY POLICIES.—Medicaid and CHIP eligibility policies, including a determination of the degree to which Federal and State policies provide health care coverage to needy populations.

(C) ENROLLMENT AND RETENTION PROCESSES.—Medicaid and CHIP enrollment and retention processes, including a determination of the degree to which Federal and State policies encourage the enrollment of individuals who are eligible for such programs and screen out individuals who are ineligible, while minimizing the share of program expenses devoted to such processes.

(D) COVERAGE POLICIES.—Medicaid and CHIP benefit and coverage policies, including a determination of the degree to which Federal and State policies provide access to the services enrollees require to improve and maintain their health and functional status.

(E) QUALITY OF CARE.—Medicaid and CHIP policies as they relate to the quality of care provided under those programs, including a determination of the degree to which Federal and State policies achieve their stated goals and interact with similar goals established by other purchasers of health care services.

(F) INTERACTION OF MEDICAID AND CHIP PAYMENT POLICIES WITH HEALTH CARE DELIVERY GENERALLY.—The effect of Medicaid and CHIP payment policies on access to items and services for children and other Medicaid and CHIP populations other than under this title or title XXI and the implications of changes in health care delivery in the United States and in the general market for health care items and services on Medicaid and CHIP.

(G) INTERACTIONS WITH MEDICARE AND MEDICAID.— Consistent with paragraph (11), the interaction of policies under Medicaid and the Medicare program under title XVIII, including with respect to how such interactions affect access to services, payments, and dual eligible individuals.

(H) OTHER ACCESS POLICIES.—The effect of other Medicaid and CHIP policies on access to covered items and services, including policies relating to transportation and language barriers and preventive, acute, and long-term services and supports.

(3) RECOMMENDATIONS AND REPORTS OF STATE-SPECIFIC DATA.—MACPAC shall—

(A) review national and State-specific Medicaid and CHIP data; and

(B) submit reports and recommendations to Congress, the Secretary, and States based on such reviews.

(4) CREATION OF EARLY-WARNING SYSTEM.—MACPAC shall create an early-warning system to identify provider shortage areas, as well as other factors that adversely affect, or have the potential to adversely affect, access to care by, or the health care status of, Medicaid and CHIP beneficiaries. MACPAC shall include in the annual report required under paragraph (1)(D) a description of all such areas or problems identified with respect to the period addressed in the report.

(5) COMMENTS ON CERTAIN SECRETARIAL REPORTS AND REGULATIONS.—

(A) CERTAIN SECRETARIAL REPORTS.—If the Secretary submits to Congress (or a committee of Congress) a report that is required by law and that relates to access policies, including with respect to payment policies, under Medicaid or CHIP, the Secretary shall transmit a copy of the report to MACPAC. MACPAC shall review the report and, not later than 6 months after the date of submittal of the Secretary's report to Congress, shall submit to the appropriate committees of Congress and the Secretary written comments on such report. Such comments may include such recommendations as MACPAC deems appropriate.

(B) REGULATIONS.—MACPAC shall review Medicaid and CHIP regulations and may comment through submission of a report to the appropriate committees of Congress and the Secretary, on any such regulations that affect access, quality, or efficiency of health care.

(6) AGENDA AND ADDITIONAL REVIEWS.—MACPAC shall consult periodically with the chairmen and ranking minority members of the appropriate committees of Congress regarding MACPAC's agenda and progress towards achieving the agenda. MACPAC may conduct additional reviews, and submit additional reports to the appropriate committees of Congress, from time to time on such topics relating to the program under this title or title XXI as may be requested by such chairmen and members and as MACPAC deems appropriate.

(7) AVAILABILITY OF REPORTS.—MACPAC shall transmit to the Secretary a copy of each report submitted under this subsection and shall make such reports available to the public.

(8) APPROPRIATE COMMITTEE OF CONGRESS.—For purposes of this section, the term 'appropriate committees of Congress' means the Committee on Energy and Commerce of the House of Representatives and the Committee on Finance of the Senate.

(9) VOTING AND REPORTING REQUIREMENTS.—With respect to each recommendation contained in a report submitted under paragraph (1), each member of MACPAC shall vote on the recommendation, and MACPAC shall include, by member, the results of that vote in the report containing the recommendation.

(10) EXAMINATION OF BUDGET CONSEQUENCES.—Before making any recommendations, MACPAC shall examine the budget consequences of such recommendations, directly or through consultation with appropriate expert entities, and shall submit with any recommendations, a report on the Federal and State-specific budget consequences of the recommendations.

(11) CONSULTATION AND COORDINATION WITH MEDPAC.—

(A) IN GENERAL.—MACPAC shall consult with the Medicare Payment Advisory Commission (in this paragraph referred to as 'MedPAC') established under section 1805 in carrying out its duties under this section, as appropriate and particularly with respect to the issues specified in paragraph (2) as they relate to those Medicaid beneficiaries who are dually eligible for Medicaid and the Medicare program under title XVIII, adult Medicaid beneficiaries (who are not dually eligible for Medicare), and beneficiaries under Medicare. Responsibility for analysis of and recommendations to change Medicare policy regarding Medicare beneficiaries, including Medicare beneficiaries who are dually eligible for Medicare and Medicaid, shall rest with MedPAC.

(B) INFORMATION SHARING.—MACPAC and MedPAC shall have access to deliberations and records of the other such entity, respectively, upon the request of the other such entity.

(12) CONSULTATION WITH STATES.—MACPAC shall regularly consult with States in carrying out its duties under this section, including with respect to developing processes for carrying out such duties, and shall ensure that input from States is taken into account and represented in MACPAC's recommendations and reports.

(13) COORDINATE AND CONSULT WITH THE FEDERAL COORDINATED HEALTH CARE OFFICE.—MACPAC shall coordinate and consult with the Federal Coordinated Health Care Office established under section 2081 of the Patient Protection and Affordable Care Act before making any recommendations regarding dual eligible individuals.

(14) PROGRAMMATIC OVERSIGHT VESTED IN THE SECRETARY.—MACPAC's authority to make recommendations in accordance with this section shall not affect, or be considered to duplicate, the Secretary's authority to carry out Federal responsibilities with respect to Medicaid and CHIP.

(c) MEMBERSHIP.—

(1) NUMBER AND APPOINTMENT.—MACPAC shall be composed of 17 members appointed by the Comptroller General of the United States.

(2) QUALIFICATIONS.—

(A) IN GENERAL.—The membership of MACPAC shall include individuals who have had direct experience as enrollees or parents or caregivers of enrollees in Medicaid or CHIP and individuals with national recognition for their expertise in Federal safety net health programs, health finance and economics, actuarial science, health plans and integrated delivery systems, reimbursement for health care, health information technology, and other providers of health services, public health, and other related fields, who provide a mix of different professions, broad geographic representation, and a balance between urban and rural representation.

(B) INCLUSION.—The membership of MACPAC shall include (but not be limited to) physicians, dentists, and other health professionals, employers, third-party payers, and individuals with expertise in the delivery of health services. Such membership shall also include representatives of children, pregnant women, the elderly, individuals with disabilities, caregivers, and dual eligible individuals, current or former representatives of State agencies responsible for administering Medicaid, and current or former representatives of State agencies responsible for administering CHIP.

(C) MAJORITY NONPROVIDERS.—Individuals who are directly involved in the provision, or management of the delivery, of items and services covered under Medicaid or CHIP shall not constitute a majority of the membership of MACPAC.

(D) ETHICAL DISCLOSURE.—The Comptroller General of the United States shall establish a system for public disclosure by members of MACPAC of financial and other potential conflicts of interest relating to such members. Members of MACPAC shall be treated as employees of Congress for purposes of applying title I of the Ethics in Government Act of 1978 (Public Law 95–521).

(3) TERMS.—

(A) IN GENERAL.—The terms of members of MACPAC shall be for 3 years except that the Comptroller General of the United States shall designate staggered terms for the members first appointed.

(B) VACANCIES.—Any member appointed to fill a vacancy occurring before the expiration of the term for which the member's predecessor was appointed shall be appointed only for the remainder of that term. A member may serve after the expiration of that member's term until a successor has taken office. A vacancy in MACPAC shall be filled in the manner in which the original appointment was made.

(4) COMPENSATION.—While serving on the business of MACPAC (including travel time), a member of MACPAC shall be entitled to compensation at the per diem equivalent of the rate provided for level IV of the Executive Schedule under section 5315 of title 5, United States Code; and while so serving away from home and the member's regular place of business, a member may be allowed travel expenses, as authorized by the Chairman of MACPAC. Physicians serving as personnel of MACPAC may be provided a physician comparability allowance by MACPAC in the same manner as Government physicians may be provided such an allowance by an agency under section 5948 of title 5, United States Code, and for such purpose subsection (i) of such section shall apply to MACPAC in the same manner as it applies to the Tennessee Valley Authority. For purposes of pay (other than pay of members of MACPAC) and employment benefits, rights, and privileges, all personnel of MACPAC shall be treated as if they were employees of the United States Senate.

(5) CHAIRMAN; VICE CHAIRMAN.—The Comptroller General of the United States shall designate a member of MACPAC, at the time of appointment of the member as Chairman and a member as Vice Chairman for that term of appointment, except that in the case of vacancy of the Chairmanship or Vice Chairmanship, the Comptroller General of the United States may designate another member for the remainder of that member's term.

(6) MEETINGS.—MACPAC shall meet at the call of the Chairman.

(d) DIRECTOR AND STAFF; EXPERTS AND CONSULTANTS.—Subject to such review as the Comptroller General of the United States deems necessary to assure the efficient administration of MACPAC, MACPAC may—

(1) employ and fix the compensation of an Executive Director (subject to the approval of the Comptroller General of the United States) and such other personnel as may be necessary to carry out its duties (without regard to the provisions of title 5, United States Code, governing appointments in the competitive service);

(2) seek such assistance and support as may be required in the performance of its duties from appropriate Federal and State departments and agencies;

(3) enter into contracts or make other arrangements, as may be necessary for the conduct of the work of MACPAC (without regard to section 3709 of the Revised Statutes (41 U.S.C. 5));

(4) make advance, progress, and other payments which relate to the work of MACPAC;

(5) provide transportation and subsistence for persons serving without compensation; and

(6) prescribe such rules and regulations as it deems necessary with respect to the internal organization and operation of MACPAC.

(e) POWERS.—

(1) OBTAINING OFFICIAL DATA.—MACPAC may secure directly from any department or agency of the United States and, as a condition for receiving payments under sections 1903(a) and 2105(a), from any State agency responsible for administering Medicaid or CHIP, information necessary to enable it to carry out this section. Upon request of the Chairman, the head of that department or agency shall furnish that information to MACPAC on an agreed upon schedule.

(2) DATA COLLECTION.—In order to carry out its functions, MACPAC shall—

(A) utilize existing information, both published and unpublished, where possible, collected and assessed either by its own staff or under other arrangements made in accordance with this section;

(B) carry out, or award grants or contracts for, original research and experimentation, where existing information is inadequate; and

(C) adopt procedures allowing any interested party to submit information for MACPAC's use in making reports and recommendations.

(3) ACCESS OF GAO TO INFORMATION.—The Comptroller General of the United States shall have unrestricted access to all deliberations, records, and nonproprietary data of MACPAC, immediately upon request.

(4) PERIODIC AUDIT.—MACPAC shall be subject to periodic audit by the Comptroller General of the United States.

(f) FUNDING.—

(1) REQUEST FOR APPROPRIATIONS.—MACPAC shall submit requests for appropriations (other than for fiscal year 2010) in the same manner as the Comptroller General of the United States submits requests for appropriations, but amounts appropriated for MACPAC shall be separate from amounts appropriated for the Comptroller General of the United States.

(2) AUTHORIZATION.—There are authorized to be appropriated such sums as may be necessary to carry out the provisions of this section.

(3) FUNDING FOR FISCAL YEAR 2010.—

(A) IN GENERAL.—Out of any funds in the Treasury not otherwise appropriated, there is appropriated to MACPAC to carry out the provisions of this section for fiscal year 2010, $9,000,000.

(B) TRANSFER OF FUNDS.—Notwithstanding section 2104(a)(13), from the amounts appropriated in such section for fiscal year 2010, $2,000,000 is hereby transferred and made available in such fiscal year to MACPAC to carry out the provisions of this section.

(4) AVAILABILITY.—Amounts made available under paragraphs (2) and (3) to MACPAC to carry out the provisions of this section shall remain available until expended.

Biographies of Commissioners

Sharon L. Carte, M.H.S., has served as executive director of the West Virginia Children's Health Insurance Program since 2001. From 1992 to 1998, Ms. Carte was deputy commissioner for the Bureau for Medical Services overseeing West Virginia's Medicaid program. Prior to that, she was administrator of skilled and intermediate care nursing facilities and before that a coordinator of human resources development in the West Virginia Department of Health. Ms. Carte's experience includes work with senior centers and aging programs throughout the state of West Virginia and policy issues related to behavioral health and long-term care services for children. She received her master of health science from the Johns Hopkins University School of Public Health.

Richard Chambers is president of Molina Healthcare of California, a health plan serving 340,000 Medicaid, CHIP, and Medicare Advantage Special Needs Plan (SNP) members in five counties in California. Nationally, Molina Healthcare arranges for the delivery of health care services or offers health information management solutions for nearly 4.2 million individuals and families who receive their care through Medicaid, CHIP, Medicare Advantage, and other government-funded programs in 15 states. Before joining Molina Healthcare in 2012, Mr. Chambers was chief executive officer for nine years at CalOptima, a County Organized Health System providing health coverage to 410,000 low-income residents in Orange County, California, through Medicaid, CHIP, and Medicare Advantage SNP programs. Prior to CalOptima, Mr. Chambers spent over 27 years working for the Centers for Medicare & Medicaid Services (CMS). He served as the director of the Family and Children's Health Programs Group, responsible for national policy and operational direction of Medicaid and CHIP. While at CMS, Mr. Chambers also served as associate regional administrator for Medicaid in the San Francisco regional office and as director of the Office of Intergovernmental Affairs in the Washington, DC office. He received his bachelor's degree from the University of Virginia. Mr. Chambers is a member of the Congressional Budget Office's Panel of Health Advisers.

Donna Checkett, M.P.A., M.S.W., is vice president of state government relations at Aetna, where she is responsible for overseeing state legislative and regulatory strategies. Prior to that, she was the vice president of business development for Aetna's Medicaid division as well as the chief executive officer of Missouri Care, a managed Medicaid health plan owned by University of Missouri–Columbia Health Care, one of the largest safety net hospital systems in the state. For eight years, Ms. Checkett served as the director of the Missouri Division of Medical Services (Medicaid), during which time she was the chair of the National Association of State Medicaid Directors and a member of the National Governors Association Medicaid Improvements Working Group. She served as chair of the advisory board for the Center for Health Care Strategies, a non-profit health policy resource center dedicated to improving health care quality for low-income children and adults. Ms. Checkett also served as chair of the National Advisory Committee for Covering Kids, a Robert Wood Johnson Foundation program fostering outreach and eligibility simplification efforts for Medicaid and CHIP beneficiaries. She received a master of public administration from the University of Missouri–Columbia and a master of social work from the University of Texas at Austin.

Andrea Cohen, J.D., is the director of health services in the New York City Office of the Mayor, where she coordinates and develops strategies to improve public health and health care services for New Yorkers. She serves on the board of the Primary Care Development Corporation and represents the deputy mayor for health and human services on the board of the Health and Hospitals Corporation, the largest public hospital system in the country. From 2005 to 2009, Ms. Cohen was counsel with Manatt, Phelps & Phillips, LLP, where she advised clients on issues relating to Medicare, Medicaid, and other public health insurance programs. Prior professional positions include senior policy counsel at the Medicare Rights Center, health and oversight counsel for the U.S. Senate Committee on Finance, and attorney with the U.S. Department of Justice. She received her law degree from Columbia University School of Law.

Burton L. Edelstein, D.D.S., M.P.H., is a board-certified pediatric dentist and professor of dentistry and health policy and management at Columbia University. He is founding president of the Children's Dental Health Project, a national non-profit Washington, DC-based policy organization that promotes equity in children's oral health. Dr. Edelstein practiced pediatric dentistry in Connecticut and taught at the Harvard School of Dental Medicine for 21 years prior to serving as a 1996–1997 Robert Wood Johnson Foundation health policy fellow in the office of U.S. Senate leader Tom Daschle, with primary responsibility for the State Children's Health Insurance Program. Dr. Edelstein worked with the U.S. Department of Health and Human Services on its oral health initiatives from 1998 to 2001, chaired the U.S. Surgeon General's Workshop on Children and Oral Health, and authored the child section of *Oral Health in America: A Report of the Surgeon General*. His research focuses on children's oral health promotion and access to dental care, with a particular emphasis on Medicaid and CHIP populations. He received his degree in dentistry from the State University of New York at Buffalo School of Dentistry, his master of public health from Harvard University School of Public Health, and completed his clinical training at Boston Children's Hospital.

Patricia Gabow, M.D., was chief executive officer of Denver Health from 1992 until her retirement in 2012, transforming it from a department of city government to a successful, independent governmental entity. She is a trustee of the Robert Wood Johnson Foundation, serves on the Institute of Medicine (IOM) Roundtable on Value and Science Driven Health Care and the National Governors Association Health Advisory Board, and was a member of the Commonwealth Commission on a High Performing Health System throughout its existence. Dr. Gabow is a professor of medicine at the University of Colorado School of Medicine and has authored over 150 articles and book chapters. She received her medical degree from the University of Pennsylvania School of Medicine. Dr. Gabow has received the American Medical Association's Nathan Davis Award for Outstanding Public Servant, the Ohtli Award from the Mexican government, the National Healthcare Leadership Award, the David E. Rogers Award from the Association of American Medical Colleges, the Health Quality Leader Award from the National Committee for Quality Assurance (NCQA), and election to the Association for Manufacturing Excellence Hall of Fame for her work on Toyota Production Systems in health care.

Herman Gray, M.D., M.B.A., is president of the Children's Hospital of Michigan (CHM) and senior vice president of the Detroit Medical Center. At CHM, Dr. Gray served previously as pediatrics vice chief for education, director of the Pediatric Residency Program, chief of staff, and then chief operating officer. He also served as associate dean for graduate medical education (GME) and vice president for GME at Wayne State University School of Medicine and the Detroit Medical Center, respectively. Dr. Gray has also served as the chief medical consultant for the Michigan Department of Public Health Division of Children's Special Health Care Services and as vice president and medical director of clinical affairs for Blue Care Network. During the 1980s, he pursued private medical practice in Detroit. Dr. Gray serves on the board of trustees of the National Association of Children's Hospitals and the board of directors of the Child Health Corporation of America, now merged and known as Children's Hospital Association. He received his medical degree from the University of Michigan in Ann Arbor, and a master of business administration from the University of Tennessee.

Denise Henning, C.N.M., M.S.N., is clinical director for women's health at Collier Health Services, a federally qualified health center in Immokalee, Florida. A practicing nurse midwife, Ms. Henning provides prenatal and gynecological care to a service population that is predominantly uninsured or covered by Medicaid. From 2003 to 2008, she was director of clinical operations for Women's Health Services at the Family Health Centers of Southwest Florida, where she supervised the midwifery and other clinical staff. Prior to this, Ms. Henning served as a certified nurse midwife in Winter Haven, Florida, and as a labor and delivery nurse in a Level III teaching hospital. She is a former president of the Midwifery Business Network and chair of the business section of the American College of Nurse-Midwives. She received her master of science in nurse midwifery from the University of Florida in Jacksonville and her bachelor of science in nursing from the University of Florida in Gainesville. She also holds a degree in business management from Nova University in Fort Lauderdale, Florida.

Mark Hoyt, F.S.A., M.A.A.A., was the national practice leader of the Government Human Services Consulting group of Mercer Health & Benefits, LLC, until his retirement in 2012. This group helps states purchase health services for their Medicaid and CHIP programs and has worked with over 30 states. He joined Mercer in 1980 and worked on government health care projects starting in 1987, including developing strategies for statewide health reform, evaluating the impact of different managed care approaches, and overseeing program design and rate analysis for Medicaid and CHIP programs. Mr. Hoyt is a fellow in the Society of Actuaries and a member of the American Academy of Actuaries. He received a bachelor of arts in mathematics from UCLA and a master of arts in mathematics from the University of California at Berkeley.

Judith Moore is an independent consultant specializing in policy related to health, vulnerable populations, and social safety net issues. Ms. Moore's expertise in Medicaid, Medicare, long-term services and supports, and other state and federal programs flows from her career as a federal senior executive who served in the legislative and executive branches of government. At the Health Care Financing Administration (now CMS), Ms. Moore served as director of the Medicaid program and of the Office of Legislation and Congressional Affairs. Her federal service was followed by more than a decade as co-director and senior fellow at George Washington University's National Health Policy Forum, a non-partisan education program serving federal legislative and regulatory health staff. In addition to other papers and research, she is co-author with David G. Smith of a political history of Medicaid: *Medicaid Politics and Policy*.

Trish Riley, M.S., is a senior fellow and adjunct professor of health policy and management at the Muskie School of Public Service, University of Southern Maine, and was the first distinguished visiting fellow and lecturer in state health policy at The George Washington University, following her tenure as director of the Maine Governor's Office of Health Policy and Finance. She was a principal architect of the Dirigo Health Reform Act of 2003, which was enacted to increase access, reduce costs, and improve quality of health care in Maine. Ms. Riley previously served as executive director of the National Academy for State Health Policy and as president of its corporate board. Under four Maine governors, she held appointed positions including executive director of the Maine Committee on Aging, director of the Bureau of Maine's Elderly, associate deputy commissioner of health and medical services, and director of the Bureau of Medical Services responsible for the Medicaid program and health planning and licensure. Ms. Riley served on Maine's Commission on Children's Health, which planned the S-CHIP program. She is a member of the Kaiser Commission on Medicaid and the Uninsured and has served as a member of the IOM's Subcommittee on Creating an External Environment for Quality and its Subcommittee on Maximizing the Value of Health. Ms. Riley has also served as a member of the board of directors of the NCQA. She received her master of science in community development from the University of Maine.

Norma Martínez Rogers, Ph.D., R.N., F.A.A.N., is a professor of family nursing at the University of Texas (UT) Health Science Center at San Antonio, where she has served on the faculty since 1996. Dr. Martínez Rogers has held clinical and administrative positions in psychiatric nursing and at psychiatric hospitals, including the William Beaumont Army Medical Center in Fort Bliss during Operation Desert Storm. She has initiated a number of programs at the UT Health Science Center in San Antonio, including a support group for women transitioning from prison back into society and the Martínez Street Women's Center, a non-profit organization designed to provide support and educational services to women and teenage girls. Dr. Martínez Rogers is a fellow of the American Academy of Nursing and is the former president of the National Association of Hispanic Nurses. She received a master of science in psychiatric nursing from the UT Health Science Center at San Antonio and her doctorate in cultural foundations in education from the UT at Austin.

Sara Rosenbaum, J.D., is founding chair of the Department of Health Policy and the Harold and Jane Hirsh Professor of Health Law and Policy at the George Washington (GW) University School of Public Health and Health Services. She also serves on the faculties of the GW Schools of Law and Medicine. Professor Rosenbaum's research has focused on how the law intersects with the nation's health care and public health systems, with a particular emphasis on insurance coverage, managed care, the health care safety net, health care quality, and civil rights. She is a member of the IOM and has served on the boards of numerous national organizations, including AcademyHealth. Professor Rosenbaum is a member of the Centers for Disease Control and Prevention's (CDC) Advisory Committee on Immunization Practices and also serves on the CDC Director's Advisory Committee. She has advised the Congress and presidential administrations since 1977 and served on the staff of the White House Domestic Policy Council during the Clinton administration. Professor Rosenbaum is the leading author of *Law and the American Health Care System,* published by Foundation Press (2012). She received her law degree from Boston University School of Law.

Diane Rowland, Sc.D., has served as chair of MACPAC since December 2009. She is the executive vice president of the Henry J. Kaiser Family Foundation and the executive director of the Kaiser Commission on Medicaid and the Uninsured. She is also an adjunct professor in the Department of Health Policy and Management at the Johns Hopkins Bloomberg School of Public Health. Dr. Rowland has directed the Kaiser Commission since 1991 and has overseen the foundation's health policy work on Medicaid, Medicare, private insurance, HIV, women's health, and disparities since 1993. She is a noted authority on health policy, Medicare and Medicaid, and health care for low-income and disadvantaged populations, and frequently testifies as an expert witness before the U.S. Congress on health policy issues. A nationally recognized expert with a distinguished career in public policy and research—focusing on health insurance coverage, access to care, and health care financing for low-income, elderly, and disabled populations—Dr. Rowland has published widely on these subjects. She is an elected member of the IOM, a founding member of the National Academy for Social Insurance, and past president and fellow of the Association for Health Services Research (now AcademyHealth). Dr. Rowland holds a bachelor's degree from Wellesley College, a master of public administration from the University of California at Los Angeles, and a doctor of science in health policy and management from The Johns Hopkins University.

Robin Smith and her husband Doug have been foster and adoptive parents for many children covered by Medicaid, including many children with special needs. Her experience seeking care for these children has included working with an interdisciplinary Medicaid program called the Medically Fragile Children's Program, a national model partnership between the Medical University of South Carolina Children's Hospital, South Carolina Medicaid, and the South Carolina Department of Social Services. Ms. Smith serves on the Family Advisory Committee for the Children's Hospital at the Medical University of South Carolina. She has testified at congressional briefings and presented at the 2007 International Conference of Family Centered Care and at grand rounds for medical students and residents at the Medical University of South Carolina.

David Sundwall, M.D., serves as vice chair of MACPAC. He is a clinical professor of public health at the University of Utah School of Medicine, Division of Public Health, where he has been a faculty member since 1978. He served as executive director of the Utah Department of Health and commissioner of health for the state of Utah from 2005 through 2010. He currently serves on numerous government and community boards and advisory groups in his home state, including as chair of the Utah State Controlled Substance Advisory Committee. Dr. Sundwall was president of the Association of State and Territorial Health Officials from 2007 to 2008. He has chaired or served on several committees of the IOM and is currently on the IOM Standing Committee on Health Threats Resilience. Prior to returning to Utah in 2005, he was president of the American Clinical Laboratory Association and before that was vice president and medical director of American Healthcare Systems. Dr. Sundwall's federal government experience includes serving as administrator of the Health Resources and Services Administration, assistant surgeon general in the Commissioned Corps of the U.S. Public Health Service, and director of the health staff of the U.S. Senate Labor and Human Resources Committee. He received his medical degree from the University of Utah School of Medicine, and completed his residency in the Harvard Family

Medicine Program. He is a licensed physician, board-certified in internal medicine and family practice, and works as a primary care physician in a public health clinic two half-days each week.

Steven Waldren, M.D., M.S., is senior strategist for health information technology at the American Academy of Family Physicians. He also serves as vice chair of the American Society for Testing Materials' E31 Health Information Standards Committee. Dr. Waldren sits on several advisory boards dealing with health care information technology (health IT), and he was a past co-chair of the Physicians Electronic Health Record Coalition, a group of more than 20 professional medical associations addressing issues around health IT. He received his medical degree from the University of Kansas School of Medicine. While completing a post-doctoral National Library of Medicine medical informatics fellowship, he completed a master of science in health care informatics from the University of Missouri, Columbia. Dr. Waldren is a co-founder in two start-ups dealing with health IT systems design: Open Health Data, Inc., and New Health Networks, LLC.

Biographies of Staff

Annie Andrianasolo, M.B.A., is executive assistant. She previously held the position of special assistant for global health at the Public Health Institute and was a program assistant at the World Bank. Ms. Andrianasolo has a bachelor of science degree in economics and a master of business administration from the Johns Hopkins Carey Business School.

Amy Bernstein, Sc.D., M.H.S.A., is senior advisor for research. She manages and provides oversight and guidance for all MACPAC research, data, and analysis projects, including statements of work, research plans, and all deliverables and products. She also directs analyses on Medicaid dental and maternity care policies. Her previous positions have included director of the Analytic Studies Branch at the Centers for Disease Control/National Center for Health Statistics, and senior analyst positions at the Alpha Center, the Prospective Payment Assessment Commission, the National Cancer Institute, and the Agency for Healthcare Research and Quality. Dr. Bernstein earned a master of health services administration degree from the University of Michigan School of Public Health and a doctor of science degree from the School of Hygiene and Public Health at The Johns Hopkins University.

Vincent Calvo is an administrative assistant. Previously, he was an intern at Financial Executives International where he focused on researching the effects of health and tax laws on Fortune 500 companies. Mr. Calvo holds a bachelor of science degree from Austin Peay State University.

Mathew Chase is chief information officer. He is responsible for the technology strategy, information architecture, security, and operations at MACPAC. Mr. Chase previously served as the information technology (IT) manager for the Medicare Payment Advisory Commission (MedPAC) from 2004 to 2005 where he was responsible for all aspects of technology: strategic planning, budget, security, data reliability, support, and administration. Mr. Chase has also provided IT expertise and leadership in the private sector to organizations such as Cirque du Soleil, *The Las Vegas Review-Journal,* and several internet start-ups. He received his bachelor of science degree in decision sciences and management information systems from George Mason University.

Laura Diamond is communications director. Previously, she served as social media director at Enroll America, focusing on the organization's public launch and communications planning. Prior to that, she held positions as communications director for health care-related organizations including the Partnership for Prevention, the American Nurses Association, and the Blue Cross and Blue Shield Association. Ms. Diamond earned her bachelor of science degree from Boston University.

Benjamin Finder, M.P.H., is a senior analyst. His work focuses on benefits and payment policy. Prior to joining MACPAC, he served as an associate director in the Health Care Policy and Research Administration at the District of Columbia Department of Health Care Finance, and as an analyst at the Henry J. Kaiser Family Foundation. Mr. Finder holds a master of public health degree from The George Washington University, where he concentrated in health policy and health economics.

Moira Forbes, M.B.A., is director of payment and program integrity, focusing on issues relating to payment policy and the design, implementation, and effectiveness of program integrity activities in Medicaid and the Children's Health Insurance Program (CHIP). Previously, Ms. Forbes served as director of the division of health and social service programs in the Office of Executive Program Information at the U.S. Department of Health and Human Services (HHS) and as a vice president in the Medicaid practice at The Lewin Group. At Lewin, Ms. Forbes worked with every state Medicaid and CHIP program on issues relating to program integrity and eligibility quality control. She also has extensive experience with federal and state policy analysis, Medicaid program operations, and delivery system design. Ms. Forbes has a master of business administration degree from The George Washington University and a bachelor's degree in Russian and political science from Bryn Mawr College.

April Grady, M.P.Aff., is director of data development and analysis. In 2011, she was temporarily detailed to the Joint Select Committee on Deficit Reduction to provide Medicaid policy expertise during its deliberations. Prior to joining MACPAC, Ms. Grady worked at the Congressional Research Service and the Congressional Budget Office, where she provided non-partisan analyses of Medicaid, private health insurance, and other health policy issues. She has also held positions at the LBJ School of Public Affairs at The University of Texas at Austin and Mathematica Policy Research. Ms. Grady received a master of public affairs degree from the LBJ School of Public Affairs at The University of Texas and a bachelor of arts in policy studies from Syracuse University.

Benjamin Granata is a finance/budget specialist. His work focuses on reviewing financial documents to ensure completeness and accuracy for processing and recording in the financial systems. Mr. Granata graduated from Towson University with a bachelor's degree in business administration, specializing in project management.

Lindsay Hebert, M.S.P.H., is special assistant to the executive director. Previously, she was a research assistant at The Johns Hopkins School of Medicine, focusing on patient safety initiatives in the department of pediatric oncology. Prior to that, she was a project coordinator in the Pediatric Intensive Care Unit at The Johns Hopkins Hospital. Ms. Hebert holds a master of science in public health degree from The Johns Hopkins Bloomberg School of Public Health and a bachelor of arts degree from the University of Florida.

Angela Lello, M.P.Aff., is a senior analyst. Her work focuses on Medicaid for people with disabilities, particularly long-term services and supports (LTSS). Previously she was a Kennedy Public Policy Fellow at the U.S. Department of Health and Human Services, Administration on Intellectual and Developmental Disabilities, conducting policy research and analysis on a variety of HHS initiatives. Her prior work included analyzing and developing LTSS for people with disabilities while at the Texas Department of Aging and Disability Services and the Texas Council for Developmental Disabilities. Ms. Lello received a master of public affairs degree from the LBJ School of Public Affairs at The University of Texas.

Molly McGinn-Shapiro, M.P.P., is a senior analyst. Her work focuses on issues related to individuals dually eligible for Medicaid and Medicare. Previously, she was the special assistant to the executive vice president of the Henry J. Kaiser Family Foundation and to the executive director of the Kaiser Commission on Medicaid and the Uninsured. Ms. McGinn-Shapiro holds a master of public policy degree from Georgetown University's Georgetown Public Policy Institute.

Chris Park, M.S., is a senior analyst. His work focuses on issues related to managed care payment and Medicaid drug policy and provides data analyses using Medicaid administrative data. Prior to MACPAC, he was a senior consultant at The Lewin Group. At Lewin, he provided quantitative analyses and technical assistance on Medicaid policy issues, including Medicaid managed care capitation rate setting and pharmacy reimbursement and cost-containment initiatives. Mr. Park has a master of science degree in health policy and management from the Harvard School of Public Health and a bachelor of science degree in chemistry from the University of Virginia.

Chris Peterson, M.P.P., is director of eligibility, enrollment, and benefits. Prior to joining MACPAC, he was a specialist in health care financing at the Congressional Research Service, where he worked on major health legislation. Prior to that, he worked for the Agency for Healthcare Research and Quality and the National Bipartisan Commission on the Future of Medicare. Mr. Peterson has a master of public policy degree from Georgetown University's Georgetown Public Policy Institute and a bachelor of science degree in mathematics from Missouri Western State University.

Ken Pezzella is chief financial officer. He has more than 10 years of federal financial management and accounting experience in both the public and private sectors. Mr. Pezzella also has broad operations and business experience, and is a proud veteran of the U.S. Coast Guard. He holds a bachelor of science degree in accounting from Strayer University.

Anne L. Schwartz, Ph.D., is executive director. Dr. Schwartz previously served as deputy editor at *Health Affairs;* vice president at Grantmakers In Health, a national organization providing strategic advice and educational programs for foundations and corporate giving programs working on health issues; and special assistant to the executive director and senior analyst at the Physician Payment Review Commission, a precursor to the Medicare Payment Advisory Commission. Earlier, she held positions on committee and personal staff for the U.S. House of Representatives. Dr. Schwartz earned a doctorate in health policy from the School of Hygiene and Public Health at The Johns Hopkins University.

Lois Simon, M.H.S., is director of managed care. Prior to joining MACPAC, she served as director of the Bureau of Program Planning and Implementation in the Division of Managed Care at the New York State Office of Health Insurance Programs and was director of compliance at HIP Health Plan of New York (now EmblemHealth) where she was instrumental in the implementation of the plan's compliance program, the Health Insurance Portability and Accountability Act (HIPAA), and disaster recovery efforts. Ms. Simon has also held positions with the Commonwealth Fund and the Kaiser Commission on the Future of Medicaid (now the Kaiser Commission on Medicaid and the Uninsured). She began her career working in the Congressional Budget Office and in the office of U.S. Representative Joseph P. Addabbo. Ms. Simon received her master of health science degree from the School of Hygiene and Public Health at The Johns Hopkins University.

Anna Sommers, Ph.D., M.P.Aff., M.S., is director of access and quality. Dr. Sommers has conducted health services research related to Medicaid programs for over 15 years. Previously, she was a senior health researcher at the Center for Studying Health System Change in Washington, D.C. Prior to that, she was a senior research analyst at The Hilltop Institute, University of Maryland,

Baltimore County, and a research associate at the Urban Institute. Dr. Sommers received a doctorate and master of science in health services research, policy and administration from the University of Minnesota School of Public Health, and a master of public affairs degree from the University of Minnesota's Hubert H. Humphrey Institute of Public Affairs.

Mary Ellen Stahlman, M.H.S.A., is senior advisor for congressional affairs. In addition to managing MACPAC's congressional affairs, she assists in directing MACPAC's policy agenda and editing and producing the Commission's reports to the Congress. Previously, she held positions at the National Health Policy Forum, focusing on Medicare issues including private plans and the Medicare drug benefit. She served at the Centers for Medicare & Medicaid Services and its predecessor agency—the Health Care Financing Administration—for 18 years, including as deputy director of policy. Ms. Stahlman received a master of health services administration from The George Washington University and a bachelor of arts from Bates College.

James Teisl, M.P.H., is a principal analyst focused on issues related to Medicaid payment and financing. Previously, he was a senior consultant with The Lewin Group and has also worked for the Greater New York Hospital Association and the Ohio Medicaid program. Mr. Teisl received a master of public health degree from The Johns Hopkins Bloomberg School of Public Health.

Ricardo Villeta, M.B.A., is deputy director of operations, finance, and management with overall responsibility for management of the MACPAC budget and resources. Mr. Villeta directs all operations related to financial management and budget, procurement, human resources, information technology, and contracting. Previously, he was the senior vice president and chief management officer for the Academy for Educational Development, a private, non-profit educational organization which provided training, education and technical assistance throughout the United States and in more than 50 countries. Mr. Villeta holds a master of business administration degree from The George Washington University and a bachelor of science degree from Georgetown University.

Eileen Wilkie is the administrative officer and is responsible for human resources, office maintenance, and coordinating travel and Commission meetings. Previously, she held similar roles at National Public Radio and the National Endowment for Democracy. Ms. Wilkie has a bachelor of science in political science from the University of Notre Dame.

www.ingramcontent.com/pod-product-compliance
Lightning Source LLC
Chambersburg PA
CBHW081722170526
45167CB00009B/3665